DRUGS IN USE

Clinical Case Studies for Pharmacists

DRUGS IN USE

Clinical Case Studies for Pharmacists

Edited by

Linda J. Dodds

Clinical Pharmacy Trainer, Kent and Canterbury Hospital

London
THE PHARMACEUTICAL PRESS
1991

Copyright © 1991 by The Pharmaceutical Press, London

British Library Cataloguing in Publication Data
Drugs in use: Clinical case studies for pharmacists
 1. Drugs
 I. Dodds, Linda
 615.1

 ISBN 0-85369-233-5

Copies of this book may be obtained through any good bookseller or, in any case of difficulty, direct from the publisher or the publisher's agents:

 The Pharmaceutical Press
 (Publications division of the Royal Pharmaceutical Society of Great Britain)
 1 Lambeth High Street, London SE1 7JN, England

Australia

 The Australian Pharmaceutical Publishing Co. Ltd.
 40 Burwood Road, Hawthorn, Victoria 3122, *and*
 Pharmaceutical Society of Australia
 Pharmacy House, P.O. Box 21, Curtin, ACT 2605

Germany, Austria, Switzerland

 Deutscher Apotheker Verlag
 Birkenwaldstrasse 44, D-7000 Stuttgart 1

India

 Arnold Publishers (India) Pte. Ltd.
 AB/9 Safdarjung Enclave, New Delhi 110029

Japan

 Maruzen Co. Ltd
 3–10 Nihonbashi 2-chome, Chuo-ku, Tokyo 103

New Zealand

 The Pharmaceutical Society of New Zealand
 124 Dixon Street, P.O. Box 11–640, Wellington 1

U.S.A.

 Rittenhouse Book Distributors, Inc.
 511 Feheley Drive, King of Prussia, Pennsylvania 19406

*For Peter, Graham and Elizabeth
and my parents Alan and Jean Birdsell*

Contents

Preface

Pharmacists working in hospitals and in the community are increasingly being asked to contribute to drug therapy decisions and to offer critical comment on the suitability of prescribed drug regimens. Many of us feel ill-prepared to carry out these roles effectively and one of the reasons for this is the way we have been taught about diseases and their treatment. At both undergraduate and postgraduate levels, disease states are presented to pharmacists as distinct entities, with lists of the signs and symptoms that contribute to the diagnosis, the drugs used to treat them, and the side-effects associated with such treatment. Commonly used reference sources reinforce this simplistic approach. However, as soon as any pharmacist begins to care for patients it becomes apparent that many additional factors influence the choice of therapy, such as the patient's other diseases and therapies, his or her previous medical and drug history, and recent changes in clinical opinion about the use of various agents. Without an appreciation of these factors it can be difficult for a pharmacist to comprehend the reason for a particular therapy decision, to respond appropriately to questions regarding the choice of therapy for an individual, or even to know when it is useful to offer drug-related information. If it is not clear why a drug has been prescribed, it is also more difficult to monitor its usage appropriately, or to counsel the patient on how to take it.

One way of acquiring the extra knowledge and skills needed to contribute effectively to the care of individual patients is to work with, and learn from, experienced clinical pharmacists; unfortunately, such rôle models are not accessible to all. This book was therefore conceived as an alternative method of helping pharmacists to "bridge the gap" between the acquisition of theoretical knowledge about drugs and its practical application to individual patients.

Pharmacists with considerable experience of the clinical use of drugs were asked to share their expertise by contributing a case study in an area of special interest to them. The topics chosen for inclusion in the book are ones which are either commonly encountered, associated with particular difficulties in dosage individualisation, or in which major advances in therapeutics have occurred in recent years. By presenting a case and using a question and answer format, the authors demonstrate how they would select the most appropriate therapy for the patient under discussion and how they would monitor that therapy by observing the patient and interpreting the results of laboratory tests, including serum drug concentrations. They also illustrate how skills such as formulation, the taking of medication histories and counselling can be used by pharmacists to improve patient care.

I should like to take this opportunity to thank all the pharmacists who have contributed material for this book. Preparing case studies requires an enormous amount of time and effort and everyone involved has given unstintingly of both. They also contrived to adhere to the tight schedule that was set in order to ensure the shortest possible time between the preparation of material and its publication. The reward for all this is largely the hope that the book will be of use to pharmacists who are committed to improving their clinical skills.

Linda J. Dodds
October 1990

Notes on the Use of This Book

This book has been written to help demonstrate how the specialised knowledge and skills possessed by pharmacists can be applied to the care of individual patients. It is a teaching aid and should not be regarded, or used, as a pharmacology textbook.

The case studies and questions have been kept separate from the answers in order to encourage readers to formulate their own answers before reading the author's. A short reading list can be found at the end of each case study to help pharmacists unfamiliar with the topic to acquire any necessary background knowledge.

The background information provided on each patient has been kept to the level that should be easily accessible to the pharmacist, either by consulting the medical notes, or from discussions with the patient's physician. Although all the patients in this book are presented as hospital inpatients, the problems suffered by many of them, and the consequent need for pharmacist input, could as easily occur if they were living in the community and consulting their GPs.

The questions interspersing the case presentation have been designed to cover a number of important areas. They primarily reflect those most frequently posed by other health professionals together with those that should be considered by a pharmacist when a particular prescription is seen. However, they are also designed to ensure that the reader understands the reasoning behind a therapy decision that pharmacists may not usually be directly involved in, and to indicate which therapy decisions pharmacists can and should be involved in.

The observant reader will notice that the reference ranges for some laboratory indices vary between case studies. This reflects the normal practice of an individual laboratory setting its own reference ranges.

The answer sections illustrate how the questions should be approached and what factors should be taken into consideration when resolving them. The answers are based on clinical opinion current at the time of writing but they also represent, to some degree, the opinions of the authors themselves. It is thus highly likely that after studying the literature and also taking into account new drugs and new information which may have become available since the case studies were prepared, some readers will disagree with decisions arrived at by the authors. This is entirely appropriate in a book endeavouring to teach decision-making skills in complex areas where there is rarely an absolute right or wrong answer. Indeed, it is hoped that the questions raised in the case studies will generate discussion and argument between groups of pharmacists as it is through such debate that communication skills are developed. The ability to put forward and defend drug therapy decisions to medical colleagues is almost as important a skill to the pharmacist wishing to develop his or her clinical involvement as the ability to formulate such decisions.

Finally, as this book is intended for teaching purposes and not as a reference work, it has been indexed to disease states and drug names only.

CASE STUDY *1*

CARDIAC FAILURE

Stephen A. Hudson

Principal Pharmacist, Western General Hospital, Edinburgh; and Lecturer, University of Strathclyde, Glasgow

Day 1 Mrs A, a 68-year-old former schoolteacher, was admitted by referral from her general practitioner. She was a small, thin woman who had been healthy up until four months ago. Since then she had suffered increasing tiredness, difficulty in sleeping, and shortness of breath on exertion. She was anxious and had lost about 6 kg during this period of ill health, weighing 51 kg on admission. Mrs A also said she experienced periods of discomfort in the chest, which she described as "palpitations" rather than tightness or pain.

On examination she was pale and rather tense. Her temperature was 37.3°C, pulse 130 beats per minute (bpm) and irregular, and blood pressure (lying) 155/80 mmHg. Her jugular venous pulse was elevated 3 cm, and pitting oedema was present in both feet and ankles. The apex of the beat was difficult to locate, and crepitations were present in both lung fields. There was slight enlargement of the liver beyond the costal margin but no tenderness. She had a fine tremor of the hands and an increase in the limb reflexes.

The results of serum biochemistry and haematology investigations on admission were:

Sodium 137 mmol/L (reference range 135–150)
Potassium 3.7 mmol/L (3.5–5.0)
Urea 10.4 mmol/L (2.6–6.6)
Creatinine 120 micromol/L (80–150)
Haemoglobin 10.5 g/dL (12–16)
MCV 71 fL (77–91)
MCHC 0.30 g/dL (0.32–0.36)
Total T_4 260 nanomol/L (58–156)

An electrocardiogram (ECG) demonstrated rapid atrial fibrillation without ischaemic changes or signs of infarction.

The diagnosis was thyrotoxicosis and atrial fibrillation associated with cardiac failure, and complicated by anaemia of an iron-deficiency picture.

1. Which of the possible causes of cardiac failure are relevant in the case of Mrs A?

2. What symptoms of cardiac failure does she exhibit?

3. What are the therapeutic aims for Mrs A?

4. What role could digoxin play in controlling her cardiac failure?

5. How should digoxin therapy be instituted in this patient?

6. Would diuretic therapy benefit Mrs A? If so, which diuretic(s) would you recommend?

Day 5 Mrs A was discharged home on the following medication:

Digoxin 250 micrograms once daily
Bendrofluazide 5 mg each morning
Propranolol 40 mg three times daily
Carbimazole 10 mg three times daily
Ferrous sulphate 200 mg three times daily after food

A two-week follow-up appointment was arranged.

7. How long will this dose of carbimazole be required, and how should carbimazole therapy be monitored?

8. Is propranolol therapy appropriate for Mrs A?

Day 20 Mrs A was seen in clinic. She still seemed to be a little restless at home and had some difficulty in climbing stairs. Oedema was still present in both ankles and her pulse was 108 bpm.

9. Why is Mrs A's cardiac failure still uncontrolled?

10. What symptoms might lead you to suspect digoxin toxicity?

11. Would you recommend a plasma digoxin assay?

12. When should blood samples be drawn for digoxin assay?

13. What strategies could be adopted to control Mrs A's continuing atrial fibrillation? Which of these would you recommend?

Mrs A's digoxin dose was increased to 375 micrograms daily and she was asked to return to clinic in two weeks.

Day 35 Mrs A was visited at home by her general practitioner after a week-long deterioration in her condition. She felt unwell, tired, and nauseated. She had been unsociable and had not been out of the house for three days. She was readmitted to hospital with suspected digoxin toxicity.

14. What clinical factors predispose patients to digoxin toxicity?

15. Why do you think Mrs A has developed digoxin toxicity?

On examination in hospital Mrs A's pulse was found to be 72 bpm and regular. She was still nauseated, withdrawn, and a little confused. An ECG demonstrated sinus rhythm with no abnormalities. Blood was sampled for urea, electrolytes and plasma digoxin. Her plasma potassium was 3.1 mmol/L (3·5–5.0) and her plasma digoxin concentration was 3·4 microgram/L (1.0–2.0).

16. What are the cardiac effects of digoxin toxicity?

17. Apart from stopping the drug, how can digoxin toxicity be managed?

Mrs A was prescribed oral potassium chloride (Slow K® 1200 mg [16 mmol] four times daily), and her digoxin was discontinued. She improved mentally within 24 hours and became mobile over the following two days. She was discharged after five days on the following therapy:

Frusemide 40 mg each morning
Slow K® 600 mg (8 mmol) four times daily
Carbimazole 15 mg each morning
Propranolol 40 mg three times daily

Day 70 Mrs A was clinically euthyroid and in sinus rhythm. However, she was complaining of increasing shortness of breath and further ankle swelling.

18. What treatment options can you recommend to manage Mrs A's cardiac failure now?

19. How can vasodilators benefit a patient in heart failure?

20. What factors affect the choice of an angiotensin-converting enzyme (ACE) inhibitor from the products available at present?

Answers

1. Hyperthyroidism, anaemia, and atrial fibrillation.

The heart fails when its output falls short of the perfusion needs of the tissues.

Hyperthyroidism and anaemia can lead to "high output" failure, where the heart may be otherwise healthy but delivery of blood to the tissues is insufficient. In the case of hyperthyroidism, blood delivery cannot meet the exaggerated metabolic demand; while anaemia, if it severely depletes the blood of oxygen, requires the cardiac output to compensate by increasing the blood supply to the tissues.

"Low output" failure occurs when the heart pump is compromised by ventricular damage (e.g. ischaemia or infarction), persistent arrhythmia, valve disorder, or outflow obstruction. Hyperthyroidism can lead to impaired ventricular function as a result of atrial fibrillation (AF), an arrhythmia that commonly accompanies thyrotoxicosis. In AF, the contractions of atria are disorganised, and frequent electrical impulses (more than 600 per minute) pass down the conducting fibres. The ventricles cannot contract at this rate, owing to the refractoriness of the conducting system (the atrio-ventricular node); instead, they contract irregularly, at a rate usually between 100 and 200 bpm. The cardiac output is reduced as a result of reduced ventricular filling arising from:

(a) loss of normal atrial contraction,

(b) short diastole (owing to the high ventricular rate).

Thus, Mrs A's atrial fibrillation is likely to be the result of her thyrotoxicosis. Her cardiac failure may be reversed by treatment of her thyroid condition, but further complicated by her iron-deficiency anaemia.

2. Dyspnoea, oedema and raised jugular venous pulse, pallor, and tiredness.

Reduced output from the left ventricle causes impaired blood supply to the tissues and organs, which particularly affects the function of muscle, kidney, and nervous system. Shortness of breath arises from congestion of blood in the lungs, which produces increased pulmonary capillary pressure, and leads to pulmonary oedema. Owing to the reduced compliance of the congested lungs, more effort is required to expand them. Failure of the right ventricle leads to congestion and oedema in the peripheral tissues. The venous congestion may be demonstrated in the reclining patient by visible elevation of the jugular venous pulse in the neck.

Dyspnoea occurs on exertion and on lying down (orthopnoea). Muscle fatigue further diminishes tolerance to exercise because of the decreased blood supply. Symptoms are often insidious in onset, especially in the elderly, as patients may adjust their lifestyle to accommodate a loss of tolerance to exercise.

When the patient is lying down, oedema is redistributed and, in the lungs, this produces cough or breathlessness. Orthopnoea may progress to attacks of gasping at night, termed paroxysmal nocturnal dyspnoea, which are relieved by sitting or standing up. In cardiac failure, retention of sodium and fluid leads to oedema in the lungs, ankles, wrists, and abdomen.

Other symptoms resulting from a reduced blood supply to the tissues of the brain, kidneys, liver, and gut are confusion, renal failure, enlargement of the liver (hepatomegaly) and abdominal distension, anorexia, nausea, and abdominal pain. The patient's complexion may be pale, and the hands cold and sweaty, owing to stimulation of the sympathetic nervous system in response to reduced cardiac output. In Mrs A's case, the fact that she is suffering from thyrotoxicosis will also increase her sympathetic discharge.

3. The therapeutic aims are as follows.

(a) Treatment of the underlying thyrotoxicosis. The options for this are antithyroid drugs, surgery, or radio-iodine therapy. In the absence of a goitre, drug therapy is probably the first choice. Surgery and radio-iodine often induce hypothyroidism, which then requires long-term treatment with thyroxine.

(b) Treatment of the AF to control the ventricular rate, pending resolution of the thyrotoxicosis and return to a normal thyroid state.

(c) Investigation and treatment of Mrs A's suspected iron-deficiency anaemia. A dietary and drug history is required, together with any history of blood loss from the body (e.g. gastro-intestinal, postmenopausal, urinary). Laboratory tests should include serum iron, total iron binding capacity, and serum ferritin to confirm or refute true iron-deficiency.

(d) Control of the oedema of cardiac failure.

4. Digoxin could control Mrs A's heart failure by exerting a positive inotropic effect, and by controlling her AF.

These actions are produced by an increase in myocardial intracellular ionic calcium, secondary to the inhibition of sodium extrusion from the myocardial cell.

The positive inotropic effect secures the contractile force of the myocardium; however, this effect of digoxin may not be maintained during long-term administration. Studies have shown that the drug can be discontinued in many patients in sinus rhythm without any worsening of symptoms. Only a trial of digoxin discontinuation can demonstrate whether a patient is continuing to benefit from the drug.

Levels of digoxin above 1.5 microgram/L usually result in a reduction in electrical discharge from the sino-atrial node, with slowing of conduction and increasing refractoriness of the atrio-ventricular node. Digoxin's effects on the atrio-ventricular node are relevant to AF and the control of ventricular rate. Digoxin is often highly effective in controlling AF.

5. Mrs A requires an initial loading dose of 750 micrograms digoxin orally, given as three 250 microgram aliquots at six-hourly intervals. Additional 250 microgram loading doses may be required, depending on her response. A maintenance dose of 250 micrograms once daily should then be prescribed.

Digoxin pharmacokinetics are relevant to the selection of a dosage regimen. The drug is slowly absorbed, and bioavailability is incomplete. Digoxin is only 25% bound to plasma proteins, and the drug distributes slowly into a large apparent volume of distribution (approximately 7 L/kg bodyweight). Therapeutic serum levels of digoxin (1-2 micrograms/L) will not be achieved until the body compartments are saturated. Thus, to ensure a rapid onset of the drug's therapeutic effects, Mrs A must be given a loading dose of digoxin. As 99% of digoxin in the body is tissue-bound, primarily to skeletal and cardiac muscle and minimally within body fat, a suitable oral loading dose is calculated from the patient's lean body weight on the basis of 12-15 micrograms/kg. As Mrs A is a thin woman, her actual body weight can be used; so a suitable loading dose would be 765 micrograms (51×15 micrograms) orally, given as three doses of 250 micrograms at six-hourly intervals to reduce side-effects of nausea and vomiting.

Mrs A's thyrotoxicosis may increase her digoxin requirements, partly by increasing the apparent volume of distribution of the drug, and its clearance, but mainly by reducing cardiac sensitivity to digoxin. An additional one or two doses in the loading regimen may therefore be needed to control her ventricular rate, prior to instituting a daily maintenance dose.

If Mrs A had been in urgent need of digitalisation, for example if she had been suffering from acute dyspnoea as a result of her cardiac failure, intravenous digoxin therapy might have been more appropriate to control her tachycardia. An intravenous dosage regimen must, however, take account of the increased bioavailability of the drug by this route; the dose should be 70% of that calculated for oral administration, and the total dose should, whenever possible, be divided into aliquots with an interval of one to two hours between injections to allow proper clinical evaluation.

Several factors must be taken into account when calculating an appropriate maintenance dose (MD) of digoxin for Mrs A. The first is her renal function. The half-life of digoxin is normally 36-40 hours. Since the drug is excreted approximately 70% unchanged in the urine, any impairment of renal function will extend the half-life and must therefore be taken into account. The plasma creatinine level can be used to estimate Mrs A's creatinine clearance (CrCl). When the equation of Cockcroft and Gault is used, it can be calculated that Mrs A has a CrCl of 31 mL/min, which indicates that caution must be taken in choosing an MD. The extension of digoxin half-life can be calculated from:

$$\text{Extension in half-life} = \frac{1}{(1 - F_e) + (R_f . F_e)}$$

where F_e = fraction of drug excreted unchanged in urine (for digoxin, 0.7), and R_f = fraction of normal renal function (patient's CrCl/100; for Mrs A = 0.31).

For Mrs A, extension in half-life = 2; i.e. her predicted digoxin half-life is double that of a person with normal renal function; as a guide, her renal impairment should be compensated for by a 50% reduction in MD.

If a loading dose were NOT given to Mrs A, then the maximum clinical effect of an MD would only be seen after the serum digoxin level was at steady state (i.e. when digoxin input = digoxin excretion), which is usually after four or five half-lives. In Mrs A's case, this would be 12-15 days.

The choice of an MD can also be guided by estimating the proportion of the loading dose that will be excreted each day, and which must therefore be replaced, using the formula:

% loading dose excreted each day =
$$(14\% + \text{patient's CrCl/5}).$$

For Mrs A, this gives a figure of 20% of the loading dose being excreted each day. If the loading dose were 750 micrograms, then the MD would be 150 micrograms.

Unfortunately, these dosing recommendations can only be a guide to Mrs A's requirements, since interindividual variations in clinical response limit the usefulness of pharmacokinetic methods. In particular, doses needed to control AF may produce plasma levels that would be judged excessive (i.e. greater than 2.5–3.5 micrograms/L), compared with the usually quoted therapeutic range of 1–2 micrograms/L. Furthermore, AF in the context of thyrotoxicosis may only respond to doses that would usually be avoided in euthyroid patients. The presence of thyrotoxicosis may allow tolerance to the toxic effects of these larger doses. Although in Mrs A the MD needs to be reduced because of her renal function, her dose requirement may increase as her renal function improves following control of her cardiac failure.

In summary, after loading, a daily MD of 250 micrograms is probably most appropriate for Mrs A, but this should be modified according to clinical response in terms of ventricular rate and symptomatic control. Careful observation will be required for clinical or ECG signs of digoxin toxicity.

6. Yes. Bendrofluazide 5 mg daily would be the most appropriate first choice.

Mrs A's oedema may eventually resolve, once her AF and associated cardiac failure are successfully controlled; however, short-term diuretic therapy may help reduce the oedema and any associated discomfort. A thiazide diuretic, such as bendrofluazide, should suffice. More vigorous diuresis from a loop diuretic carries a greater risk of hypokalaemia in the short term, although thiazides pose the greater long-term risk of hypokalaemia and hyponatraemia, particularly in elderly patients. A further advantage to prescribing a thiazide for Mrs A is the long duration of action (average 12–24 hours) of this class of drugs. Loop diuretics act within six hours. A rapid or profound diuresis can exacerbate cardiac failure by reducing blood volume, or it can increase the patient's uraemia (pre-renal azotaemia). Maximum diuresis with a thiazide occurs at low doses (with bendrofluazide, 10 mg); further increases in dose offer no benefit and add to the risk of metabolic side-effects, notably hyperglycaemia and hyperuricaemia. Thiazide diuretics lose effectiveness when CrCl rates drop below 25 mL/min. Mrs A's potassium level must be monitored closely as she is on digoxin, and hypokalaemia increases the risk of digoxin side-effects. If required, potassium-sparing diuretics or adequate potassium supplements (e.g. 40–80 mmol/day) should be prescribed.

Combination diuretic + potassium products, such as Neo-NaClex-K® (bendrofluazide 2.5 mg + potassium 8.4 mmol), are not suitable as their potassium content is so low.

7. This dose will be required until Mrs A is clinically euthyroid. Apart from plasma T_4 estimations, no routine monitoring is required whilst Mrs A is receiving carbimazole therapy.

The most common cause of thyrotoxicosis (Graves' disease) may eventually remit spontaneously; however, active treatment of thyrotoxicosis is usually necessary to achieve rapid control of symptoms.

Carbimazole (first choice) or propylthiouracil are used to control hyperthyroidism but about 50% of patients do eventually relapse. Carbimazole 30–60 mg daily is given in divided doses, and an objective clinical response (slowing of pulse, and weight gain) usually occurs after three to six weeks. A clinically euthyroid state can be confirmed by the plasma T_4 concentration; once this is achieved the dose of carbimazole can be reduced to a single daily maintenance dose of 5–15 mg.

Side-effects of carbimazole therapy include reversible leucopenia (which occurs in up to 12% of patients), and agranulocytosis (which occurs in less than 0.5%). Both these dyscrasias can occur suddenly, usually during the first three months of therapy, so routine white cell counts are not useful, although they are indicated if the patient complains of persistent cough, sore throat, or mouth ulceration.

8. Yes. Propranolol therapy can provide symptomatic control of thyrotoxicosis, pending remission of the condition using antithyroid agents.

Unselective beta-adrenergic blockade reduces symptoms of sympathetic overactivity, such as tremor, nervousness, fatigue, sinus tachycardia, and associated anxiety. Although beta-blockers do not affect the thyroid, they may beneficially reduce the conversion of thyroxine to the more active triiodothyronine in the liver and tissues. Beta-blockers can, however, exacerbate cardiac failure by negative chronotropic and inotropic effects. In Mrs A, the negative chronotropic effect of propranolol is potentially beneficial because of her AF, while the negative inotropic effect should be counteracted by the effects of digoxin.

9. Mrs A's pulse rate suggests inadequate digitalisation.

Inadequate digitalisation could have resulted because the dose prescribed is too small or because of the failure of Mrs A to comply; however, loss of control of cardiac failure may also occur in digoxin toxicity, and this needs to be excluded by enquiring about other symptoms of digoxin toxicity.

10. The loss of control of her cardiac failure and her complaint of restlessness.

Digoxin toxicity may easily go unrecognised. It is commonly signalled by gastro-intestinal and/or central nervous system symptoms. These may be vague and insidious in onset, such as fatigue, apathy or restlessness, insomnia, confusion, abdominal discomfort, or change in bowel habits (especially diarrhoea). More overt signs are anorexia, nausea, vomiting, lethargy, and psychosis. Visual disturbances (blurring, haloed or yellow vision, red-green colour blindness) are well documented but are not often among the first symptoms volunteered by the patient.

In the absence of other symptoms, Mrs A's restlessness is probably the result of her underlying thyroid condition rather than digoxin toxicity.

11. No. The target plasma concentration for controlling AF in thyrotoxicosis is not defined, so a digoxin assay is unlikely to be of help in Mrs A's management.

Overuse of the digoxin plasma assay is both common and wasteful. In addition, assay results cannot be interpreted if the sampling times are unrecorded or inappropriate.

12. Blood should be sampled for digoxin between six and 24 hours after a dose.

The slow distribution of the drug confers two-compartment pharmacokinetic characteristics. The equilibration between drug in the plasma and that in the myocardium (and other tissues) continues for up to six hours after a dose. Before six hours, the change in the plasma digoxin is disproportional to the change in the amount of digoxin in the tissues, and therefore its effect on the myocardium.

13. (a) Optimise the digoxin dose,
(b) add verapamil to Mrs A's therapy,
(c) increase the dose of beta-blocker.

For Mrs A, optimisation of the digoxin dose is probably preferable; however, before her dose is increased it must be ensured that she is complying with her present digoxin regimen.

Verapamil alone is at least as effective as digoxin in controlling AF. Also, AF unresponsive to digoxin alone may be controlled by the addition of verapamil; however, verapamil affects digoxin pharmacokinetics, and the addition of this drug to

Mrs A's regimen risks an unpredictable gradual increase in plasma digoxin concentration.

Since propranolol is already indicated in Mrs A, an increase in the dose of this beta-blocker could be considered.

14. Hypokalaemia, hypomagnesaemia, hypercalcaemia, alkalosis, hypoxia, and hypothyroidism.

Hypokalaemia, hypercalcaemia, and hypomagnesaemia all lead to an increase in responsiveness of tissues to digoxin's cardiac effects, and to toxic symptoms in general. The most common contributor to digoxin toxicity is hypokalaemia, and plasma digoxin concentrations can only be interpreted in conjunction with a plasma potassium measurement.

Alkalosis and hypoxia also potentiate digoxin toxicity, while hypothyroidism increases responsiveness to digoxin and elevates plasma concentrations by decreasing the drug's clearance and apparent volume of distribution.

15. Mrs A may have become increasingly vulnerable to digoxin toxicity because of an increased sensitivity to the drug as her thyrotoxicosis goes into remission.

16. Arrhythmias and loss of control of cardiac failure.

Digoxin increases the automaticity and slows conduction in all cardiac cells. Cardiotoxicity may occur without other warning symptoms and the cells of the atrio-ventricular and sino-atrial nodes are affected in particular. Common arrhythmias include atrio-ventricular block with supraventricular tachycardias, junctional or escape rhythms, ventricular ectopic beats, and ventricular tachycardia. Sinus bradycardia and sino-atrial arrest may occur. Loss of control of cardiac failure may also be a feature of digoxin toxicity.

17. (a) Correct any underlying factors contributing to digoxin toxicity,
(b) use resins or digoxin-specific antibody fragments to increase digoxin elimination.

If present, hypokalaemia should be corrected, unless the presence of atrio-ventricular block contra-indicates potassium use. When heart block persists, lignocaine and similar anti-arrhythmic agents (such as propranolol and phenytoin) are recommended, and cardiac pacing is indicated.

Attempts to reduce digoxin concentrations by dialysis are ineffective, as 99% of drug in the body is tissue-bound and not in the plasma. The use of oral resins such as cholestyramine and colestipol (bile-acid-chelating agents which also bind digoxin) can increase elimination by interrupting enterohepatic circulation of the drug; however, severe toxicity requires the use of digoxin-specific antibody fragment preparations (by the intravenous route). These act as a specific, rapid antidote, but they are expensive. The antibody fragments are non-immunogenic and the complex formed with digoxin is readily excreted by the kidney.

18. (a) Discontinue propranolol,
    (b) adjust Mrs A's diuretic therapy,
    (c) consider prescribing a vasodilator,
    (d) consider anticoagulation.

A euthyroid state has now been achieved and Mrs A no longer has the benefit of digitalisation; furthermore, she no longer has the symptoms for which propranolol was originally indicated. Her symptoms of cardiac failure suggest an underlying low cardiac output to which her propranolol therapy may be contributing. Propranolol should therefore be discontinued.

Should further treatment be needed, the absence of AF and Mrs A's recent episode of digoxin toxicity argue against redigitalisation. Instead, there is scope for modestly increasing the diuretic effect by substituting a potassium-sparing diuretic for the potassium supplement (e.g. amiloride 5 mg each morning), and increasing the dose of frusemide. Following these measures, consideration should be given to prescribing a vasodilator.

Finally, Mrs A has a heart rhythm which has ranged from AF to sinus rhythm over the three months of observation. Some clinicians would consider oral anticoagulation, to prevent embolic complications such as stroke.

19. Vasodilation on the arterial side reduces the pressure against which the heart must work. Vasodilation on the venous side reduces the rate of return of blood to the heart and the tendency of the ventricles to overfill.

Directly acting agents such as hydralazine and organic nitrates exert a selective action on arteries and veins respectively. Alpha-adrenoceptor blockers (such as prazosin), calcium-channel blockers (such as nifedipine), and ACE inhibitors (such as captopril) act on both the arterial and the venous circulations.

ACE inhibitors produce vasodilation by blocking the sequence of events leading to hyperaldosteronism, which involves the circulating vasoconstrictor angiotensin II. Through impairment of aldosterone formation, ACE inhibitors also benefit heart failure by reducing sodium and water retention. ACE inhibitors are therefore able to interrupt a cycle of secondary physiological events in cardiac failure.

20. The choice of an ACE inhibitor will be affected by its onset and duration of action, and side-effect profile.

At the time of writing, three ACE inhibitors are marketed for oral administration in chronic cardiac failure: captopril, enalapril, and lisinopril.

Captopril acts in one hour and the effect on arterial pressure lasts three to six hours. Enalapril acts in one to two hours and lasts 12–24 hours. Lisinopril acts in two to four hours and lasts 24–30 hours. In cardiac failure, captopril may be given in two or three doses daily, whereas enalapril may be given once or twice daily, and lisinopril once daily.

All three drugs are eliminated predominantly by the kidney and require dosage adjustment in renal failure (CrCl less than 60 mL/min). The risk of hyperkalaemia precludes the use of potassium supplements or potassium-sparing diuretics with ACE inhibitors, unless plasma potassium is carefully monitored.

The major problems with all ACE inhibitors are first-dose hypotension (worsened by an upright posture), skin rashes, and renal toxicity signified by proteinuria. First-dose hypotension is particularly marked in patients who have recently received high doses of diuretics. The sensitivity of blood pressure to the introduction of an ACE inhibitor follows from high circulating angiotensin levels which maintain the blood pressure in circumstances of reduced blood volume secondary to diuresis. To minimise acute hypotension, high diuretic doses should be curtailed, if possible for a few days prior to starting treatment with the ACE inhibitor, and a small first dose of the drug should be administered at bedtime. Other patients at particular risk of this first-dose effect include patients who have activation of the renin-angiotensin system and secondary hyperaldosteronism (e.g. patients with liver disease). In patients at risk of hypotension, captopril has the disadvantage of a faster onset of effect, but the advantage of a shorter duration of action in the event of an exaggerated response.

Unwanted immunological effects on the skin, and proteinuria, occur more often with captopril than with the other agents but are rare in the usual therapeutic dose range, unless the patient has a connective tissue disorder such as rheumatoid arthritis. Alteration or loss of taste, cough, and mouth ulcers are also recognised side-effects of ACE inhibitors, but are not specific to any one agent.

References and Further Reading

Cohn J.N., Current therapy of the failing heart, *Circulation*, 1988, **78**, 1097–1107.

Halpern J.L. and Hart R.G., Atrial fibrillation and stroke, new ideas, persisting dilemmas, *Stroke*, 1988, **19,** 937–941.

Lewis R. and McClay J., Clinical pharmacology of chronic atrial fibrillation, *J. R. Coll. Physn. (London)*, 1988, **22**, 252–256.

Mooradian A.D., Digitalis: an update of clinical pharmacokinetics, therapeutic monitoring techniques and treatment recommendations, *Clin. Pharmacokinet.*, 1988, **15,** 165–179.

Stockigt J.R. and Topliss D.J., Hyperthyroidism, current drug therapy, *Drugs*, 1989, **37**, 375–381.

Timmis A.D., Modern treatment of heart failure, *Br. med. J.*, 1988, **297,** 83–84.

HYPERTENSION

Ros L. Batty

Principal Pharmacist (Clinical Services, Training and Development), Clinical Pharmacy Unit, Northwick Park Hospital, Harrow, Middlesex

Day 1 (August 1984) Mr Y, a 58-year-old man, was admitted to hospital complaining of left-sided weakness following a stroke. His previous medical history was unremarkable. He did not smoke and drank only socially. He had not been taking any drugs prior to admission. He was obese (weight 95 kg) and on examination was found to be hypertensive (resting blood pressure [BP] 170/120 mmHg) with a pulse rate of 72 beats per minute.

He was prescribed bendrofluazide 5 mg in the morning, and put on a weight-reducing diet. Regular physiotherapy was started to improve movement in his left arm and leg.

His serum biochemistry and haematology results were:

Sodium 139 mmol/L (reference range 135–148)
Potassium 4.2 mmol/L (3.5–5.0)
Urea 5.6 mmol/L (2.9–7.0)
Glucose 5.6 mmol/L (3.9–10.0)
Haemoglobin 14.1 g/dL (12–18)

One week later Mr Y's BP was still raised (165/115 mmHg), and his dose of bendrofluazide was increased to 10 mg daily. After a further six days his hypertension was unchanged, so atenolol 50 mg in the morning was added to his drug therapy.

1. What are the aims of treating hypertension and how can they be achieved?

2. Was the treatment prescribed for Mr Y appropriate? Comment on the doses prescribed.

3. How should thiazide and beta-blocker therapy be monitored?

Day 28 Mr Y's BP was controlled at 135/85 mmHg. However, routine urinalysis showed traces of sugar, but no protein or ketones.

4. Why might Mr Y have sugar in his urine?

5. What action would you have recommended?

The team treating Mr Y decided to stop the bendrofluazide and increase the dose of atenolol to 100 mg in the morning. A random blood glucose measurement was 11.2 mmol/L (3.9–10) and his serum potassium was 3.9 mmol/L (3.5–5.0).

Day 42 Mr Y's mobility had improved sufficiently to allow him to go home. His blood sugar was normal and his BP was 130/90 mmHg. He was discharged on atenolol 100 mg daily.

Month 8 (March 1985) Mr Y attended a routine out-patient appointment. He claimed he was still taking atenolol 100 mg daily, but his BP was 160/120 mmHg.

It was decided to add prazosin to his regimen, starting with a dose of 500 micrograms at bedtime, then 500 micrograms twice daily. He was asked to return to the clinic at weekly intervals, so that the dose of prazosin could be adjusted according to his BP. He was eventually stablised on atenolol 100 mg daily and prazosin 1 mg three times daily.

6. Was the dosage regimen of prazosin appropriate? How should the dose be increased and by what increments?

7. Would you have recommended prazosin? What other vasodilators could have been used?

Month 56 (March 1989) Over the last four years, Mr Y had remained well on the same drug therapy, but at a routine out-patient visit, he was found to be hypertensive (BP 175/120 mmHg). He was complaining of "tired legs"; on further questioning, he admitted he had not been taking his tablets recently as he had "run out of them and they weren't doing me any good, and it is difficult to remember to take them three times a day".

The prazosin was stopped and nifedipine 20 mg tablets twice daily added to the atenolol. Mr Y was counselled by the clinic doctor regarding the importance of his drug therapy.

8. What are the differences between the calcium-channel blockers used for hypertension? Which would you have recommended for Mr Y?

Month 58 Mr Y returned to out-patients complaining of headaches and lightheadedness. His BP was 150/95 mmHg and it was decided to admit Mr Y for review and rationalisation of his antihypertensive therapy.

His serum biochemistry and haematology results were:

Sodium 138 mmol/L (135–148)
Potassium 3.9 mmol/L (3.5–5.0)
Urea 7.1 mmol/L (2.9–7.0)
Glucose 6.0 mmol/L (3.9–10.0)
Haemoglobin 14.5 g/dL (12–18)

The medical team decided to use an angiotensin-converting enzyme (ACE) inhibitor.

9. How do ACE inhibitors work?

10. What appear to be the advantages of ACE inhibitors in the treatment of hypertension?

11. Which ACE inhibitor would you recommend and at what dose?

12. Would you recommend any adjustments to his existing therapy?

13. What parameters would you want to monitor whilst Mr Y is receiving an ACE inhibitor?

It was also decided to start aspirin 75 mg daily to prevent a further stroke, as Mr Y had had a transient ischaemic attack on the second day of the admission.

Mr Y's BP was eventually controlled on atenolol 100 mg once daily and enalapril 10 mg in the morning.

14. What points would you cover when counselling Mr Y on discharge?

Answers

1. The aims of antihypertensive therapy are to prevent premature death and morbidity by lessening the incidence of stroke, heart failure, and other complications of hypertension. These aims may be achieved by maintaining the BP within "normal limits".

For a man of Mr Y's age, diastolic pressure should ideally be 95 mmHg or less; however, in practice achievement of this goal must be weighed against the side-effects of the drugs used because hypertension, as in Mr Y's case, is often symptomless. Also, since therapy is likely to be long-term, the regimen should be as simple as possible to encourage compliance.

2. The treatment prescribed for Mr Y was appropriate.

Drug therapy is usually initiated using a "stepped care" approach. The current view is that a thiazide diuretic or a beta-blocker should be used as first-line therapy. The dose of the chosen agent is then adjusted until BP control is achieved, side-effects develop, or the maximum dose is reached.

The antihypertensive effect of thiazides is due mainly to a decrease in extracellular fluid volume, but direct vasodilation may also occur. The antihypertensive mechanism of the beta-blockers is unclear, but contributory factors include a reduction in cardiac output, reduced renin release and a mechanism involving the central nervous system (CNS). The usual contra-indications to both beta-blockers and thiazides apply. If one class of drug alone does not achieve BP control, then a combination of the two classes is tried. If the combination is not effective, a third agent is added; this traditionally has been a direct or alpha-blocking vasodilator, but now other agents such as calcium-channel blockers or ACE inhibitors are being used. There are some claims that ACE inhibitors and calcium-channel blockers should be used as first-line agents, but as yet long-term experience with these drugs is limited.

The choice of a thiazide diuretic as first-line therapy was appropriate for Mr Y for two reasons. Firstly, the Medical Research Council (MRC) treatment trial of mild hypertension has shown older patients respond better to diuretic therapy. The reason for this is uncertain, but may be related to the low circulating levels of plasma renin that occur in the elderly. Secondly, Mr Y did not suffer either type II diabetes or gout, both of which would contra-indicate the use of a thiazide diuretic.

Bendrofluazide was a suitable choice of thiazide for Mr Y, as it is safe, easy to use, and can be given once daily, which may help his compliance. In addition the MRC data showed patients receiving this agent suffered fewer strokes. Small doses (2.5–5 mg) are as effective as large ones, and it is thus not surprising that Mr Y's BP was not affected by increasing the dose to 10 mg. Large doses cause more biochemical side-effects.

The addition of a beta-blocker as a second-line agent was logical. Mr Y does not suffer from airways obstruction, cardiac failure, or heart block, all of which can contra-indicate the use of beta-blockers. Most beta-blockers lower BP to a similar extent when given at the recommended doses; the choice of agent should thus be made after considering the patient's clinical condition and the properties of the drug, e.g. cardioselectivity and lipid solubility. For a patient such as Mr Y, with no additional complicating diseases, the choice of beta-blocker should be based on cost, and the practising doctor's familiarity with the particular drug. Atenolol was a suitable choice for Mr Y, as it can be given once daily, only rarely causes sleep disturbance, and is moderately cheap. The more lipid-soluble beta-blockers (e.g. propranolol) can accumulate in the CNS, and may be responsible for causing nightmares in some patients. Water-soluble beta-blockers such as atenolol may accumulate in patients with renal failure; however, Mr Y's urea level does not suggest renal impairment.

Most beta-blockers need only be given once or twice daily to treat hypertension as their antihypertensive properties outlast their elimination half-lives. Intrinsic sympathomimetic and membrane-stabilising activity are not thought to have any practical value in antihypertensive therapy. Atenolol in normal doses acts mainly on the $beta_1$-receptors in the heart, without blocking the $beta_2$-receptors; this cardioselectivity reduces the drug's effects on extracardiac tissues, and may be useful in patients with insulin-dependent diabetes mellitus or peripheral vascular disease. Although Mr Y does not need this cardioselective property, the other properties of this beta-blocker (ease of dosing, relative lack of CNS effects, moderate cost) make it suitable for him.

3. The following points should be considered.

Thiazide diuretics
Thiazides can cause a fall in serum potassium concentration, a rise in urate levels, impairment of glucose tolerance, and hypercholesterolaemia. There is much controversy about the significance of these metabolic effects with regard to long-term

morbidity and mortality. Most clinicians still do not routinely monitor urate or lipid levels. Potassium supplementation is usually only given if the serum potassium falls to less than 3.5 mmol/L (unless the patient is on digoxin), or if symptoms of hypokalaemia occur. It would, however, be prudent to monitor Mr Y's serum potassium. Changes in serum potassium are usually noticeable after a week and reach a nadir after a month or two. Other side-effects of thiazide diuretic therapy include impotence, constipation, and lethargy.

Beta-blockers

No specific biochemical monitoring is required for beta-blockers, although they can sometimes affect blood glucose and adversely alter lipid levels. Mr Y should be questioned about subjective complaints such as fatigue, and cold or painful extremities. His heart rate should be monitored. Patients on the more lipid-soluble beta-blockers should be asked about nightmares and hallucinations. Patients at risk should be monitored for signs and symptoms of bronchospasm and heart failure.

Finally, and obviously, Mr Y's BP should be monitored to ensure that the thiazide and beta-blocker therapies are effective.

4. As a side-effect of his drug therapy.

Beta-blockers have been reported to cause hyperglycaemia; they inhibit insulin secretion, but their effects on glycogenolysis, growth hormone, and glucose utilisation may contribute to raising the blood glucose.

As mentioned earlier, impaired glucose tolerance is a well recognised side-effect of thiazide therapy, particularly when high doses are used. The mechanism of this effect is unclear, but potassium is likely to be involved, since potassium supplementation can partly reverse the hyperglycaemia in hypokalaemic patients.

The reported incidence of hyperglycaemia is higher with thiazides than with cardioselective beta-blockers such as atenolol, and it thus seems more likely that Mr Y's glycosuria is a consequence of his bendrofluazide therapy.

5. Discontinue bendrofluazide therapy and start treatment with a third-line agent.

Diuretic-induced hyperglycaemia is reversible, though it may take weeks or months for the blood sugar to return to normal after stopping the drug. In 1984, when Mr Y was being treated, the accepted third-line agents were vasodilators. ACE inhibitors were not often prescribed then, as captopril had been on the market for less than a year and severe

side-effects (such as neutropenia and proteinuria) were being described.

The alternative approach was to stop the thiazide and raise the dose of atenolol to 100 mg daily. However, this is a less commendable option: it must be borne in mind that single drug therapy fails to control BP in at least 20% of patients with mild hypertension, and Mr Y's BP had not been well controlled when bendrofluazide had been used as a single agent. Increasing the dose of atenolol above 100 mg would be unlikely to provide additional benefit and may cause more side-effects.

6. The starting dosage regimen of prazosin was appropriate, but once the regular dose had been established, it could have been given twice daily.

Prazosin causes a "first dose syncope", due to hypotension, in up to 40% of patients. To prevent this, the lowest dose (500 micrograms) should be taken on retiring to bed, and then 500 micrograms should be taken two or three times daily for three to seven days, increasing to 1 mg two or three times daily for a further three to seven days. It was particularly important for Mr Y to follow the low initial dosage regimen, as adding prazosin to beta-blocker treatment has been reported to cause hypotension. Further dose adjustments should then be made according to BP response. Once the optimum dosage had been determined, Mr Y's prazosin dose could have been adjusted to allow twice daily administration. This strategy may encourage compliance. Although it was not available in 1985, the manufacturers of Hypovase® now make a "b.d. starter" pack for patients commencing on prazosin.

7. Of the vasodilators available in 1985 (prazosin, minoxidil, hydralazine, and the calcium-channel blocker, nifedipine) prazosin was an appropriate choice, although nifedipine would also have been suitable.

Prazosin is an effective antihypertensive, being particularly effective when used in combination with a beta-blocker. It does not cause electrolyte or metabolic changes or fluid retention. In addition, unlike thiazides and beta-blockers (which can raise total plasma lipids), prazosin lowers low density lipoprotein cholesterol and raises high density lipoprotein cholesterol. The main disadvantages of prazosin, and the newer related alpha-blocker, terazosin, are first-dose and orthostatic hypotension, although tolerance to the hypotensive effects can occur with long-term treatment. The most recently marketed quinazoline alpha-blocker, doxazosin, is reported not to cause first-dose hypotension, and its long elimination half-life and duration of action allow once daily dosage which may aid patient compliance. However, this drug was not available in 1985. Doxazosin is more expensive than prazosin.

Nifedipine combines well with beta-blockers, offsetting the bradycardia. It causes few symptomatic effects although flushing, headache and fluid retention may be troublesome to some patients. Like prazosin, it can be given twice daily.

Alternative vasodilators available in 1985 included minoxidil and hydralazine. Both these agents are less likely to cause postural hypotension than prazosin, but more likely to cause tachycardia and fluid retention. Minoxidil should be reserved for hypertension refractory to other agents, as side-effects may be severe. Concomitant diuretic and beta-blocker therapy may be required with hydralazine, and are essential with minoxidil, and diuretic therapy had already induced hyperglycaemia in Mr Y. Hydralazine, particularly in doses over 100 mg, may cause a lupus-like syndrome.

8. The calcium-channel blockers indicated for hypertension are nifedipine, nicardipine, isradipine and verapamil. They differ primarily in their side-effect profiles. Nifedipine was the most appropriate choice for Mr Y.

All the calcium-channel blockers listed above block the slow influx of calcium into the cells of vascular smooth muscle, causing vasodilation. The first three are dihydropyridines. They cause reflex tachycardia, flushing, and headaches, and also peripheral oedema. Combination with a beta-blocker reduces the incidence of palpitations and oedema. Nifedipine is a negative inotrope and is contra-indicated in heart failure. Nicardipine has less of a negative inotropic effect, but experience with its use is limited. Isradipine has a higher affinity for calcium channels in arterial smooth muscle than in the heart, and so has only a small effect on heart function. Isradipine theoretically causes less tachycardia than nifedipine and nicardipine as it selectively inhibits the sinus node, while not affecting atrio-ventricular node conduction. All three drugs can be given twice daily, though during initial dosage titration nicardipine is given three times daily. Nifedipine has to be given as tablets (Adalat Retard®) to be effective twice daily. These tablets are not formulated for sustained release, but they do have a different release profile from the capsules (Adalat®) which contain nifedipine in solution and have to be given three times daily.

Verapamil prolongs atrio-ventricular node conduction, and it does not cause reflex tachycardia. It can cause constipation. Since verapamil lowers the heart rate, combination with a beta-blocker is contra-indicated in some texts; however, many cardiology specialists use the combination successfully without undue adverse effects. Verapamil is usually given two or three times daily. There are sustained release products, and recent uncontrolled studies have shown that, given once daily, they lower the blood pressure over a 24-hour period. However, clinically equivalent sustained release formulations are expensive compared to conventional formulations and should be reserved for patients who are poorly compliant.

Nifedipine was the most appropriate agent for Mr Y, as clinical experience with the other dihydropyridines is limited, and verapamil combined with atenolol might have caused heart failure.

9. ACE inhibitors are thought to reduce BP by decreasing peripheral vascular resistance.

They competitively block angiotensin-converting enzyme, which converts angiotensin I to angiotensin II. The latter is a potent vasoconstrictor, which also stimulates aldosterone release. ACE inhibitors also block the metabolism of bradykinin, a vasodilator, but the significance of this effect is unclear.

10. ACE inhibitors are effective without causing many adverse effects that might cause the patient to discontinue therapy.

One study has suggested that therapy with an ACE inhibitor has less effect on the patient's quality of life than therapy with propranolol and methyldopa. However, quality of life indexes are subjective. There is evidence that ACE inhibitors slow the decline in renal function that occurs in hypertensive patients with renal impairment.

11. Enalapril at a starting dose of 5 mg daily.

The ACE inhibitors currently on the market are captopril, enalapril, lisinopril, and quinapril. All four agents are similar in efficacy. When used in high doses (over 100 mg daily), captopril produced serious side-effects, such as agranulocytosis and nephrotic syndrome. These effects are seen infrequently with the currently recommended doses of captopril, as they are with the other ACE inhibitors. Captopril has to be given twice daily, which may affect Mr Y's compliance. Enalapril is a pro-drug which is rapidly converted to the active enalaprilat by ester hydrolysis in the liver. Its long half-life usually allows for once daily administration. Lisinopril, the lysine analogue of enalaprilat, is not a pro-drug, and is rapidly hydrolysed in plasma. Quinapril can also be given once daily, as its active metabolite quinaprilat has a long half-life. Enalaprilat and quinaprilat accumulate in renal failure. All the ACE inhibitors have similar side-effects, which include headache, dizziness, gastro-intestinal upset, and cough.

Since there is little to choose in terms of efficacy and side-effects between the ACE inhibitors that can be administered once daily, and Mr Y had no evidence of hepatic problems, it would seem appropriate to choose enalapril, which costs slightly less. Since Mr Y is not taking a diuretic, the recommended starting dose is 5 mg daily. The dose can be doubled every three to five days until adequate BP control is achieved.

12. Stop nifedipine; continue with atenolol.

On admission, Mr Y was taking atenolol 100 mg daily and nifedipine 20 mg twice daily. Since he was complaining of dizziness and headaches, which are common side-effects of nifedipine therapy, it would be logical to stop this drug.

ACE inhibitors can be effective antihypertensives when given on their own, but it is recommended that beta-blocker therapy should not be discontinued abruptly. Once enalapril therapy has been started, it may be possible to reduce the dose of atenolol. Mr Y's compliance may be improved if his BP could be controlled on a single drug; however, combinations of ACE inhibitors and beta-blockers are successfully used in hypertension. Against this is a theoretical argument that the combination is not logical, as beta-blockers have an anti-renin effect and ACE inhibitors appear to be most effective in patients with high renin states.

13. (a) BP regularly;
(b) renal function (serum urea and, if possible, serum creatinine and/or creatinine clearance) initially, then every few months;
(c) serum potassium every week initially, then periodically;
(d) temperature and other signs of infection (if any of these symptoms occur, then his white blood cell count should be monitored).

14. (a) Stress the importance of continuing to take his medication in the prescribed doses, even if he feels well.
(b) Tell Mr Y to go to his general practitioner if he has fever, sore throat or other symptoms of infection.
(c) Tell Mr Y to report to his general practitioner any cough or taste disturbance.
(d) Warn Mr Y that some prescription and non-prescription drugs may interfere with his "blood pressure" drugs, so he must always tell the doctor and/or the pharmacist what he is taking.
(e) Advise Mr Y that he is taking a small dose of aspirin and that he should not take any more aspirin or aspirin-containing medication.

References and Further Reading

Anon., The treatment of mild hypertension, *Drug Ther. Bull.*, 1988, **26**, 5–8.

Anon., Alpha-blockade for hypertension: indifferent past, uncertain future, *Lancet*, 1989, **1**, 1055–1056.

Anon., Drugs for hypertension, *Med. Lett.*, 1989, **39**, 25–30.

Baker P., Hypertension and its treatment, *Pharm. J.*, 1987, **239**, 12–14.

Ramsay L.E., Managing mild hypertension, *Prescribers J.*, 1987 , **27**, 1–8.

Simpson F.O., Hypertensive disease, in *Avery's Drug Treatment: Principles and Practice of Clinical Pharmacology and Therapeutics*, 3rd edn, Speight T.M. (ed.), Auckland, ADIS Press, 1987, 676–731.

ANGINA

Linda Stephens

Pharmacy Services Manager, Leicester General Hospital

Day 1 Mrs M, a 69-year-old woman, was admitted onto the coronary care unit. Earlier that day, at 7 a.m., she had experienced a sudden chest pain which radiated down her left arm, into her hand, and up into her throat. She had associated nausea but did not feel sweaty. She had a three-year history of angina, for which she had been prescribed a glyceryl trinitrate (GTN) spray. Using the spray had given her some relief from the pain.

At 9 p.m. the same day she had experienced the same gripping pain, although this time it had increased in severity. It had radiated to her back and caused more nausea. Her family contacted her general practitioner, and she was admitted into the hospital at 11.45 p.m.

In addition to her history of angina, Mrs M had had a pulmonary embolus in the previous year, and was a non-insulin-dependent diabetic. There was nothing else of note in her medical history or her family history. Mrs M was a non-smoker, and did not drink alcohol.

Mrs M's regular drug therapy included:

GTN spray when required
Isosorbide mononitrate (ISMN) 20 mg twice daily
Nifedipine slow release tablets 20 mg twice daily

Her diabetes was controlled by diet alone.

On examination, Mrs M was found not to be in obvious distress. Her pulse was 90 beats per minute (bpm) and regular, her blood pressure (BP) was 140/90 mmHg, and her jugular venous pulse was not raised. Heart sounds 1 and 2 could be heard with no added sounds. Examination of her chest showed no abnormalities: the trachea was central, the percussion note resonant and the breath sounds were vesicular. Abdominal examination was also unremarkable: bowel sounds were present, the abdomen was soft and non-tender, and she was slightly obese. She had no evidence of anaemia, jaundice, clubbing, cyanosis, oedema, or lymphadenopathy, and all peripheral pulses were present. A diagnosis of exacerbation of her angina was made, but blood was taken for cardiac enzyme measurement to exclude acute myocardial infarction (MI).

Mrs M was given a Suscard® 5 mg buccal tablet (GTN sustained release). This did not relieve her pain, so an intravenous infusion of isosorbide dinitrate (ISDN) was prepared and administered at a dose of 2–10 mg/hour via a syringe pump. Mrs M was also prescribed her usual dose of nifedipine slow release tablets, sublingual GTN tablets 500 micrograms when required, 36 mmol of oral potassium per day, and 5000 units of subcutaneous heparin twice daily.

Her serum biochemistry and haematology results were:

Sodium 139 mmol/L (reference range 133–144)
Potassium 3.3 mmol/L (3.3–5.3)
Urea 4.7 mmol/L (2.5–6.5)
Creatinine 78 micromol/L (60–120)
Glucose 7.0 mmol/L (4.0–6.6)
White cell count 8.5×10^9/L (4–11×10^9)
Haemoglobin 14.5 g/dL (11.5–16.5)
Platelets 244×10^9/L (150–400×10^9)

1. What are the advantages of GTN spray over GTN sublingual tablets? How would you counsel Mrs M on the use of her spray?

2. What is the main indication for prescribing buccal, oral, or percutaneous GTN? What are the advantages and disadvantages of buccal GTN, compared with percutaneous or oral formulations of the drug?

3. Would you have recommended Suscard® buccal therapy for Mrs M?

4. What are the pharmaceutical precautions that would need to be taken into account when preparing ISDN for infusion? Given that Mrs M was prescribed 2–10 mg/hour, how should the dose be titrated?

5. *Would you have recommended GTN infusion rather than ISDN infusion for Mrs M?*

6. *Does Mrs M have any risk factors for coronary artery disease? Are there any aggravating or precipitating factors present?*

Day 2 Mrs M's serum biochemistry results were:

Creatine kinase (CPK) 106 iu/L (25–200)
Hydroxybutyric dehydrogenase (HBD) 114 iu/L (100–240)
Sodium 138 mmol/L (133–144)
Potassium 3.8 mmol/L (3.3–5.5)
Urea 4.3 mmol/L (2.5–6.5)
Creatinine 81 micromol/L (60–120)
Glucose 6.9 mmol/L (4.0–6.6)

Mrs M was now pain-free, but she felt weak. Q waves were present on the electrocardiogram (ECG). Mrs M was prepared for transfer to a medical ward; however, at 3 p.m. she once again complained of severe, tight, gripping pain at rest. Her ECG showed ST segment depression but there was no clinical evidence of left ventricular failure. A diagnosis of unstable angina was made.

Mrs M was given a single 50 mg dose of atenolol, her dose of nifedipine was increased from 20 mg twice daily to 40 mg twice daily, the ISDN infusion rate was increased, and 150 mg aspirin was given. Mrs M was monitored for the next hour; her ECG showed changes in leads V1–V3 with a rise in the ST segment. An infusion of 1.5 million units of streptokinase in 100 mL of 0.9% sodium chloride was administered over one hour. The ISDN infusion had been continued at 5 mg/hour over this period. It was decided to decrease the infusion rate gradually over the next 12 hours, and prescribe oral isosorbide mononitrate (ISMN) therapy instead.

7. *Why was Mrs M given a dose of atenolol?*

8. *Why was Mrs M given streptokinase and aspirin?*

9. *Do you agree that ISMN is more appropriate than ISDN as oral therapy for Mrs M?*

10. *What oral dose of ISMN would be appropriate for Mrs M when the ISDN infusion is discontinued?*

11. *Are there any advantages to the controlled release ISMN preparations?*

12. *What problems arise if oral nitrates are given at regular intervals through the day?*

Mrs M's serum biochemistry results were:

1st sample (3 p.m. Day 2)   CPK 422 iu/L (25–200)
                            HBD 180 iu/L (100–240)
2nd sample (12 hours later) CPK 129 iu/L (25–200)
                            HBD 103 iu/L (100–240)
3rd sample (24 hours later) CPK 106 iu/L (25–200)
                            HBD 114 iu/L (100–240)
Sodium 138 mmol/L (133–144)
Potassium 3.9 mmol/L (3.3–5.3)
Urea 4.5 mmol/L (2.5–6.5)
Creatinine 90 micromol/L (60–120)

Day 3 Mrs M was now free from pain. As she had no signs of heart failure, it was decided to continue therapy with atenolol 50 mg orally daily. Her pulse was 80 bpm, and she was in sinus rhythm with a BP of 110/60 mmHg. Heart sounds 1 and 2 were heard with no added sounds. Mrs M was transferred from the coronary care unit to the general medical ward.

13. *Would you have recommended long-term beta-blocker therapy for Mrs M? Was atenolol an appropriate choice?*

14. *What are the main therapeutic goals with respect to Mrs M's treatment now?*

15. *How would you monitor the effectiveness of her therapy?*

16. *Is nifedipine slow release an appropriate choice of calcium-channel blocker for Mrs M?*

17. *If Mrs M did show signs of heart failure, which calcium-channel blocker might be more appropriate?*

Day 5 At 8.20 p.m. Mrs M once again complained of chest pain which radiated down her left arm. The pain had been brought on by mild exertion. She was given two GTN sublingual tablets 500 micrograms, which slightly relieved the pain. Her pulse was found to be 80 bpm, she was still in sinus rhythm, and her BP was 136/58 mmHg. However, her ECG showed ST segment depression in leads V4, V5 and V6, and Q waves in leads V1 and V2. The doctor monitoring Mrs M diagnosed a return of her unstable angina and re-started an ISDN infusion on her transfer back to the coronary care unit.

In view of Mrs M's history of angina at rest, with ECG changes following a recent dose of streptokinase, she was referred for cardiac catheterisation.

Day 6 Mrs M's catheterisation showed that the left anterior descending artery was blocked.

18. *What additional therapy could be added to Mrs M's regimen?*

19. *What alternatives to drug therapy exist for Mrs M?*

Answers

1. Sublingual GTN is a relatively cheap and convenient preparation. The major disadvantage is the unstable nature of the tablets. GTN spray is a useful economic option for patients who need to use GTN infrequently. In addition, some patients may find a spray more convenient than sublingual tablets. GTN sprays are stable for up to three years. Both preparations are useful in the treatment of an anginal attack. They have a quick onset of action (one to two minutes), and a short duration of action (five to ten minutes).

The following points should be covered when counselling Mrs M.
(a) She should rest, ideally in a sitting position.
(b) The canister should not be shaken. It should be held vertically with the valve head uppermost and the spray orifice as close to the mouth as possible.
(c) The dose should be sprayed under the tongue, and the mouth closed immediately after each dose.
(d) A second 400 microgram metered dose can be administered after ten minutes if the first dose is ineffective. No more than three metered doses are generally recommended at any one time. If the chest pain persists, Mrs M should contact her general practitioner.
(e) For the prevention of exercise-induced angina, or in other precipitating conditions, a metered dose can be sprayed under the tongue immediately prior to the event.
(f) Do not inhale the spray.
(g) If Mrs M had not previously used a GTN spray, she should be warned about the possibility of side-effects, especially facial flushing and headache.

2. Sublingual preparations of GTN are useful in the treatment of angina attacks; however, if the incidence of angina necessitates frequent dosing with these preparations, the use of a longer-acting preparation should be considered.

Buccal, percutaneous and oral GTN preparations all have a longer duration of action than sublingual formulations.

Percutaneous GTN can be administered as a controlled release patch, or as an ointment. The former may have some psychological benefit as the patch can be placed directly over the heart, whereas the latter is messy, and dosing can be inaccurate.

There is some doubt about the clinical effectiveness of the slow release GTN tablet preparations, and generally they are little used.

Buccal GTN has an extremely rapid onset of action which is nearly comparable to sublingual GTN; however, unlike a sublingual formulation, the buccal preparation has a longer duration of action (it persists while the tablet is in contact with the buccal mucosa).

A disadvantage to longer acting formulations of GTN is that tolerance can occur with all the available preparations, particularly GTN patches.

3. Yes. There is some merit in trying Suscard® buccal tablets for Mrs M's condition. Administration does not involve the introduction of an intravenous line, and the tablets are considerably cheaper than parenteral preparations.

The data sheet recommends starting with a 1 mg buccal tablet; however, in practice, the 5 mg tablet is usually used. If, as in Mrs M's case, this preparation is insufficient to render the patient pain-free, an intravenous infusion of ISDN can be started.

4. It must be remembered that nitrate solutions suffer loss of potency if used in conjunction with PVC infusion bags and giving sets. Mrs M's dose should be increased gradually until she is pain-free.

Nitrate preparations for intravenous use are compatible with commonly used infusion solutions, for example, dextrose 5%, and sodium chloride 0.9%. However, nitrate solutions in contact with PVC may lose up to 40% on prolonged contact. Viaflex® and Steriflex® bags should therefore be avoided. In practice, administration is usually via an infusion pump.

Mrs M's dose of ISDN infusion should be gradually increased until she is pain-free. The dose range of 2–10 mg/hour is of necessity a broad band, reflecting the wide patient-to-patient dose requirement for effective therapy. During administration her BP and pulse must be monitored. The dose should be reviewed after 24 hours as tolerance can occur. In practice, it has been found that the majority of patients need comparatively high doses, but for a short period of time, and tachyphylaxis is not a problem.

5. Yes. A GTN infusion would have been preferable.

GTN infusions should be diluted to a concentration of 400 micrograms/mL or less. Although it is recommended that ISDN infusion is diluted prior to administration, it is usually given as a slow intravenous infusion via a syringe pump. There are obvious advantages to using ISDN infusion in patients who have cardiac failure, where fluid intake may be restricted; however, in patients like Mrs M who are not so restricted, GTN is an equally effective but cheaper alternative.

The half-life of intravenous GTN is 10–15 seconds, compared with approximately ten minutes for ISDN. Some studies suggest that GTN is predominantly a venous vasodilator, as it affects mainly the systemic venous bed, and lowers pulmonary capillary pressure. ISDN reduces peripheral vascular resistance and increases cardiac output, suggesting that, when given intravenously, ISDN has the haemodynamic properties of a mixed – rather than a purely venous – vasodilator. ISDN may thus also be more appropriate when there is a combination of lowered cardiac output and normal pulmonary capillary pressure, as during acute myocardial infarction (MI).

6. No. Mrs M does not appear to have any risk factors for coronary artery disease.

The major risk factors are hypercholesterolaemia, hypertension, and cigarette smoking. Family history, age, male gender, and obesity may also have an effect. As Mrs M is normotensive and a non-smoker, her only possible risk factor is her weight. She shows no signs of clinical hypercholesterolaemia, and is not being investigated further in this respect. Anaemia, thyrotoxicosis or myxoedema can all aggravate angina, but Mrs M is not suffering from any of these conditions.

7. Atenolol has been prescribed with the aim of controlling Mrs M's unstable angina.

Unstable angina is usually defined as angina at rest or on minimal exertion. It has also been described as pre-infarction angina, and the condition should thus be regarded as an urgent medical problem. Treatment includes bedrest, administration of nitrates, and careful monitoring. The presence of recurrent pain at rest raises the possibility of coronary vasospasm. When coronary vasospasm is the main problem, treatment should be coronary vasodilation, suitable agents being calcium-channel blockers, and nitrates.

Beta-blockers may exacerbate the condition by inhibiting coronary artery dilation; however, they also inhibit the actions of catecholamines on the heart and the peripheral arterioles. This leads to a decrease in myocardial oxygen consumption by:

(a) reducing heart rate, especially the increases associated with exercise and stress,

(b) reducing BP, and

(c) reducing the force of contraction of the heart.

For these reasons, beta-blockers are of value in unstable angina.

8. To limit cardiac damage as she has suffered an MI.

ECG changes, later confirmed by her laboratory results, indicate she has suffered an MI. The Second International Study of Infarct Survival (ISIS-2), in 1988, showed that concurrent administration of 1.5 million units of streptokinase and 150 mg of aspirin, could significantly limit cardiac damage if given within 24 hours, but ideally within 6 hours of an MI.

9. Yes. ISMN has several advantages over ISDN as oral therapy for Mrs M.

ISDN is completely absorbed, and rapidly metabolised to two active metabolites, isosorbide-2-mononitrate, and isosorbide-5-mononitrate (approved name isosorbide mononitrate, or ISMN). Approximately 50% of an oral dose of ISDN circulates as the 5-mononitrate metabolite, but this can vary between individuals from 22 to 68%. The elimination half-life of the dinitrate, and the 2- and 5-mononitrate metabolites are 0.5, 1.5, and 4.5 hours respectively.

The advantages of ISMN over ISDN are:

(a) Oral ISMN is not subject to the variable first-pass metabolism of ISDN, and therefore provides a more predictable, and reproducible plasma concentration, and hence clinical effect. Blood levels achieved are similar to those after intravenous infusion of an equal dose.

(b) The duration of action of ISMN is longer than that of ISDN. Because of its short half-life, ISDN is available in various sustained release preparations.

(c) Bioavailability problems that have been noted between different brands of sustained release ISDN are not apparent with the mononitrate preparations; therefore, there are fewer problems with generic prescriptions.

(d) ISMN is cheaper than clinically equivalent doses of ISDN.

10. Mrs M should be started on 20 mg of ISMN twice daily after the infusion is discontinued.

The choice of this dose is empirical, and is not related to the intravenous dose over 24 hours. The intravenous dose range of 2–10 mg/hour is of necessity high, while a patient like Mrs M is at risk. The intravenous dose should be tailed off over a period of 8–12 hours to avoid any rebound vasoconstriction. In a patient who had not previously taken ISMN, a lower dose – 10 mg twice daily – would have been preferable to avoid nitrate side-effects, particularly headache.

11. No clear advantages have yet become apparent.

The controlled release ISMN preparations that are currently available, Imdur® and Elantan LA®, seem to be effective in angina. Studies have shown that they are formulated to give a "low-nitrate" period, and in clinical practice tolerance does not seem to be a problem. In theory, because the initial nitrate level is lower than that produced by a non-controlled release tablet of ISMN, headaches should be less of a problem for patients. In practice, however, there seems little evidence of this, and thus, overall clinical advantages are equivocal.

12. Tolerance.

Before addressing this phenomenon it is necessary to discuss the mode of action of organic nitrates in angina. GTN, ISDN, and isosorbide-2- and 5-mononitrate are all organic nitro-esters, containing the chemical moiety $R-O-NO_2$. The ester bond is important for the vascular smooth-muscle-relaxing effect of these drugs.

Nitrates relieve the symptoms of angina through a combination of their indirect effects on pre-load and after-load, and their direct effects on coronary circulation. It has been suggested that dilation of the venous capacitance vessels may be the most important mechanism for the anti-anginal effect of nitrates. The reduction of pre-load by venous vasodilation is both immediate and pronounced. This causes a reduction in both right- and left-sided pressures during diastole, thereby bringing about a fall in right atrial pressure as well as pulmonary capillary wedge pressure. As a result, cardiac oxygen demands are reduced. In addition, as the intramural pressure on sub-endocardial vessels falls during diastole, blood flow increases to these deeper levels of the myocardium. Nitrates also have a direct anti-ischaemic effect on coronary vessels. Dilation of coronary stenoses occurs, as does an increase in inter-coronary collateral flow.

There are a number of proposed mechanisms for the vasodilating effects of organic nitrates:

(a) interaction with a specific sulphydryl nitrate receptor,

(b) stimulation of guanylate cyclase and synthesis of cyclic guanosine monophosphate,

(c) lowering of intracellular calcium,

(d) stimulation of vasodilating prostaglandins.

Chronic and continuous administration of all nitrates, regardless of formulation or route of administration, will result in tolerance. Tolerance can be described as a reduction in, or the attenuation of, the haemodynamic or anti-ischaemic effects. However, the majority of patients still respond to a bolus dose of nitrate, for example a sublingual GTN tablet.

Tolerance is thought to develop because of oxidation of sulphydryl groups. It is postulated that there is a specific sulphydryl nitrate receptor. Organic nitrates are converted to nitric oxide with the production of nitrosothiols by reaction with these sulphydryl-containing compounds in receptors in vascular smooth muscle. The nitrosothiols will in turn augment the production of cyclic guanosine monophosphate. It is possible by the concurrent administration of sulphydryl donors, such as acetylcysteine or captopril, that tolerance may be avoided or minimised. However, further studies are required before these strategies are employed regularly. The number of sulphydryl groups can be restored simply by allowing nitrate concentrations to fall to a low level during part of the dosing regimen.

Thus, a nitrate-free period seems to be an effective way of avoiding the development of tolerance. This can be achieved in practice by having low nitrate levels for periods of between eight and 16 hours per day. Patients should be told to remove transdermal patches before retiring to bed, and the last dose of long-acting nitrates should be taken with the evening meal, and not at bedtime. Patients who experience regular angina attacks throughout the day should be given a beta-blocker or calcium-channel blocker to cover the "low-nitrate" period.

13. Yes. Although beta-blockers should be used with caution in patients with type II diabetes (see full discussion in Case Study 24), the severity of Mrs M's angina warrants the inclusion of this agent as third-line treatment in her drug regimen.

In patients with angina who do not have contra-indications to beta-blockers, these agents would be regarded as first- or second-line agents. Atenolol is an appropriate choice for Mrs M because it is cardioselective. Beta-blockers can interfere with the metabolic and autonomic responses to hypoglycaemia, but the cardioselective agents appear to have less effect than the non-selective agents.

14. (a) Prevent further ischaemic episodes.
    (b) Ensure that Mrs M remains pain-free.
    (c) Prevent further MIs.

15. The effectiveness of the regimen can be assessed in a number of ways.

Mrs M's exercise tolerance can be measured, although this cannot be done until she has fully recovered from her MI. Mrs M herself can be questioned about her exercise capabilities, bearing in mind the fact that she would be more active at home than in hospital. Another way is to count the number of GTN tablets consumed each day. Usage of more than ten per day would indicate a need to reassess the preventative therapy.

16. Yes, provided Mrs M's blood glucose is monitored regularly, initially and after dose increases, as nifedipine can interfere with insulin release in some patients.

In patients like Mrs M with unstable angina, coronary spasm is felt to be an important factor leading to myocardial ischaemia. In these patients, calcium-channel blockers are thought to be beneficial because of their vasodilatory effects on coronary arteries. The three major drugs in this category are nifedipine, verapamil, and diltiazem. These drugs relieve angina mainly by inhibiting the influx of calcium into the excited myocardial fibre, thus reducing ATP consumption by the contractile system. This in turn leads to a reduction in myocardial oxygen consumption, and also has the effect of depressing myocardial contractility. Similar mechanisms lead to a reduction in vascular smooth muscle tone, and the dilation of coronary arteries and peripheral resistance vessels. The net effect is a change in myocardial oxygen supply/demand ratio. The anti-anginal effect of these drugs is comparable with that of beta-blocker therapy.

Some of the side-effects are related to the vasodilator action, and include headache, flushing, palpitations, and ankle swelling. Nifedipine has a more pronounced peripheral effect than verapamil or diltiazem, and may be more likely to cause these symptoms. Nifedipine may also cause reflex sinus tachycardia, and as a result the occasional patient may actually complain of worsening angina.

Verapamil and diltiazem both depress cardiac conduction, and must be avoided in sick sinus syndrome or atrio-ventricular block. Neither of these drugs should be given parenterally with a beta-blocker, as this can result in severe bradycardia. However, the combination can be used orally as long as the patient is advised to report any symptoms suggestive of hypotension, bradycardia, or cardiac failure. Verapamil is also known to cause constipation, and as such would not be recommended for an elderly patient such as Mrs M.

17. Diltiazem.

Diltiazem appears to have less negative inotropic affect than nifedipine because it has a less pronounced peripheral effect. If Mrs M develops cardiac failure, it may be prudent to substitute diltiazem for nifedipine in her regimen and to discontinue her atenolol therapy. Beta-blockers also have a negative inotropic effect, and combination with calcium-channel blockers can lead to an increased risk of bradycardia and atrio-ventricular block.

18. Mrs M is now on triple therapy for the control of her angina. She is taking a beta-blocker, a long-acting nitrate, and a calcium-channel blocker. There is little else that could be added to Mrs M's regimen. However, the regimen could be manipulated as follows.

(a) The dose of ISMN could be increased. The maximum dose is dependent on the patient's tolerance to side-effects, particularly headache.

(b) The dose of nifedipine slow release could be doubled, but careful monitoring would be required.

(c) The dose of beta-blocker could be doubled, but as Mrs M is a Type II diabetic this would be the least satisfactory manoeuvre.

19. Coronary artery bypass surgery would be an alternative for Mrs M. However, there would have to be a suitable time lapse to allow her to recover fully from her MI.

References

Anon., Is isosorbide mononitrate better than the dinitrate?, *Drug Ther. Bull.*, 1984, **22**, 7–8.

Anon., The calcium antagonists: an important new group of drugs, *Drug Ther. Bull.*, 1984, **22**, 65–68.

Anon., Nitrates in heart disease, *Drug Ther. Bull.*, 1984, **22**, 77–79.

Anon., Nitrates: the problem of tolerance, *Drug Ther. Bull.*, 1988, **26**, 57–59.

Anon., Nitrates and angina, *Lancet*, 1984, **1**, 998–999.

Anon., Transdermal nitrates: effective or not?, *Lancet*, 1985, **2**, 594–595.

Anon., Prevention of coronary heart disease, *Lancet*, 1987, **1**, 601–602.

Balcon R., Angina, in *Oxford Textbook of Medicine*, 2nd edn, Weatherall D.J., Ledingham J.G.G. and Warrell D.A. (eds), Oxford, Oxford University Press, 1987, 13.163–13.166.

Bray C. and Ward C., *Ischaemic Heart Disease*, Update, Postgraduate Centre Series, 1986, 16–25.

Cowan C. *et al.*, Tolerance to glyceryl trinitrate patches: prevention by intermittent dosing, *Br. med. J.*, 1987, **294**, 544–545.

Ectuzen H. and Eichelbaum M., Clinical pharmacokinetics of verapamil, nifedipine and diltiazem, *Clin. Pharmacokinet.*, 1986, **11**, 425–449.

Fuster V., Cohen M. and Halperin J. Aspirin in the prevention of coronary artery disease, *New Engl. J. Med.*, 1989, **321**, 183–185.

Opie L.H., *Drugs for the heart*, 2nd edn., New York, Grune Stratten, 1987.

Petch M.C., Aspirin for unstable angina?, *Br. med. J.*, 1986, **293**, 1–2.

Raehl C.L. and Nolan P.E., Angina pectoris, in *Applied Therapeutics – the Clinical Use of Drugs*, 4th edn, Young L.Y. and Koda-Kimble M.A. (eds), Vancouver, WA, Applied Therapeutics, 1988, 271–288.

Thadani U. and Whitsett T., Relationship of pharmacokinetic and pharmacodynamic properties of organic nitrates, *Clin. Pharmacokinet.*, 1988, **15,** 32–43.

Theroux P., Talymans Y. and Water D.D., Calcium antagonists, clinical use in the treatment of angina, *Drugs*, 1983, **25,** 178–195.

MYOCARDIAL INFARCTION

P. Julie Cannon

Clinical Pharmacist, Intensive Care and Coronary Care Units, Derbyshire Royal Infirmary

Day 1 Mr B, a 58-year-old managing director of a printing company, presented to the casualty department of the local district general hospital complaining of a severe pain in his chest which had started about two hours ago and had not been relieved by two paracetamol tablets. He had also experienced a tingling sensation in his left arm. His wife had called the ambulance when the pain worsened and her husband had looked pale and sweaty. He had vomited twice while waiting for the ambulance. On questioning by the casualty officer, Mr B said that he had been previously fit and well. However, in the last two weeks he had experienced some chest discomfort while walking up stairs, but had not consulted his general practitioner about this. He admitted to smoking between 10 and 15 cigarettes a day and to social drinking. He had two children who no longer lived at home. His father had died at the age of 60 of a heart attack and his older brother suffered from angina.

The doctor in casualty performed an electrocardiogram (ECG), took a blood sample, and explained to Mr B that he may have suffered a heart attack and that he was being sent to the coronary care unit for close observation. An intravenous bolus of 2.5 mg of diamorphine hydrochloride was given, which relieved the pain. Mr B had no contra-indications to thrombolytic therapy and therefore a streptokinase infusion was prescribed to be started as soon as possible.

His serum biochemistry results on admission were:

Sodium 141 mmol/L (reference range 133–145)
Potassium 3.3 mmol/L (3.5–5.0)
Glucose 5.7 mmol/L (4.0–5.8, fasting)
Urea 4.2 mmol/L (2.5–6.6)
Creatinine 105 micromol/L (60–130)

1. What risk factors did Mr B have for developing an acute myocardial infarction?

2. What blood tests could be carried out to confirm the diagnosis of myocardial infarction?

3. What is the rationale for giving thrombolytic therapy in acute myocardial infarction?

4. When should thrombolytic therapy commence if maximum benefit is to be obtained?

5. What are the contra-indications to giving thrombolytic therapy?

6. What other agents, apart from thrombolytics, have been used clinically to reduce infarct size?

7. Would you have recommended thrombolytic therapy or an alternative for Mr B? Defend your decision.

8. Is streptokinase the thrombolytic of choice for Mr B?

9. Is Mr B's serum potassium level likely to be a cause for concern over the next 24 hours?

On admission to the coronary care unit, Mr B was connected to a three-lead ECG to monitor his heart rate and rhythm. Subsequently, a 12-lead ECG was performed which showed sinus rhythm (heart rate 70 beats per minute) with ST segment elevation and T wave inversion in leads II, III, and aVF, and reciprocal ST depression in leads aVL and V_2–V_4, which suggested an inferior myocardial infarction. His blood pressure was 170/90 mmHg.

His prescribed therapy was:

Diamorphine hydrochloride 2.5–5 mg intravenously when required
Metoclopramide hydrochloride 10 mg intravenously when required
Glyceryl trinitrate 500 micrograms–1 mg sublingually when required
Hydrocortisone sodium succinate 100 mg intravenously prior to streptokinase
Streptokinase 1.5 million units in 100 ml normal saline by intravenous infusion over one hour

Aspirin 150 mg orally at once, then 150 mg orally once daily
Lactulose 10 mL orally when required
Oxygen 35% via mask

Mr B's serum biochemistry results 24 hours after admission were:

Sodium 140 mmol/L (133–145)
Potassium 3.4 mmol/L (3.5–5.0)
Glucose 5.4 mmol/L (4.0–5.8, fasting)
Urea 4.1 mmol/L (2.5–6.6)
Creatinine 96 micromol/L (60–130)

10. Is diamorphine hydrochloride appropriate for Mr B? Is the dose appropriate? Which other narcotic analgesic agents could be used?

11. Why is it normally advisable to avoid intramuscular injections after an acute myocardial infarction?

12. Why has metoclopramide hydrochloride been prescribed? What is the maximum dose that can be administered in 24 hours to a patient like Mr B?

13. What is the rationale for prescribing hydrocortisone sodium succinate prior to the administration of streptokinase?

14. What advice would you give to the coronary care nurse regarding the preparation and administration of the streptokinase infusion?

15. How should Mr B be monitored during administration of the streptokinase infusion?

16. Would you have recommended aspirin therapy for Mr B? Was the dose appropriate?

17. Comment on the appropriateness of prescribing lactulose for Mr B.

About two hours after commencing the streptokinase infusion, Mr B's heart rate fell to 35 beats per minute. His blood pressure at this time was 70/50 mmHg. After he was given atropine 600 micrograms by an intravenous bolus, his heart rate returned to 65 beats per minute and his blood pressure increased to 120/70 mmHg.

18. What are the likely causes of bradycardia in this patient?

19. If Mr B had not responded to atropine, what would you have recommended as alternative treatment(s) for bradycardia?

20. What advice would you give to a doctor who asked if it was safe to place a temporary pacing wire in Mr B three hours after giving a streptokinase infusion?

Day 2 Mr B complained of chest pain which was worse on breathing. He was examined by the doctor who diagnosed pericarditis and prescribed indomethacin 50 mg orally three times a day for two days only.

Mr B had three further episodes of chest pain in the coronary care unit which were unlike his previous pain and which responded to 500 micrograms of sublingual glyceryl trinitrate. He was prescribed isosorbide dinitrate 10 mg orally three times a day.

The serum cardiac enzyme results were:

CK 171 iu/L (on admission) (24–195)
CK 3190 iu/L (12 hours after admission)
CKMB 328 iu/L (12 hours after admission)
CKMB% 10% (12 hours after admission) (0–5%)

These results, together with the ECG, confirmed a diagnosis of myocardial infarction.

21. How is angina pain distinguished from pericarditic pain?

22. What are the problems associated with prescribing indomethacin for Mr B?

23. How should Mr B be monitored while on indomethacin?

Day 3 Mr B was transferred to a medical ward. He had no further chest pain on the ward. He was prescribed timolol maleate 5 mg orally twice daily on day 5. During his stay, Mr B was counselled by the ward sister regarding his heart attack and was given advice about changing his diet and lifestyle. Prior to discharge, the sister requested that the ward pharmacist speak to the patient about his discharge medication.

Day 7 Mr B was discharged home, feeling well.
His medication on discharge was:

Glyceryl trinitrate 500 micrograms–1 mg sublingually when required
Isosorbide dinitrate 10 mg orally three times a day
Aspirin 150 mg orally once daily
Timolol maleate 10 mg orally twice daily

A seven-day supply of medication was dispensed.

24. What points would you cover when counselling Mr B on his discharge medication?

25. How long should his aspirin therapy be continued after discharge from the hospital?

26. What is the rationale for prescribing timolol maleate for Mr B? Is the dosage regimen appropriate? How long would you recommend treatment be continued?

27. Could another beta-blocker have been used instead of timolol maleate?

Answers

1. Mr B's major risk factors for sustaining a myocardial infarction were his sex, age, and the fact that he smoked cigarettes.

(a) Sex – males are about twice as likely to develop ischaemic heart disease as females, although with increasing age the risk is about the same in both sexes.

(b) Age – increasing age is a risk factor for developing myocardial infarction.

(c) Cigarette smoking – smoking greatly increases the risk of myocardial infarction.

Other factors which may be of some importance in this case are:

(a) Family history – Mr B's older brother had angina and his father had died at an early age of a heart attack; thus there is a history of ischaemic heart disease in his family which increased Mr B's risk of the same.

(b) A possible history of angina – Mr B had experienced some chest pain in the weeks preceding his admission, which may have been angina. A history of angina is a risk factor for developing a myocardial infarction (MI). Epidemiological data have shown that about one-quarter of male patients and one-eighth of women with angina will have an infarct within five years of the date of diagnosis.

Mr B admitted to social drinking. While a high alcohol intake is a possible risk factor for the development of ischaemic heart disease, a small or moderate intake may actually be of benefit. Alcohol ingestion is associated with an increase in high density lipoprotein (HDL) cholesterol in the blood, and there is a strong correlation between HDL cholesterol levels and the absence of ischaemic heart disease.

Mr B is a managing director, which indicates that his job may be stressful. However, stress has not been proved to be a risk factor for MI. It is a common misbelief that individuals in the higher social classes, such as Mr B, are at greater risk of developing ischaemic heart disease than those in the lower social classes. However, epidemiological data show that it is those in the lower social classes who are at greatest risk, probably because their tobacco and alcohol intake is higher.

2. Determination of the so-called "cardiac enzymes".

A blood sample is taken on admission and again 12–24 hours later to measure cardiac enzymes. The three most commonly measured cardiac enzymes are:

(a) creatine kinase (CK) (and the isoenzyme specific for myocardium, CK-MB),

(b) lactate dehydrogenase (LDH), and

(c) aspartate aminotransferase (AST).

These enzymes are liberated by the myocardium (heart muscle) in response to damage. Each enzyme has a particular time course of release following acute MI. CK is increased within 6–8 hours of an MI, reaches a peak in 24 hours, and declines to normal within 3–4 days. AST is increased within 12 hours of infarction and the peak activity occurs between 18 and 36 hours after infarction. Normal levels are resumed within 2–4 days. LDH is increased within 24–48 hours of the onset of pain, the peak activity occurs within 3–6 days, and the level is back to normal between 8 and 14 days after infarction. LDH is used in the retrospective diagnosis of infarction.

For Mr B, CK and possibly AST measurements are the most appropriate, as his history suggests that his infarct occurred about two hours prior to admission. LDH measurement is not necessary. It must be remembered when interpreting results that the enzymes are not specific for heart muscle. CK may also be found in skeletal muscle; and for this reason, the isoenzyme specific for myocardium is also measured, and expressed as a percentage of the total CK. LDH is also liberated from haemolysed red blood cells. AST is also a hepatic enzyme and levels may rise after hepatic congestion due to cardiac failure.

3. To limit heart muscle damage.

In about 90% of patients who suffer an MI, the cause is obstruction of one or more of the major coronary arteries by a clot (thrombosis). This clot comprises platelets, white cells and fibrin. It is known that the area of myocardium normally supplied by the obstructed coronary artery does not die immediately, but takes up to six hours. During this time it is possible to halt the process by dissolving the clot that is causing the blockage, and reperfusing the ischaemic myocardium. Thrombolytic agents dissolve the clot and may salvage some of the myocardium, reducing the amount of heart muscle damage and thereby improving long-term prognosis.

4. Within six hours of the onset of symptoms.

In the major thrombolytic trials, thrombolytic therapy was usually commenced within five to six hours of the onset of symptoms suggestive of an MI. A significant reduction in mortality was demonstrated in all these trials in patients receiving thrombolytic agents, compared with controls. One of the major thrombolytic trials (ISIS-2) demonstrated a reduction in mortality and re-infarction rate in patients given streptokinase up to 24 hours after the onset of symptoms suggestive of an MI. However, this trial clearly showed that the greatest benefit was achieved if streptokinase was given within the first six hours. It is therefore generally agreed that the maximum benefit is obtained when thrombolytic agents are commenced within six hours of the onset of symptoms.

5. The contra-indications to thrombolytic therapy are as follows (reasons given in brackets).

(a) History of bleeding, e.g. gastric bleeding, cerebral haemorrhage, pulmonary haemorrhage (streptokinase causes depletion of fibrinogen and other clotting factors and hence impairs the ability to clot, thus bleeding may be precipitated);

(b) uncontrolled hypertension (since this may increase the risk of stroke due to cerebral haemorrhage);

(c) known or suspected active peptic ulceration (increases the risk of gastric bleeding);

(d) pregnancy or lactation (unknown effects in foetus/infant);

(e) streptokinase or anistreplase therapy within the previous six months (previous exposure to these drugs induces the production of antibodies, and subsequent doses can cause anaphylactic shock);

(f) possible allergy to streptokinase (risk of anaphylaxis);

(g) recent intracranial haemorrhage or stroke (further risk of haemorrhage);

(h) any recent invasive procedure such as insertion of a central, arterial or venous line (increased risk of bleeding);

(i) recent surgery, including tooth extraction (increased bleeding from wound site);

(j) patients with defective haemostasis (increased risk of bleeding);

(k) those who have had prolonged cardiopulmonary resuscitation (risk of bleeding into liver or organs ruptured by rib fractures);

(l) anticoagulant therapy (increased risk of bleeding).

6. Other agents that have been shown to reduce infarct size are the beta-blockers, nifedipine and nitrates; however not all of these agents have been shown to reduce mortality after an MI.

A number of trials have been performed where beta-blockers were given shortly after the onset of symptoms in an attempt to reduce infarct size and subsequent mortality. One trial using atenolol demonstrated a 15% reduction in mortality (ISIS-

1). In another study using metoprolol (MIAMI), just under 6,000 patients were randomised to receive either metoprolol or placebo, first intravenously then orally. The mortality reduction at 15 days was 13%, which was similar to that in the ISIS-1 trial but was not statistically significant.

While nifedipine has been shown to reduce infarct size in animal models and in minor clinical trials, the benefit was not demonstrated in a large mortality study (Wilcox, 1986). In this trial, patients with suspected MI were randomised to receive either nifedipine or placebo immediately after assessment in the coronary care unit. The overall one-month mortality rates were 6.3% in the placebo-treated group and 6.7% in the nifedipine-treated group. There was thus a possible increase in mortality in the group of patients who received nifedipine, but the difference in mortality rates was not statistically significant.

Intravenous glyceryl trinitrate has been shown to reduce cardiac enzyme levels and to improve left ventricular function, suggesting limitation of infarct size, but has not been shown to reduce mortality.

7. Thrombolytic therapy plus aspirin was the most appropriate treatment for Mr B.

The agents that have been shown in clinical trials to reduce infarct size and mortality are the thrombolytic agents streptokinase, anistreplase and alteplase, and atenolol and aspirin.

Whilst beta-blockers have been shown to reduce mortality when given in the early stages after an MI, the benefit is not great. In a very large controlled study (ISIS-1; 16,000 patients), atenolol 5–10 mg was given intravenously within five hours of onset of symptoms, followed by 100 mg daily by mouth for up to seven days. This dosage regimen was shown to reduce mortality by 15%. In real terms this means that it would be necessary to treat 200 patients to avoid one re-infarction, one cardiac arrest and one death during the first seven days post-MI. In addition, beta-blockers do carry certain risks in patients with suspected MI. They are contra-indicated in those with bradycardia, heart block, uncontrolled heart failure, or hypotension, and therefore cannot be given to up to 50% of possible candidates. On admission, Mr B had no contra-indications to administration of a beta-blocker, and therefore he was a potential candidate for atenolol therapy. However, a later ECG showed that he had suffered an inferior MI. Such patients have an increased risk of bradycardia, which may be potentiated by the use of a beta-blocker. A course of treatment with atenolol, given intravenously initially and followed by seven days' oral therapy, costs approximately £2.50.

Aspirin was shown to reduce mortality and re-infarction rate significantly in the ISIS-2 trial, both when given alone and when combined with strep-tokinase. There appears to be an additive benefit when streptokinase is given with aspirin: the five-week vascular mortality reduction compared with placebo, in patients treated up to 24 hours after the onset of symptoms, was 25% for streptokinase alone, 23% for aspirin alone, and 42% for strepto-kinase plus aspirin.

Thrombolytic agents do have serious complica-tions: in the ISIS-2 trial, 0.5% of patients receiving streptokinase had bleeds requiring transfusion compared with only 0.2% of those receiving pla-cebo; furthermore, 0.1% of streptokinase-treated patients had confirmed cerebral haemorrhage com-pared with none receiving placebo. There was therefore a small risk involved in giving streptoki-nase to Mr B. However, he was relatively young, had been previously fit and well, and had no contra-indications to thrombolytic or aspirin therapy on admission, so the benefits of an improved prognosis probably outweigh the risks in his case.

The cost of aspirin is small but streptokinase costs approximately £60 per treatment. Despite the greater cost of streptokinase compared with ateno-lol, streptokinase plus aspirin is the first choice of therapy for Mr B, because it can offer increased benefit and fewer complications. In hospitals where the drug budget is limited, aspirin alone or atenolol therapy would be a second choice.

8. Yes. Apart from streptokinase, the other throm-bolytic agents that are currently available are anistreplase (APSAC, anisoylated plasminogen streptokinase activator complex) and alteplase (rt-PA, recombinant tissue-type plasminogen ac-tivator).

In clinical trials all three agents have been shown to reduce mortality significantly after MI. Anistrep-lase and alteplase have some selectivity for fibrin-bound plasminogen and therefore produce less systemic fibrinolysis than streptokinase. In theory this "clot-specificity" should reduce haemorrhagic complications; however, in clinical trials the inci-dence of major bleeds is similar in patients given alteplase or anistreplase to those given strepto-kinase.

At the time of writing, there have been no large studies on the comparative effects of thrombolytics after an acute MI. The trials already published do not indicate any clear advantage of one thromboly-tic agent over the others. The choice of agent for Mr

B is likely to be governed by local hospital prescrib-ing policies. At the time of writing, streptokinase is the least expensive agent at £60 per dose, anistrep-lase costs around £495 per dose, and alteplase costs about £550 per dose. Thus, in the absence of a clear clinical advantage, streptokinase is probably the agent of choice for Mr B, based on cost.

9. Mr B's low serum potassium is unlikely to be a cause for concern over the next 24 hours, unless a further fall is noted.

Patients who have suffered an acute MI are at increased risk of developing arrhythmias, and hypokalaemia further increases this risk. The cause of hypokalaemia in Mr B is probably excess catecholamine release in response to the pain and anxiety caused by the infarction. Unless Mr B is prescribed diuretics, his serum potassium is not likely to be a problem.

10. Yes.

The pain caused by an MI is severe and a strong analgesic such as a narcotic agent is appropriate. It should be given by the intravenous route for a rapid effect. Diamorphine is the narcotic agent of choice as, in addition to its analgesic properties, it allays the anxiety caused by the severe chest pain and the admission to hospital.

The dose prescribed for Mr B was also appro-priate. An initial dose of 2.5–5 mg can be supple-mented by doses of 2.5 mg at 10-minute intervals until pain relief is adequate. Thereafter, doses can be repeated every four to six hours. Relatively low doses of diamorphine should be prescribed initially in a patient with an MI, to avoid respiratory depression.

Morphine sulphate (5–10 mg) may be given intravenously as an alternative to diamorphine. Pethidine is inappropriate in a patient who has suffered an MI, since it may cause hypertension. In addition, it is shorter acting than diamorphine or morphine and needs to be given every three hours to be effective.

11. To avoid obscuring the diagnosis by interfer-ing with CK estimation, and to ensure rapid and predictable drug absorption.

Administration of drugs by the intramuscular route may cause some muscle damage, which results in liberation of the enzyme CK from muscle cells. This enzyme is also released from damaged heart muscle following an MI and, as discussed earlier, a rise in the level of CK is used to confirm the diagnosis. Intramuscular injections may thus cause a rise in the CK level in the blood, which can lead to confusion over the diagnosis.

The absorption of drugs given by the intramuscular route in a patient who has suffered an MI is also likely to be impaired, owing to a reduced peripheral circulation as a result of pain or reduced cardiac function. The intravenous route ensures faster and more predictable drug absorption, and this is therefore the preferred method of administration.

12. Nausea and vomiting are often experienced by a patient like Mr B, as a result of both the MI itself and the administration of an opioid analgesic. Metoclopramide is used intravenously in doses of 10 mg up to eight-hourly to prevent or treat nausea and vomiting.

13. To reduce the possibility of an allergic or anaphylactic reaction to streptokinase.

Streptokinase is produced from haemolytic streptococci, and patients who have had a streptococcal infection in the past are likely to have antibodies to streptokinase. Thus, allergy or anaphylaxis may occur after administration of streptokinase to these patients. It may also occur in those who have been previously exposed to streptokinase or anistreplase. This risk is theoretically reduced by pre-treatment with an intravenous corticosteroid or an H_1-receptor blocker, although there is no evidence that the use of either offers any such benefit.

14. The nurse who is preparing the streptokinase infusion should be advised as follows.

(a) Observe aseptic precautions during preparation.

(b) Dissolve streptokinase by adding an appropriate volume of diluent to the vial(s) and then gently rolling the vial(s) between the hands, being careful not to shake the vials vigorously.

(c) Add the streptokinase solution to a 100 mL infusion of normal saline.

(d) Administer the infusion over one hour; after completion, flush the intravenous line with at least 30 mL of normal saline to ensure the total dose is administered.

(e) Avoid administering other intravenous drugs at the same time as the streptokinase, since there are no compatibility data available at present.

15. During the administration of streptokinase, Mr B should be observed for signs of an allergic reaction to the drug. Typical signs and symptoms of minor allergy include urticaria, itching, headache, musculoskeletal pain, flushing, nausea, and pyrexia. A major allergic reaction is indicated by bronchospasm, hypotension and angioneurotic oedema.

His ECG should be closely monitored for any changes in heart rate or rhythm, as reperfusion arrhythmias or bradycardia may follow the administration of streptokinase. His blood pressure should also be checked regularly, since hypotension is frequently observed during the administration of streptokinase. Any changes in blood pressure should be reported to the doctor. His temperature should be monitored frequently, since a mild pyrexia of short duration may occur in some patients. Finally, Mr B should be observed for signs of bleeding, e.g. gum bleeding, epistaxis, haematoma, oozing at the catheter site, or pain from internal bleeding. The infusion site should be observed frequently for signs of bleeding or phlebitis. Patients are at risk of post-thrombolytic bleeding for two to four days after treatment.

16. Yes.

Aspirin has been shown in clinical trials to be effective in reducing mortality and re-infarction rate when given alone or in combination with streptokinase. There is an additive benefit when the two drugs are given in combination, and thus patients such as Mr B who have received streptokinase should also be given aspirin, unless there is evidence of allergy, recent epigastric pain, or other symptoms of aspirin intolerance. The mechanism of action of low doses of aspirin is the irreversible inhibition of cyclo-oxygenase-dependent platelet aggregation. Aggregation of platelets is partly responsible for the formation of the thrombus that causes obstruction of one of the coronary arteries in acute MI. The dose of aspirin used in the ISIS-2 trial was 160 mg daily. This preparation is not commercially available; two 75 mg tablets or half a 300 mg tablet daily may be taken instead.

17. Fibre or senna tablets would have been more appropriate.

Laxatives are often required to prevent constipation in patients who have had an MI, for the following reasons: they are bed-ridden for at least 24 hours and are less mobile thereafter, there is a change in diet as a result of hospital food, and administration of diamorphine or other opiate agents may cause constipation. A regularly scheduled laxative is therefore appropriate in those in whom constipation is a problem; however, lactulose may take up to 48 hours to act, and it would, therefore have been more appropriate to prescribe it on a regular basis rather than "as required" to ensure its effectiveness. Alternatively, a regular dose of fibre in the form of additional bran in the diet, or ispaghula husk (one sachet of Regulan® or Fybogel® twice daily), is as effective and less expensive than lactulose, as are senna tablets in doses of two to four at night as required.

18. Streptokinase therapy.

Mr B had suffered an inferior MI, and such a patient is likely to develop bradycardia. However, in this instance the episode occurred two hours after giving the streptokinase infusion. It is well documented that streptokinase therapy may cause bradycardia. It is thus most likely that it was the streptokinase therapy that precipitated Mr B's episode.

19. Isoprenaline is an alternative treatment for bradycardia if atropine fails to have an effect.

Isoprenaline may be given as an initial intravenous bolus of 100–200 micrograms; thereafter, an infusion of isoprenaline in glucose 5% may be given at a rate of 1–10 micrograms per minute. Isoprenaline should only be used as a short-term measure because of the danger of arrhythmias with long-term treatment. If the bradycardia persists, it may be appropriate for the doctor to consider inserting a temporary pacing wire and artificially pacing the heart.

20. It would not be advisable to insert a pacing wire three hours after giving streptokinase therapy.

Streptokinase has intrinsic anticoagulant activity and impairs clotting factors for up to 48 hours after the infusion has been given. There would therefore be an increased risk of bleeding from this procedure, which involves insertion of a wire into the subclavian vein. If it is absolutely necessary to insert a pacing wire in the first 48 hours, a femoral or antecubital route is recommended, to allow pressure to be applied if bleeding occurs, but this has to be a medical decision. After 48 hours it should be safe to insert a central line, but it is advisable to monitor the patient's clotting factors first.

21. The two types of pain are primarily differentiated by considering when and where they occur.

Angina causes central chest pain which radiates to the left arm, back, neck or jaw. The pain usually occurs after exertion or emotion, although some cases may occur at rest. It is relieved within a few minutes by rest or sublingual glyceryl trinitrate.

Pericarditic pain is caused by an acute inflammation of the pericardial membrane. It occurs at the same sites as angina-type pain and may radiate to the shoulders or neck. Pericarditic pain is distinguished from angina pain in that it is typically sharp and is worse or only appears on inspiration. In addition, it is altered by changes of position. The diagnosis of pericarditis is confirmed by the presence of a friction rub heard on auscultation of the chest.

22. Indomethacin inhibits platelet aggregation and may increase the risk of bleeding into the pericardium, which could result in cardiac tamponade.

Mr B has received streptokinase, which is known to deplete clotting factors; this may further increase his risk of systemic bleeding and pericardial haemorrhage. In addition, indomethacin has effects that are undesirable in the presence of infarction: for example, it causes fluid retention, systemic vasoconstriction, and (perhaps) coronary vasoconstriction.

23. While receiving indomethacin Mr B should be monitored for signs and symptoms of gastric complications and bleeding from any site. Since indomethacin may cause salt and water retention, his weight should also be monitored, and he should be observed for signs of oedema.

24. The following points should be covered during counselling of Mr B by the pharmacist.

Glyceryl trinitrate sublingual tablets

(a) Glyceryl trinitrate (GTN) tablets are for the relief of the type of chest pain that has been experienced in hospital.

(b) The tablets should be placed underneath the tongue and allowed to dissolve naturally. A burning or tingling sensation in the mouth is common after sublingual administration of GTN.

(c) Initially one tablet should be used, but if no relief is obtained a second and then a third tablet may be taken at five-minute intervals. If no relief is obtained after three tablets, Mr B should seek medical attention.

(d) It is advisable to sit down while taking the tablets, since this will help to relieve the pain and also avoid postural hypotension (feeling dizzy).

(e) The tablets are not addictive and there is no limit to how many can be taken in one day. However, Mr B should consult his general practitioner if his daily usage exceeds his usual requirements.

(f) The tablets may cause a headache and/or facial flushing. If the headache persists after relief from chest pain has been obtained, the remains of the tablet should be spat out or swallowed.

(g) Correct storage of GTN tablets is vital. They should be stored in a cool place in the original container and should not be transferred to other receptacles. No cotton wool wadding or other tablets or capsules should be added to the container. The tablets should be available at all times.

(h) The date on which the bottle of tablets was first opened should be noted, and the tablets should be replaced within eight weeks of this date.

(i) It may be appropriate to advise Mr B that GTN tablets can be purchased from a community pharmacist without a prescription.

Isosorbide dinitrate

These tablets are to prevent chest pain and therefore should be taken regularly. They should reduce the number of occasions on which sublingual GTN will be required. Isosorbide dinitrate tablets are likely to cause a headache in the first few days of treatment; however, this effect will wear off after continual use and Mr B should be encouraged to continue with the treatment. If headache is a problem he can take paracetamol. Aspirin-containing products should not be used since they interfere with the antiplatelet effect of the low-dose aspirin. Mr B should be advised to consult his community pharmacist before purchasing any over-the-counter medication. A prescription for a further supply of isosorbide dinitrate tablets should be obtained from his general practitioner (GP) before the hospital supply runs out.

Aspirin

Low doses of aspirin will reduce the chance of another heart attack occurring by preventing some of the blood cells from sticking together. Products containing the usual (higher) doses of aspirin do not have this effect, thus other aspirin-containing products (which can be purchased over the counter) should not be taken. Further supplies of low-dose aspirin should be obtained on a GP's prescription, or may be purchased from a community pharmacist. The course of treatment usually lasts one year. Aspirin is best taken with a meal to avoid gastric irritation.

Timolol

These tablets reduce the chance of Mr B having another heart attack (although this risk is very small). Depending on what information has been given to Mr B by the doctor already, it may be appropriate to advise him of possible side-effects. For example, if he experiences any breathlessness he should consult his doctor. Information about other side-effects, such as lethargy, low heart rate, and impotence, may be given at the discretion of the pharmacist.

Various information leaflets are available from the British Heart Foundation which may be given to patients such as Mr B. Some of the topics covered include "Back to Normal (Heart Attacks)", "What is Angina?", "Diet and Your Heart", "Smoking and Your Heart", and "The Heart and its Problems: A Layman's Guide." Alternatively, some hospital consultants produce their own guidelines regarding lifestyle changes following a heart attack.

25. Aspirin is normally continued for one year after discharge.

In the ISIS-2 trial, aspirin was continued for one month; however, other studies have investigated the benefits of giving aspirin over longer periods. In these trials aspirin was given to patients who had suffered an MI, in an attempt to reduce subsequent mortality and re-infarction rates (secondary prophylaxis). None of these studies individually has shown a conclusive reduction in mortality, but analysis of the pooled data from all relevant large trials suggests that aspirin prophylaxis reduces mortality by about 10% and re-infarction by about 21% (Anon., 1987). Most of the benefit occurs during the first year of treatment; it would thus be reasonable for Mr B to continue the aspirin for this period, provided he does not experience any side-effects, such as gastro-intestinal bleeding.

26. Beta-blockers have been shown to reduce the re-infarction and mortality rates when given within 28 days of an acute MI.

The mechanism by which beta-blockers prevent re-infarction is uncertain, but it may be a result of lowering blood pressure and heart rate on exercise, thus reducing myocardial oxygen consumption. Alternatively it may be related to their inherent anti-arrhythmic activity reducing the incidence of fatal arrhythmias such as ventricular fibrillation or ventricular tachycardia; or to their effect of lowering plasma free fatty acids, thereby reducing the risk of the development of further atheroma and hence another heart attack.

The dose of timolol maleate used in Mr B is the same as that used in the Norwegian trial, which demonstrated a significant reduction in mortality and re-infarction rate in patients given timolol maleate (10 mg orally twice daily) within 28 days of an acute MI, compared with the control group. In clinical practice it is usual for the patient to be commenced on a reduced dose of timolol maleate, such as 5 mg orally twice daily. This dose is increased to 10 mg orally twice daily a few days later, unless side-effects are experienced. Treatment with a beta-blocker is usually continued for up to two years; however, there is no published evidence regarding the optimum time to stop therapy. Treatment should be discontinued if troublesome side-effects occur.

27. Propranolol 80 mg twice daily could have been prescribed.

Several large studies have been performed which have attempted to demonstrate that beta-blockers, when prescribed within 7–28 days of an acute MI, reduce the rate of re-infarction and mortality in comparison with placebo. These trials are known as the "late entry" beta-blocker trials in MI, in contrast to the "early entry" trials where beta-blockers are started within 24 hours of the onset of symptoms. All the beta-blockers studied (propranolol, oxprenolol, practolol, alprenolol, timolol, and sotalol) appear to reduce mortality and re-infarction rate. However, taking into consideration the 95% confidence interval of the percentage reduction in mortality, only two of these "late entry" trials have demonstrated a conclusive reduction in mortality. The beta-blockers used in these two trials were timolol maleate (10 mg orally twice daily) and propranolol (80 mg orally twice daily) (Hampton, 1982). Of the two agents, propranolol is less expensive.

Acknowledgment

I should like to acknowledge the helpful comments on this paper received from Professor J. R. Hampton, Professor of Cardiology, University Hospital, Nottingham.

References and Further Reading

Anon., Aspirin and myocardial infarction, *Drug Ther. Bull.* 1987, **25,** 17–19.

Cannon J., Treatment of heart attacks, *Pharm. J.*, 1987, **239,** 497–499.

Hampton J.R., Should every survivor of a heart attack be given a beta blocker? Part 1: Evidence from trials, *Br. med. J.*, 1982, **285,** 33–36.

Hampton J.R., Secondary prevention of myocardial infarction, *Med. Educ. (Int.)*, 1985, **2,** 848–852.

ISIS-1 collaborative group, Randomised trial of intravenous atenolol among 16,027 cases of suspected acute myocardial infarction: ISIS-1 (First international study of infarct survival), *Lancet*, 1986, **2,** 57–66.

ISIS-2 collaborative group, Randomised trial of intravenous streptokinase, oral aspirin, both or neither among 17,187 cases of suspected acute myocardial infarction: ISIS-2, *Lancet*, 1988, **2,** 349–360.

Kannel W.B. and Feinleib M., Natural history of angina in the Framingham study: prognosis and survival, *Am. J. Cardiol.*, 1972, **29,** 154–163.

MIAMI trial research group, Metoprolol in acute myocardial infarction (MIAMI): a randomised placebo-controlled international trial, *Eur. Heart J.*, 1985, **6,** 199–226.

Norris R.M., The management of acute myocardial infarction, *Med. Educ. (Int.)*, 1985, **2,** 841–847.

Norwegian multicenter study group, Timolol-induced reduction in mortality and re-infarction in patients surviving acute myocardial infarction, *New Engl. J. Med.*, 1981, **304,** 801–807.

Wilcox R.G. *et al.*, Trial of early nifedipine in acute myocardial infarction: the Trent study, *Br. med. J.*, 1986, **293,** 1204–1208.

ACUTE RENAL FAILURE

Alexander Harper

Principal Pharmacist, Clinical Services, Royal United Hospital, Bath

Day 1 Mrs C, a 69-year-old woman, was admitted urgently at the request of her general practitioner. His letter detailed the following history. Mrs C had collapsed at the elderly people's home where she lived. The warden said she had been complaining of nausea and loss of appetite for two or three days (her current weight was 51 kg) and had vomited that morning. She had fallen on the previous day but had recovered quickly.

She had a long history of biventricular cardiac failure which had been controlled for some time with frusemide 80 mg in the morning, isosorbide dinitrate 20 mg three times daily, and captopril 6.25 mg twice daily, although a degree of ankle oedema had recently necessitated an increase in the dose of frusemide to 120 mg in the morning. However, this increase had precipitated gout, which had been manifested by pain in the distal interphalangeal joint of both great toes. The pain had been treated with indomethacin 50 mg three times daily for the previous 21 days.

The patient herself was a poor historian. On examination she was pale and tired-looking, with sunken eyes. Her pulse was 120 beats per minute while her blood pressure was 105/70 mmHg lying and 85/60 mmHg standing. Ankle oedema was absent and there was no evidence of pulmonary oedema. Her extremities were cold and there was a marked reduction in skin turgor.

Mrs C's serum biochemistry results were:

Sodium 131 mmol/L (reference range 135–150)
Potassium 5.5 mmol/L (3.5–5.0)
Bicarbonate 17 mmol/L (22–31)
Creatinine 312 micromol/L (60–110)
Urea 27.2 mmol/L (3.2–6.6)
Glucose 4.8 mmol/L (3.5–6.0)
MCV 71 fL (77–91)
Osmolality 306 mOsmol/kg (275–295)

A diagnosis of sodium and water depletion with consequent renal hypoperfusion was made. An infusion of one litre sodium chloride 0.9% every four to six hours was prescribed, and the following investigations were requested: full blood count; culture and sensitivity of blood and urine; 24-hour urine collection for determination of creatinine clearance; urinary sodium, urea, and osmolality; and chest x-ray, and abdominal x-ray.

1. Could Mrs C's drug therapy have contributed to her renal problems?

2. What is the aim of intravenous normal saline therapy?

3. Which methods of assessing and monitoring Mrs C's status would you recommend?

Day 2 The 24-hour urine collection yielded a volume of only 290 mL. Other data obtained from analysis of Mrs C's urine included:

Sodium 43 mmol/L
Urea 117 mmol/L
Creatinine 20.12 mmol/L
Osmolality 337 mOsmol/kg

The low urine volume obtained despite the concurrent volume expansion indicated that further measures were required to prevent the development of acute tubular necrosis. Mannitol was considered inappropriate in this patient, so 250 mg of frusemide was administered by slow intravenous infusion; a further dose of 500 mg was administered after six hours: neither dose produced an increase in urine production. An infusion of dopamine at an initial dose of 2 microgram/kg/min was started. The infusion rate was increased over the next few hours to 10 microgram/kg/min, but this again failed to produce a diuresis. A diagnosis of established acute tubular necrosis causing acute renal failure was made. The following recommendations were made: daily fluid charts; daily weights; daily serum urea and electrolyte estimations; and dietary restrictions (consult dietician).

4. Why was mannitol inappropriate for Mrs C?

5. Would you have recommended the use of high dose intravenous frusemide at this point?

6. Is the dose of dopamine critical?

7. What dietary considerations are necessary in Mrs C?

Day 4 Mrs C complained of having muscle cramps at night, with the result that quinine sulphate 300 mg at night was prescribed. She also complained of diarrhoea which was described by the nursing staff as black and tarry in appearance. A full blood count revealed a normochromic and normocytic anaemia with a haemoglobin of 8.1 g/dL (reference value 12–16 g/dL). Ranitidine 150 mg at night was prescribed.

Serum biochemistry results revealed the following:

Sodium 137 mmol/L (135–150)
Potassium 7.1 mmol/L (3.5–5.0)
Calcium 2.04 mmol/L (2.25–2.6)
Bicarbonate 19 mmol/L (22–31)
Phosphate 1.8 mmol/L (0.9–1.5)
Albumin 34 g/L (33–55)
Urea 31.7 mmol/L (3.2–6.6)
Creatinine 567 micromol/L (60–110)
pH 7.28 (7.36–7.44)

A bolus dose of 10 mL of calcium gluconate was immediately administered intravenously, followed by an intravenous injection of 10 units soluble insulin with 50 mL of 50% glucose solution; the latter was written up for three further administrations over the next twelve hours. Therapy with calcium resonium 15 g orally four times daily was also initiated. A monitor was ordered to observe for cardiac toxicity; however no electrocardiogram changes were apparent.

8. Would you have recommended quinine sulphate 300 mg at night to treat Mrs C's nocturnal cramps?

9. What factors may have contributed to Mrs C's low haemoglobin? Is ranitidine therapy appropriate?

10. Is Mrs C's hyperkalaemia being treated appropriately?

11. Should Mrs C's hypocalcaemia, hyperphosphataemia and acidosis be treated at this point?

12. What factors should be considered when initiating drug therapy for a patient in acute renal failure?

Day 7 Mrs C complained of breathlessness which was increased on lying flat, and examination showed her to have developed crepitations in both lung bases. She complained of nausea and was noted to be drowsy and to have developed a flapping tremor.

Her serum biochemistry results included:

Potassium 6.6 mmol/L (3.5–5.0)
Bicarbonate 17 mmol/L (22–31)
Urea 40.5 mmol/L (3.2–6.6)
Creatinine 588 micromol/L (60–110)
pH 7.24 (7.36–7.44)

It was decided to treat Mrs C by haemofiltration, and the femoral artery and vein were cannulated for this purpose. Once haemofiltration had been initiated it was felt that she would be a good candidate for total parenteral nutrition (TPN) and arrangements were made for a Hickmann catheter to be inserted.

13. What were the indications for dialysis and/or haemofiltration in Mrs C?

14. What forms of dialysis therapy are available, and what are their advantages and disadvantages?

15. What are the advantages of haemofiltration for Mrs C?

16. What factors affect drug therapy during haemofiltration and dialysis?

17. What factors would you take into account when formulating a TPN regimen for Mrs C?

Day 12 Mrs C developed a temperature of 39.6°C and a tachycardia of 120 beats per minute. Subjectively she complained of headache and feeling "awful". A full blood count revealed a neutrophil count of 10.5×10^9/L ($2.2–7.0 \times 10^9$/L). A diagnosis of septicaemia was made, and blood samples were sent for culture and sensitivity. All indwelling catheters were removed. The following therapy was written up:

Cefotaxime 1 g intravenously every eight hours
Gentamicin 60 mg intravenously every 24 hours
Metronidazole 500 mg intravenously every eight hours.

18. Is this therapy appropriate for Mrs C's septicaemia?

19. What are the dangers associated with prescribing gentamicin for Mrs C? How should her gentamicin therapy be monitored?

Day 14 Microbiological assays revealed the infective organism to be *Staphylococcus aureus*. Gentamicin and metronidazole therapy were discontinued and, as Mrs C was clinically much improved, cefotaxime was continued as sole antibiotic therapy.

Day 19 Mrs C, now free of infection, passed over four litres of urine. It was felt that she was over the worst and that she would continue to improve.

20. Did Mrs C follow the normal course of acute renal failure? What is her prognosis?

Answers

1. Yes. Mrs C's frusemide and/or indomethacin therapy may have contributed to her admission.

Mrs C demonstrates many of the traditional signs of sodium and water depletion, including tachycardia, hypotension, postural hypotension, reduced skin turgor, reduced ocular tension (the cause of her sunken eyes), collapsed peripheral veins, and cold extremities. Evidence that Mrs C had suffered some degree of renal impairment can be seen by the elevation in her serum urea and creatinine levels, and the other biochemical abnormalities. The symptoms that Mrs C has that cannot be explained by the sodium and water depletion – namely the nausea, loss of appetite, and vomiting – can be attributed to her high blood urea level (uraemia).

One of the physiological responses to sodium and water depletion is a reduction in renal perfusion, which may in turn lead to intrinsic renal damage with a consequent acute deterioration in renal function. The condition may be caused by any significant haemorrhage, or by septicaemia, in which the vascular bed is dilated, thereby reducing the circulating volume. It may also be caused by excessive sodium and water loss from the skin, urinary tract or gastro-intestinal tract. Excessive loss through the skin by sweating occurs in hot climates and is rare in the UK, but it also occurs after extensive burns. Gastro-intestinal losses are associated with vomiting or diarrhoea. Urinary tract losses often result from excessive diuretic therapy but may also occur with the osmotic diuresis caused by hyperglycaemia and glycosuria in a diabetic patient (for this reason a random blood glucose level was performed on Mrs C).

Mrs C had indeed been vomiting, but seemingly only once, and at a late stage in her illness, so that it was more likely to be a symptom of her condition rather than the cause. It is considerably more likely that her plight has been brought about by the diuresis induced by her recently increased frusemide therapy.

Any condition that causes the kidney to be underperfused may be associated with an acute deterioration in renal function. However, such a deterioration may also be produced by nephrotoxic agents, including drugs. Non-steroidal anti-inflammatory drugs (NSAIDs) in particular are associated with renal damage, and even a short course of an NSAID (such as indomethacin) has been associated with acute renal failure. The main cause of NSAID-induced renal damage is inhibition of prostaglandin synthesis in the kidney, particularly prostaglandins E_2, D_2 and I_2 (prostacyclin). These prostaglandins are all potent vasodilators and consequently produce an increase in blood flow to the glomerulus and the medulla. In normal circumstances they do not play a large part in the maintenance of the renal circulation; however, in patients with increased amounts of vasoconstrictor substances (such as angiotensin II or antidiuretic hormone) in the blood, vasodilatory prostaglandins become important in maintaining renal blood flow. The maintenance of blood pressure in a variety of clinical conditions, such as volume depletion (which Mrs C has), congestive cardiac failure (which she had also had), or hepatic cirrhosis with ascites, may rely on the release of vasoconstrictor substances. In these circumstances, inhibition of prostaglandin synthesis may cause unopposed renal arteriolar vasoconstriction, which again leads to renal hypoperfusion.

Angiotensin-converting enzyme (ACE) inhibitors may also produce a reduction in renal function by preventing the angiotensin II-mediated vasoconstriction of the efferent glomerular arteriole, which contributes to the high pressure gradient across the glomerulus. This problem is important only in patients with renal vascular disease, particularly those with bilateral stenoses, and is consequently rare. It is thus unlikely that Mrs C's captopril therapy has contributed to her problem.

2. The aim of therapy is to restore her extracellular fluid volume.

A diagnosis of acute deterioration of renal function due to renal underperfusion carries with it the implication that restoration of renal perfusion will reverse the renal impairment. Mrs C is depleted of both water and sodium ions. Sodium chloride 0.9% is therefore an appropriate choice of intravenous fluid, since it replaces both water and sodium ions in a concentration approximately equal to plasma. Situations occasionally arise where a patient is hyponatraemic but not water-depleted, as a result of either sodium depletion or water retention: such a condition may be treated with an infusion containing sodium chloride in excess of its physiological concentration, e.g. sodium chloride 1.8% or higher. Similarly, should water depletion with hypernatraemia occur, isotonic solutions that are either free of, or low in, sodium are available, e.g. dextrose 5%, or sodium chloride 0.18% with dextrose 4%.

The effect of fluid replacement therapy on urine flow and central venous pressure should be carefully monitored. Central venous pressure provides a guide to the degree of fluid deficit and reduces the risk of pulmonary oedema by over-rapid transfusion; it should not be allowed to rise above the normal range of 10–15 cm of water. If the kidneys do not respond to replacement treatment, the probable diagnosis is acute tubular necrosis, but it is common practice to try other measures, such as treatment with mannitol, loop diuretics, and dopamine, to try to turn the condition towards recovery.

3. (a) Creatinine clearance (CrCl).

Creatinine is a by-product of normal muscle metabolism and is formed at a rate proportional to the mass of muscle. It is freely filtered by the glomerulus, with little secretion or re-absorption by the tubule. When muscle mass is stable, any change in plasma creatinine reflects a change in its clearance by filtration. Consequently measurement of CrCl gives an estimate of the glomerular filtration rate (GFR). The ideal method of calculating CrCl is by performing an accurate collection of urine over 24 hours and taking a plasma sample midway through this period. The following equation may then be used:

$$CrCl = \frac{U \times V}{P}$$

where U = urine creatinine concentration
(micromol/L)
V = urine flow rate (mL/min)
P = plasma creatinine concentration
(micromol/L)

Using this formula, it is possible to calculate Mrs C's CrCl as 13 mL/min. A quicker and less cumbersome method is to measure the plasma creatinine concentration and collect those patient factors that affect the mass of muscle, i.e. age, sex, and weight (preferably ideal body weight). This allows an estimation of CrCl to be made from average population data. The equation of Cockroft and Gault is a useful way of making such an estimation.

$$CrCl = \frac{F \times (140 - age) \times weight\ (kg)}{plasma\ creatinine\ (micromol/L)}$$

where F = 1.0 (females) or 1.23 (males)

Assuming the normal CrCl to be 120 mL/min, this enables classification of renal impairment, as follows: mild, a GFR of 50–75 mL/min; moderate, a GFR of 20–50 mL/min; and severe, a GFR of less than 20 mL/min. Using the method of Cockroft and Gault, Mrs C's CrCl can be estimated as 12 mL/min and her renal impairment could thus be classified as severe.

(b) Urine analysis.

A healthy kidney that is underperfused will attempt to compensate for the condition by retaining sodium and water, a response mediated by aldosterone and antidiuretic hormone. Thus, the urine produced will be low in sodium (less than 10 mmol/L) but otherwise concentrated, with a high urea (greater than 250 mmol/L) and osmolality (greater than 500 mOsmol/kg). However, damaged kidneys fail to re-absorb sodium adequately, which results in high urinary sodium concentrations (greater than 30 mmol/L) while the urea concentration mechanisms also fail, which results in reduced urinary urea (less than 150 mmol/L). Urine osmolality also falls to close to that of plasma. It follows therefore that examination of the urine enables assessment of the renal state. Various indexes using these data have been produced, but their value is more theoretical than practical.

(c) Serum urea levels.

These are commonly used to assess renal function; however, the rate of production of urea is considerably more variable than that of creatinine and it fluctuates throughout the day in response to the protein content of the diet. It may also be elevated by dehydration or an increase in protein catabolism, such as occurs in haemorrhage from the gastro-intestinal tract or body tissues, severe infections, trauma (including surgery), and high-dose steroid or tetracycline therapy. The serum urea level is therefore an unreliable measure of renal function, but it is often used as a crude test since it does give information on the patient's general condition and state of hydration.

(d) Fluid charts and weight.

Fluid charts are frequently used in patients with sodium and water depletion, but they are often inaccurate and should not be relied upon exclusively. Records of daily weight are more reliable but are rarely available before renal failure is diagnosed.

(e) Central venous pressure.

This is of value in assessing circulating volume. The normal range is 10–15 cm of water.

(f) Serum electrolyte levels.

Plasma potassium should be measured regularly because hyperkalaemia, which occurs in acute renal failure, may be fatal.

4. Mannitol therapy is inappropriate because Mrs C has cardiac failure.

The rationale for using mannitol arises from the theory that tubular debris may contribute to the oliguria of acute renal failure by causing mechanical obstruction, and that the use of an osmotic diuretic may wash out the debris. A dose of 0.5–1.0 g/kg as a 10–20% infusion is recommended, but only after the circulating volume has been restored (this caution holds true for any diuretic therapy). However, intravenous mannitol will, before producing a diuresis, cause a considerable increase in the extracellular fluid volume by attracting water from the intracellular fluid. This expansion of the extracellular volume is potentially dangerous for patients with cardiac failure, especially if a diuresis is not produced.

5. Yes.

As well as producing substantial diureses, all loop diuretics have been shown to increase renal blood flow, probably by stimulating the release of renal prostaglandins (this haemodynamic effect can be inhibited by indomethacin and other NSAIDs). It is thought that the use of loop diuretics may thereby help salvage renal tissue, although evidence to support this hypothesis is difficult to find. It is, however, undeniable that any increase in urine volume produced will simplify the future management of Mrs C by reducing the risk of fluid overload and hyperkalaemia.

Doses of up to 1 g of frusemide should be given intravenously at a rate of not more than 4 mg/min, since higher infusion rates may cause transient deafness. The addition of metolazone orally may also be considered. Metolazone, which is by itself a weak diuretic, has been shown to act synergistically with loop diuretics to produce a more effective diuresis.

6. Yes.

Dopamine at low doses (e.g. 1–5 micrograms/kg/min) has a vasodilator effect on the kidney. At slightly higher doses (e.g. 5–20 micrograms/kg/min) inotropic effects on the heart produce an increase in cardiac output. This dual effect increases renal perfusion. However, at higher doses still (e.g. 20 micrograms/kg/min and above) dopamine also acts on alpha receptors, causing peripheral and renal vasoconstriction, which results in impairment of renal perfusion. An initial dose of 2 microgram/kg/min, increasing to a maximum of 10 microgram/kg/min with careful monitoring of central venous pressure is thus usually appropriate. As with frusemide, dopamine may produce increases in urine volume (which may simplify management) even in those patients who progress to acute renal failure. Dobutamine does not produce renal vasodilation but may occasionally be added at an initial dose of 2.5 microgram/kg/min for its inotropic effects.

7.

In a patient with acute renal failure the aim is to provide sufficient nutrition to prevent the breakdown of body tissue, especially protein.

The diet should provide all the essential amino acids in a total protein intake of about 30 g/day. This should reduce the symptoms of uraemia, such as nausea, vomiting, and anorexia. A higher intake of protein stimulates its use as an energy source, which results in increases in blood urea concentrations; while any further reduction in protein intake brings about endogenous protein catabolism, and this again causes blood urea to increase. Fat and carbohydrate should also be given to maintain a high energy intake of about 2000 to 3000 kcal/day, or more in hypercatabolic patients, as this helps to prevent protein catabolism and promote anabolism. To avoid the commonly encountered problem of hyperkalaemia, potassium intake should be kept as low as possible. It should be noted, however, that, as uraemia causes anorexia, nausea and vomiting, many severely ill patients are unable to tolerate a diet of any kind; in such cases TPN should be considered at an early stage.

8. No.

Muscle cramps are common in patients with renal failure, probably as a result of electrolyte imbalances, and patients are generally prescribed quinine salts in doses of 200–300 mg at night. However, the efficacy of this form of treatment is dubious and few comparative trials have been performed. Nonetheless, it is seldom difficult to find patients, and indeed prescribers, who swear by it, and its use is so firmly entrenched in common medical practice that it can be difficult to dislodge. Fortunately, at the doses used for this purpose, toxicity is not a problem, although quinine poisoning still occasionally produces tragic results, particularly in young children. The dose of quinine does not require alteration in renal failure.

9.

Mrs C's low haemoglobin may be a result of reduced erythropoietin secretion, but it is more likely to be the result of gastro-intestinal bleeding, thus ranitidine therapy is appropriate.

Erythropoietin, the hormone that stimulates production of red blood cells, is produced virtually exclusively by the kidney, and a normochromic, normocytic anaemia due to reduced erythropoietin secretion is a very common symptom in chronic renal failure. However the time course of acute renal failure is often too short for this type of anaemia to become a problem, and, although it may be present in a patient on the verge of chronic renal failure who has an acute crisis, this does not appear to be the case for Mrs C.

Anaemia may also arise if there is a haemolytic element to the condition (e.g. severe septicaemia) or if a haemorrhage occurs, either as the cause of the acute renal failure or as a result of it. Uraemic gastro-intestinal haemorrhage is a recognised consequence of acute renal failure, probably occurring as a result of reduced mucosal cell turnover owing to high circulating levels of uraemic toxins. Gastro-intestinal haemorrhage is also a well recognised consequence of treatment with NSAIDs such as indomethacin, which Mrs C had been taking before admission.

Mrs C has passed melaena (black, tarry stools) and has been diagnosed as having had a gastro-intestinal bleed. This is therefore the most likely cause of her low haemoglobin. H_2-receptor blockers are effective therapy in this condition, and it is unlikely that any one would be more advantageous than another. Ranitidine was therefore an appropriate choice of treatment, and it was also appropriate to prescribe it at a reduced dosage, as Mrs C's estimated GFR was less than 10 mL/min at this stage in her illness. Sucralfate therapy would have been an effective alternative.

10. Yes. The methods used to treat Mrs C's hyperkalaemia are appropriate.

Hyperkalaemia is a particular problem in acute renal failure, not only because of reduced urinary potassium excretion but also because of potassium release from cells. Particularly rapid rises are to be expected when there is tissue damage, as in burns, crush injuries and sepsis, although this is not the case for Mrs C. She is, however, acidotic, and acidosis aggravates the situation by provoking potassium leakage from healthy cells. Hyperkalaemia may be life-threatening by causing cardiac arrythmias and, if untreated, may result in asystolic cardiac arrest. Emergency treatment is necessary if the serum potassium is above 7.0 mmol/L (as in Mrs C's case) or if there are electrocardiogram changes. This treatment consists of:

(a) 10–20 mL of calcium gluconate 10% intravenously. This has a stabilising effect on the myocardium but no effect on serum potassium concentration.

(b) 10 units of soluble insulin plus 50 mL of 50% glucose. This stimulates potassium uptake into cells, thus removing it from the plasma.

(c) Calcium resonium 15 g three or four times a day, orally or by enema. This ion-exchange resin binds potassium in the gastro-intestinal tract, releasing calcium in exchange, and is used to lower serum potassium over a period of hours or days. It is required because the effect of insulin and glucose therapy is only temporary. Both the oral and the rectal routes of administration have disadvantages: administration of large doses by mouth may result in faecal impaction, while the manufacturers recommend that the enema be retained for nine hours, a piece of advice notoriously difficult to implement. Oral therapy is not contra-indicated after a gastro-intestinal bleed, so this is probably more appropriate for Mrs C. Using a calcium-exchange resin is also appropriate as she is hypocalcaemic.

(d) 200–300 mL of sodium bicarbonate 1.4% intravenously may be used as well as insulin and glucose therapy. As well as stimulating potassium re-uptake by cells, this helps to correct the acidosis of acute renal failure. However, it is rarely used because of the fluid and electrolyte load it contains, and is particularly inappropriate in Mrs C because of her history of cardiac failure.

11. No. Mrs C's calcium and phosphate levels and serum pH, although abnormal, are not sufficiently deranged to warrant treatment at this point.

Calcium malabsorption, probably secondary to disordered vitamin D metabolism, often occurs in acute renal failure. However, it usually remains asymptomatic, as tetany of skeletal muscles and convulsions do not normally occur until plasma concentrations are as low as 1.6–1.7 mmol/L. Should it become necessary, oral calcium supplementation with calcium gluconate or lactate is usually adequate; although vitamin D may be used to treat the hypocalcaemia of acute renal failure (see answer 12), it rarely has to be prescribed. Effervescent calcium tablets should be avoided as they invariably contain a high sodium and potassium load.

Phosphate is normally excreted by the kidney, and phosphate retention and hyperphosphataemia may also occur in acute renal failure, but usually only to a slight extent, and the condition rarely requires treatment. Should it become necessary, phosphate-binding agents may be used to retain phosphate ion in the gut. The most common agents are Titralac® (calcium carbonate 420 mg + glycine 180 mg) or aluminium hydroxide in the form of mixture or capsules. The former is the drug of choice because of the slight risk that aluminium may be absorbed from the gut and deposited in bones to give a severe form of fracturing bone disease.

The inability of the kidney to excrete hydrogen ions may result in a metabolic acidosis, which again is not in itself a serious problem, although it may contribute to hyperkalaemia. It may be treated orally with sodium bicarbonate 1–6 g/day in divided doses, although, if elevations in plasma sodium preclude the use of sodium bicarbonate, extreme acidosis (plasma bicarbonate of less than 10 mmol/L) is best treated by dialysis. Although Mrs C does not currently require treatment of her electrolyte abnormalities, it is essential that she is carefully monitored for any further derangement.

12. How the drug to be used is absorbed, distributed, metabolised, and excreted, and whether it is intrinsically nephrotoxic, are all factors that must be considered. The pharmacokinetic behaviour of many drugs may be altered in renal failure.

(a) Absorption. Oral absorption in acute renal failure may be reduced, owing to vomiting or diarrhoea, although this is of limited clinical significance.

(b) Metabolism. The main hepatic pathways of drug metabolism appear to be unaffected in renal impairment. The kidney is also a site of metabolism in the body but the effect of renal impairment is clinically important in only two cases:

(i) Vitamin D. The conversion of 25-hydroxychole-calciferol to 1,25-dihydroxycholecalciferol (the active form of vitamin D) occurs in the kidney, and the process is impaired in renal failure. Patients in acute renal failure thus occasionally require vitamin D replacement therapy, and this should be in the form of 1-hydroxycholecalciferol or 1,25-dihydroxycholecalciferol.

(ii) Insulin. The kidney is the major site of insulin metabolism and the insulin requirements of diabetic patients in acute renal failure are often reduced.

(c) Distribution. Changes in distribution may be altered by fluctuations in the degree of hydration or by alterations in tissue or plasma protein binding. The presence of oedema or ascites tends to increase the volume of distribution, while dehydration tends to reduce it. In practice these changes are only significant if the drug's volume of distribution is small (less than 50 L).

Plasma protein binding may be reduced, owing either to protein loss or to alterations in binding because of uraemia. For certain highly bound drugs the net result of reduced protein binding is an increase in free drug, so that care must be taken when interpreting plasma concentrations of such drugs. Most analyses measure total plasma concentration, that is, free plus bound drug. A drug level may therefore fall within the accepted concentration range but still result in toxicity because of the increased proportion of free drug. However, this is usually only a temporary effect. Since the unbound drug is now available for elimination, its free concentration will eventually return to its original value, albeit with a lower total bound plus unbound level; the total drug concentration may therefore fall below the therapeutic range while therapeutic effectiveness is maintained. It must be noted that the time required for the new equilibrium to be established is about four or five elimination half-lives of the drug, and this itself may be altered in renal failure. Some drugs that show reduced plasma protein binding include diazepam, morphine, phenytoin, thyroxine, theophylline and warfarin. Tissue binding may also be affected; for example, the displacement of digoxin from skeletal muscle binding sites by metabolic waste products results in a significant reduction of its volume of distribution in renal failure.

(d) Excretion. Alterations in the renal clearance of drugs in renal impairment is by far the most important parameter to consider when making dosage decisions. Generally, a fall in renal drug clearance indicates a decline in the number of functioning nephrons. The GFR, of which CrCl is an approximation, can be used as an estimate of the number of functioning nephrons. Thus, a 50% reduction in GFR will suggest a 50% decline in renal clearance.

Renal impairment often necessitates drug dosage adjustments. Loading doses of renally excreted drugs are often necessary in renal failure because the prolonged elimination half-life leads to a prolonged time to reach steady state. The equation for a loading dose is the same in renal disease as normal, thus:

Loading dose (mg) =
target concentration (mg/L) ×
volume of distribution (L)

The volume of distribution may be altered (see above) but generally remains unchanged.

It is possible to derive other formulas for dosage adjustment in renal impairment. One of the most useful is:

$$DR_{rf} = DR_n \times [(1 - F_{eu}) + (F_{eu} \times RF)]$$

Where

DR_{rf} = dosing rate in renal failure
DR_n = normal dosing rate
RF = extent of renal impairment
$= \dfrac{\text{patient's creatinine clearance (mL/min)}}{\text{ideal creatinine clearance (i.e. 120 mL/min)}}$
F_{eu} = fraction of drug normally excreted unchanged in the urine.

For example, if RF is 0.2 and F_{eu} is 0.5, DR_{rf} will be 60% of normal.

An alteration in total daily dose can be achieved by altering either the dose itself, or the dosage interval, or a combination of both as appropriate. Unfortunately for this method, it is not always possible readily to obtain the fraction of drug excreted unchanged in the urine. In practice it is thus often simpler to use the guidelines to prescribing in renal impairment found in the British National Formulary, and these are adequate for almost all cases.

(e) Nephrotoxicity. Some drugs are known to be able to damage the kidney by a variety of mechanisms. The commonest forms of damage are interstitial nephritis (hypersensitivity reaction with inflammation affecting those cells lying between the nephrons), and glomerulonephritis (thought to be caused by the passive trapping of immune complexes in the glomerular tuft eliciting an inflammatory response). The list of potentially nephrotoxic drugs is a long one, but the majority cause damage by producing hypersensitivity reactions and are quite safe in most patients. Some drugs, however, are directly nephrotoxic and their effects on the kidney are consequently more predictable. Such drugs include the aminoglycosides, amphotericin, colistin, the polymyxins, and cyclosporin. The use of any drug with recognised nephrotoxic potential should be avoided in any patient if at all possible. This is particularly true in patients with pre-existing renal impairment or renal failure, such as Mrs C. Inevitably, occasions will arise when the use of potentially nephrotoxic drugs becomes necessary, and on these occasions constant monitoring of renal function is essential.

In conclusion, the simplest solution to prescribing in renal failure is to choose a drug that is:
 (i) less than 25% excreted unchanged in the urine,
 (ii) unaffected by fluid balance changes,
 (iii) unaffected by protein binding changes,
 (iv) has a wide therapeutic margin, and
 (v) not nephrotoxic.

13. Her severe uraemic symptoms (nausea, reduced consciousness, flapping tremor) and the evidence of pulmonary oedema indicated that dialysis and/or haemofiltration would be of value for Mrs C.

Dialysis should be commenced in a patient with acute renal failure when there is: hyperkalaemia of above 7 mmol/L; increasing acidosis (pH of less than 7.1 or plasma bicarbonate of less than 10 mmol/L); severe uraemic symptoms such as impaired consciousness; fluid overload with pulmonary oedema; or any combination of the above which may threaten life. It would appear that the current trend in acute renal failure is to introduce dialysis therapy early, as complications and mortality are reduced if the serum urea level is kept below 35 mmol/L.

14. There are traditionally two types of dialysis: haemodialysis and peritoneal dialysis. Both put the patient's blood on one side, and a dialysate solution on the other, of a semipermeable membrane across which exchange of metabolites occurs. In haemodialysis, blood is diverted out of the body and passed through an artificial kidney (dialyser) and returned to the patient, while in peritoneal dialysis the fluid is run in and out of the patient's abdominal cavity and the peritoneum itself acts as the semipermeable membrane.

In haemodialysis, blood is taken from an arterial line, heparinised, actively pumped through a dialyser and returned to the patient. The dialyser contains synthetic semipermeable membranes which allow the blood to come into close proximity with the dialysate. Metabolites and excess electrolytes pass from the blood to the dialysate; by increasing the pressure of the blood, water can also be removed from the patient. Haemodialysis is performed two or three times a week and the duration of a single dialysis is usually about four hours.

The principle of peritoneal dialysis is identical to haemodialysis but the technique is simpler. A semirigid catheter is inserted into the abdominal cavity. One or two litres of warmed dialysate are run into the abdomen, left for a period (usually about 30 minutes), and then run into a collecting bag. This may be done manually or by semi-automatic equipment. The procedure may be repeated up to 20 times a day, depending on the condition of the patient.

One disadvantage of haemodialysis is its dependence on expensive technology. The capital cost is considerable and the technique requires specially trained staff, so it is seldom undertaken outside a renal unit. Haemodialysis also produces rapid fluid and electrolyte shifts which may be dangerous. It does however treat renal failure much more rapidly than peritoneal dialysis, and is therefore essential in hypercatabolic renal failure where urea is produced faster than peritoneal dialysis can remove it. Haemodialysis can also be used in patients who have recently undergone abdominal surgery, in whom peritoneal dialysis is not advisable.

Peritoneal dialysis is relatively cheap and simple, does not require specially trained staff nor the facilities of a renal unit, and its use is consequently more widespread. It does, however, have the disadvantages of being uncomfortable and tiring for the patient, producing a fairly high incidence of peritonitis, and permitting protein loss, as albumin crosses the peritoneal membrane.

15. The advantages of haemofiltration for Mrs C are its simplicity of use, the fine control of fluid balance it offers, and its low cost.

Haemofiltration is a relatively recent technique, the simplicity of which is ensuring its increasing use in the treatment of acute renal failure. Usually arterial blood is obtained from the femoral artery, heparinised, passed over a semipermeable filter, similar to the membrane used in haemodialysis, and returned to the femoral vein. The hydrostatic pressure of the blood drives a filtrate similar to interstitial fluid across the filter; the volume lost can, if necessary, then be replaced by an appropriate fluid, added to the blood on its return to the venous system. Various replacement fluids are marketed commercially for this purpose (e.g. by Geistlich and Gambro), which contain electrolytes, including sodium, potassium, calcium, magnesium and chloride in differing quantities, thereby enabling an appropriate solution to be selected for the patient's needs. In addition to avoiding the expense and complexity of haemodialysis, this system enables continuous but gradual removal of fluid, thereby allowing very fine control of fluid balance in addition to electrolyte control and removal of metabolites. Very often this control of fluid balance facilitates the use of TPN. The advantages of haemofiltration over peritoneal dialysis make it likely that continuous haemofiltration, which is becoming increasingly available, will replace peritoneal dialysis as the most appropriate form of dialysis in the majority of patients with acute renal failure.

16. Whether the drug is significantly removed by dialysis or haemofiltration.

Drugs that are not removed will require dose reductions in order to avoid accumulation, and possible toxic effects. Alternatively, drug removal by these procedures may be sufficient to require a dosage supplement to ensure adequate therapeutic efficacy. In general, since haemodialysis, peritoneal dialysis and haemofiltration depend on filtration, the processes can be considered analogous to glomerular filtration. Thus, drug characteristics which favour clearance by the glomerulus are similar to those that favour clearance by dialysis or haemofiltration, and include low molecular weight, high water solubility, low protein binding, small volume of distribution, and low metabolic clearance.

Unfortunately, a number of other factors which depend on the dialysis process itself affect clearance by dialysis. For haemodialysis, these include the duration of dialysis procedure, rate of blood flow to dialyser, surface area and porosity of dialyser, and composition and flow rate of dialysate. For peritoneal dialysis they include the rate of peritoneal exchange, and the concentration gradient between plasma and dialysate.

It is therefore usually possible to predict whether or not a drug will be removed by dialysis, but it is very difficult to quantify the process, except by direct measurement, and this is rarely practical. It is therefore not surprising that a single, comprehensive guide to drug dosage in dialysis is non-existent. However, limited data for specific drugs are available in the literature, while many drug manufacturers have information on the dialysability of their products, some of which is included in the product data sheets. Thus, the most practical method for treating patients undergoing dialysis is to accumulate appropriate dosage guidelines for a number of drugs which are likely to be used in patients with renal impairment, and then use those drugs only.

Although drug clearance by haemofiltration is relatively more predictable than by dialysis, the fact that haemofiltration is still a relatively new technique means that sufficient information to produce general guidelines is again not readily available. Therefore, a similar set of individual drug dosage guidelines is useful in practice.

17. Factors that should be considered when formulating a TPN regime for Mrs C include her fluid balance, calorie and protein requirements, electrolyte balance and requirements, and vitamin and mineral requirements.

The ease with which fluid may be removed by haemofiltration greatly facilitates the decision to start parenteral nutrition. Large volumes of fluid may be administered without producing fluid overload, always a potential problem in patients with acute renal failure like Mrs C.

Mrs C's basic calorie requirements are similar to those of a non-dialysed patient (see answer 7) although protein requirements may occasionally be increased with concurrent haemofiltration, as with haemodialysis, because of amino acid losses. (Increased amounts of protein may also be required with concurrent peritoneal dialysis because of plasma protein losses.)

Although lipid emulsions may theoretically reduce the efficiency of haemofiltration, in practice their use does not have any noticeable effect, as with both forms of dialysis. It is useful, however, to infuse the TPN solution into the blood as it is being returned to the body after haemofiltration, as with patients receiving haemodialysis, as this ensures that it is available to the patient before being presented to the filter.

Electrolyte-free amino acid solutions should be used as they allow the addition of the precise quantities of sodium and potassium required. Since potassium is removed by filtration, rigorous control of potassium intake becomes less important; potassium and sodium requirements can in fact be calculated on an individual basis depending on the patient's plasma levels. There is usually no need to try to normalise plasma calcium and phosphate as they will stabilise at acceptable levels with haemofiltration, as with dialysis. If necessary, phosphate binders may be prescribed. Water-soluble vitamins are removed by haemofiltration, as by dialysis, but the standard daily doses normally included in TPN fluids more than compensate for this. Magnesium and zinc supplementation may be required because tissue repair often increases requirements.

Once TPN is started, it will be necessary to monitor Mrs C's plasma urea, creatinine, and electrolytes daily, in order to make the appropriate alterations to her nutritional support and/or haemofiltration. Her serum glucose should also be checked at least every six hours, as patients in renal failure sometimes develop insulin resistance. Her serum pH should be checked initially to see whether the addition of amino acid solutions is causing or aggravating metabolic acidosis. It would also be worth checking her calcium, phosphate, and albumin levels regularly, in case intervention becomes necessary. When practical, daily weighing gives a useful guide to fluid balance.

18. No. Cefotaxime should be replaced by an agent with broader activity against Gram-positive organisms, such as a penicillin (e.g. ampicillin, amoxycillin, or pivampicillin).

Patients in acute renal failure are prone to infection and septicaemia, and this is a common cause of death in this condition. Bladder catheters and intravenous lines should thus be used with care to reduce the chance of bacteria gaining access to the patient. Leucocytosis is sometimes seen in acute renal failure and does not necessarily imply infection, but when seen in conjunction with pyrexia, as in Mrs C, simple caution mandates aggressive treatment. Samples of blood, urine and any other material should be sent for culture before antibiotic therapy is started, and therapy should be prescribed to cover as wide a spectrum as possible until a causative organism is identified.

Aminoglycoside therapy is appropriate for Mrs C as this class of compounds is highly active against most Gram-negative organisms as well as having useful activity against *Staphylococcus aureus*; gentamicin is also inexpensive. Metronidazole is highly active against anaerobic organisms. Cefotaxime is a "third generation" cephalosporin with increased sensitivity against Gram-negative organisms, although this is balanced by reduced activity against some Gram-positive organisms, notably *Staphylococcus aureus*. It can be useful when given in combination with an aminoglycoside, but it would be more advantageous to Mrs C to use an agent with greater activity against Gram-positive organisms, for example ampicillin or one of its analogues (such as amoxycillin, pivampicillin, or Augmentin®). All penicillins may cause renal damage, most commonly acute interstitial nephritis, but the damage is a hypersensitivity reaction and therefore unpredictable, and is not an absolute contra-indication to penicillin use.

19. Gentamicin can cause nephrotoxicity and toxicity to the eighth cranial nerve. Regular monitoring for these side-effects, and of Mrs C's gentamicin serum levels, is essential.

Treatment with an aminoglycoside is justified for the reasons given in the previous answer; however, all aminoglycosides are potentially nephrotoxic, being associated with damage to the proximal tubule. (Aminoglycosides can also precipitate acute renal failure.) Because of this, they should generally be avoided in renal impairment; however, their bactericidal activity against an extremely broad spectrum of Gram-negative organisms means that they are often prescribed for seriously ill patients with systemic infections. They are excreted solely by the kidney, so accumulation may lead to a vicious circle of increasing drug levels causing further renal deterioration, and hence further accumulation. The risk of nephrotoxicity is increased by combined treatment with other nephrotoxic drugs, notably the loop diuretics. Mrs C was prescribed the loop diuretic frusemide at an early stage of this admission, but her diuretic therapy has now been discontinued; however, if it is required again, the doses of aminoglycoside and loop diuretic must be staggered as much as possible.

In addition to being nephrotoxic, aminoglycosides are toxic to the eighth cranial nerve and may produce vestibular symptoms (i.e. loss of sense of balance) or adversely affect hearing. Such symptoms should thus be checked for regularly.

In general, it is thought that the risk of nephro-toxicity and eighth cranial nerve toxicity is associated with peak serum concentrations persistently above 10 mg/L, and, perhaps more importantly, troughs persistently above 2 mg/L, although persistently low levels do not guarantee freedom from nephrotoxicity. For this reason it is vital to monitor Mrs C's peak (one hour post-dose) and trough (immediately before dose) serum levels on a regular basis. Since aminoglycosides are excreted unchanged by glomerular filtration, dosage alterations are required in cases of reduced renal function uncorrected by dialysis or haemofiltration. (Mrs C's haemofiltration has been temporarily discontinued until her septicaemia is under control.) Methods of calculating an appropriate dosage regimen can be found in the literature. Using one such method, an appropriate loading dose would be 100 mg, and the maintenance dose should be 90 mg every 36 hours. This will give a peak of approximately 8 mg/L and a trough of 1 mg/L. A loading dose should be prescribed for the reasons discussed in answer 12.

Alternatively, a simpler method of choosing an appropriate dosage regimen is to use the dosage guidelines based on CrCl which are published in the British National Formulary and appropriate product literature. There are also a number of computer software packages available which can calculate dosage regimens from relevant patient parameters, such as age, sex, weight, and plasma creatinine concentration.

The ready removal of aminoglycosides by glomerular filtration would indicate that they should be cleared by haemofiltration, peritoneal dialysis and haemodialysis, and this has been shown to be the case. When dialysis is intermittent, as with haemodialysis, it should be assumed that each treatment clears all the aminoglycoside present in the system, so that each dialysis should be followed by a loading dose (e.g. 100 mg in the case of Mrs C). When renal replacement therapy is continuous, as with peritoneal dialysis and haemofiltration, it should be assumed, at least initially, that this is equivalent to having functionally intact kidneys and the patient should be dosed accordingly. Thus, when Mrs C's haemofiltration is restarted her dosage regimen should be adjusted.

Whether Mrs C is receiving haemofiltration or not, regular peak and trough plasma estimations are a necessity. They should be performed before and after the second dose (i.e. the dose following the loading dose, when the patient should already be at steady state). Further estimations should be performed before and after every third or fourth subsequent dose, or more frequently if plasma creatinine values increase or decrease markedly.

20. Yes, Mrs C's illness followed the typical course of acute renal failure, and her survival to this stage is a good prognostic sign.

Acute tubular necrosis, the commonest form of acute renal failure, usually occurs as a consequence of severe shock, or as a result of sodium and water depletion giving rise to hypotension and generalised vasoconstriction, which in turn give rise to renal ischaemia. This was the sequence that gave rise to Mrs C's condition. Acute tubular necrosis may also develop unattended by any circulatory disturbance, for example, through direct damage to the renal parenchyma that can result from toxic or allergic reactions to drugs or other substances.

The course of acute renal failure may be divided into two phases. The first is the oliguric phase, which is characterised by a urine volume of 200–400 mL in 24 hours, a volume at which the kidney is unable to concentrate the urine sufficiently to excrete the products of metabolism. This inevitably leads to uraemia and hyperkalaemia unless adequate management is provided. The oliguric phase is usually no longer than seven to 14 days, but it may last for up to six weeks. If the patient does not expire in this period, he or she will enter the second phase, which is characterised by a urine volume that rises over a few days to several litres. This, the diuretic phase, lasts for up to seven days and corresponds to the recommencement of tubular function. Patients who survive into this phase, as Mrs C did, have a relatively good prognosis. Recovery of renal function takes place slowly over the following months, although the GFR rarely returns completely to its initial level. The elderly recover function more slowly and less completely.

The mortality of acute renal failure varies according to the cause, but overall is about 50%. Death due to uraemia and hyperkalaemia is rare now; the major causes are septicaemia and, to a lesser extent, gastro-intestinal haemorrhage. Death is more common in patients aged over 60.

References and Further Reading

Bennett W.M., *Drugs and Renal Disease*, 2nd edn, Edinburgh, Churchill Livingstone, 1986.

Ching-San C.L. and Marbury T.C., Drug therapy in patients undergoing haemodialysis, *Clin. Pharmacokinet.*, 1984, **9**, 42–66.

Dawborn J.K., Acute renal failure, *Med. Int.*, 1986, **32**, 1309–1316.

Fotheringham G., *Dosage Adjustment in Renal Failure*, UK Clinical Pharmacy Association, Leeds University Printing Service, 1986.

Harper A., *Drug Induced Renal Impairment*, UK Clinical Pharmacy Association, Leeds University Printing Service, 1988.

Ledingham J.G.G., Acute renal failure, in *Oxford Textbook of Medicine*, 2nd edn, Weatherall, D.J., Ledingham, J.G.G. and Warrell, D.A. (eds), Oxford, Oxford University Press, 1987, 18.124–18.134.

Marsh F.P. Drugs and the kidney, *ibid.*, 18.119–18.124.

Paton T.W. *et al.*, Drug therapy in patients undergoing peritoneal dialysis, *Clin. Pharmacokinet.*, 1985, **10**, 404–426.

CHRONIC RENAL FAILURE MANAGED BY CONTINUOUS AMBULATORY PERITONEAL DIALYSIS

Raymond J. Bunn

Principal Pharmacist, St Helier Hospital, Carshalton, Surrey

Day 1 Mr F, a 45-year-old blind, insulin-dependent diabetic with end-stage renal failure which was treated by continuous ambulatory peritoneal dialysis (CAPD), was admitted to the renal ward with a two-day history of abdominal pain and malaise. His sister had noticed that his CAPD effluent had become very cloudy over the previous 24 hours. It was his first admission to the renal unit at this hospital.

Mr F had been an insulin-dependent diabetic since childhood and had required CAPD for the previous two years because of diabetic nephrosclerosis. He had been registered blind for three years because of proliferative diabetic retinopathy. He was anaemic secondary to his chronic renal failure, and moderately hypertensive despite dialysis. He also suffered from chronic back pain following an industrial injury four years earlier.

Mr F had retired from work two years prior to this admission because of ill-health. He had recently moved into the area to live with his sister, who worked full-time, as he was unable to cope alone at home.

On admission, Mr F was noted to be unwell and breathless, with a pulse of 54 beats per minute, a blood pressure of 160/100 mmHg and a temperature of 36.6°C. His weight was 61 kg, which was 4 kg above his normal 'dry' weight. Clinical examination revealed moderate hypertension, ankle oedema and abdominal tenderness.

Drug therapy at the time of admission was:

Aluminium hydroxide 475 mg, three capsules three times daily
Propranolol 40 mg three times daily
Ispaghula husk, one sachet twice daily when necessary
Lactulose liquid 20 mL twice daily when necessary
Co-proxamol, two tablets four times daily when necessary
Insulin Human Mixtard, 18 units subcutaneously each morning and 12 units subcutaneously each evening

Mr F's dialysis therapy consisted of 2 L exchanges four times daily, using Dianeal 137 System 2® (Baxter). The three daytime exchanges were with dialysate containing 1.36% glucose ("weak" bags) and the overnight exchange was with dialysate containing 3.86% glucose ("strong" bag).

His serum biochemical and haematological results were as follows:

Glucose 15.1 mmol/L (reference range 2.9–6.4)
Potassium 4.2 mmol/L (3.4–5.2)
Creatinine 566 micromol/L (50–100)
Calcium 2.08 mmol/L (2.26–2.60)
Phosphate 1.43 mmol/L (0.8–1.45)
Sodium 130 mmol/L (133–144)
Red cell count 2.91×10^9/L (4.5–6.5×10^9)
White cell count 6.16×10^9/L (4.0–11.0×10^9)
Haemoglobin 5.4 g/dL (13–18)
Haematocrit 0.205 (0.4–0.54)

A chest x-ray was taken which revealed pulmonary oedema, and a sample of dialysate effluent was sent for microbiological screening.

Mr F was diagnosed as having peritonitis with fluid overload and hyperglycaemia. He was also noted to be hypocalcaemic.

1. Should the results of the microbiological cultures be obtained before initiating antibiotic therapy?

2. What treatment would you recommend for Mr F's peritonitis and why? What alternative therapeutic options are there?

3. Will Mr F's dialysis and insulin regimen need adjustment during the initial course of treatment?

4. Is subcutaneous injection the route of choice for administering insulin in CAPD patients? What is the alternative route and what are its advantages and disadvantages?

5. Why is Mr F hypocalcaemic and how would you recommend he be treated? What therapeutic options may be available in the future?

Mr F was prescribed two rapid exchanges with "weak" bags to relieve abdominal tenderness and to flush the peritoneal dialysis catheter. This was to be followed by six dialysis exchanges daily, alternating "strong" and "weak" bags. Intravenous human soluble insulin was prescribed via a syringe pump, on a sliding scale according to blood glucose measurements. Following the two rapid exchanges, vancomycin (100 mg), ceftazidime (100 mg) and heparin (200 units) were to be added to each 2 L dialysis bag prior to instillation. The antibiotics were prescribed for seven days.

6. Why is heparin being added to Mr F's CAPD bags?

Day 2 Mr F's condition was stable and he was less breathless. His hyperglycaemia was controlled. As this was Mr F's first in-patient episode since transferring to the unit it was decided to review all his medication on the evening ward round.

7. What information and recommendations would you prepare for the review, with respect to Mr F's:
(a) Phosphate binder?
(b) Analgesia?
(c) Laxative regimen?
(d) Antihypertensive therapy?
Indicate briefly possible future prospects for therapeutic options where appropriate.

8. What recommendations would you make for the treatment of Mr F's anaemia?

Day 3 Mr F's condition was improving. His pulmonary and ankle oedema had resolved and his dialysis regimen was returned to four exchanges per

day (three "weak" and one "strong" bag). His dialysate effluent was less cloudy and his abdomen was less tender. Microbiological culture revealed the Gram-positive organism *Staphylococcus epidermidis*, sensitive to vancomycin; therefore the intraperitoneal ceftazidime was stopped. The sliding scale intravenous insulin was also stopped and subcutaneous therapy was re-instated. Therapy with recombinant human erythropoietin was commenced to treat anaemia. Calcium carbonate was prescribed as a phosphate-binder and the aluminium hydroxide therapy was stopped. Alfacalcidol treatment was initiated to correct hypocalcaemia.

Captopril was introduced as an antihypertensive agent, starting with a test dose of 6.25 mg because of the risk of hyper-reaction to this drug. Propranolol therapy was discontinued. Ispaghula husk therapy was also discontinued, and the dose of lactulose liquid was reduced. Co-proxamol was replaced by paracetamol as analgesic therapy.

Day 4 Mr F continued to improve. His CAPD effluent was now almost clear, and heparin additions to each bag were stopped.

Day 5 Mr F was discharged. His medication on discharge was:

Calcium carbonate 300 mg, three tablets three times daily after food
Captopril 12.5 mg twice daily
Alfacalcidol 250 nanograms daily
Lactulose liquid 15 mL twice daily
Paracetamol 500 mg, two tablets four times daily when necessary for pain relief
Insulin Human Mixtard, 18 units subcutaneously each morning and 12 units subcutaneously each evening.

Recombinant human erythropoietin, 3000 units three times weekly (intravenously), was prescribed to be given by the district nurse.

Mr F's dialysis regimen on discharge was four 2 L exchanges daily (three "weak" and one "strong" bag), with vancomycin 100 mg to be added to each bag for two more days, after which dialysis was to continue with drug-free bags. An out-patient clinic appointment was made for three days' time.

9. How can you help Mr F to comply with the remainder of his antibiotic course and other medication when at home?

Answers

1. Definitely not.

Delay in treatment can lead to the infection, which is usually confined to the peritoneal cavity, becoming systemic. Infection can also damage the peritoneum, reducing its efficiency as a dialysis membrane in the long term. Empirical antibiotic therapy should therefore be commenced as soon as peritonitis is clinically diagnosed.

2. The concomitant use of vancomycin 50 mg/L and ceftazidime 50 mg/L added to each dialysate bag just prior to instillation into the peritoneum. The nominal course length should be seven days. Intravenous antibiotic therapy is not warranted for Mr F as he is apyrexial, and systemic infection is therefore not suspected.

An antibiotic regimen that is effective against all the major Gram-positive and Gram-negative pathogens – in particular *Staphylococcus* and *Pseudomonas* species, and Enterobacteriaceae – is required. Evidence to date favours the intraperitoneal route of administration. This route enables precise therapeutic and non-toxic concentrations of the antibiotics to be delivered directly to the infection site. The empirical intraperitoneal regimen recommended is relatively safe and has proved to be highly effective over many years' use.

Ceftazidime, a cephalosporin with broad-spectrum antimicrobial activity, including good Gram-negative activity, has a wide therapeutic index. It is reported to be stable (less than 10% loss in potency) in CAPD fluid for 24 hours at room temperature.

Vancomycin has excellent antimicrobial activity against Gram-positive *Staphylococcus* and *Streptococcus* species, the most common causative organisms of CAPD peritonitis. It is reported to be stable (less than 10% loss in potency) in CAPD fluid for at least 24 hours (at least 48 hours in one report). Despite demonstrated clinical efficacy, the stability of vancomycin and ceftazidime mixed together in CAPD fluid has not been investigated.

When given by the intraperitoneal route, both vancomycin and ceftazidime (and most other antibiotics) are absorbed systemically, particularly through an inflamed peritoneal membrane. In addition, the serum half-life of both drugs is greatly extended in patients with renal failure. Systemically, vancomycin has a narrow therapeutic index and is potentially ototoxic; however, the dialysate concentration of 50 mg/L is below the recommended maximum safe serum concentration of 60–80 mg/L. In addition, extensive experience of serum level monitoring during intraperitoneal therapy with the recommended regimen has shown that accumulation of vancomycin to potentially toxic levels does not occur in patients with end-stage renal failure, even after ten days' therapy.

The empirical antibiotic regimen should be adjusted after the results of microbiological culture and sensitivity. If a Gram-negative organism resistant to ceftazidime is isolated as the single causative organism, vancomycin and ceftazidime therapy must be stopped and replaced by intraperitoneal netilmicin. If *Pseudomonas aeruginosa* is isolated, netilmicin must be substituted, irrespective of the organism's sensitivity to ceftazidime. *Pseudomonas aeruginosa* peritonitis can be particularly aggressive and severe, and the powerful Gram-negative activity of netilmicin is thus preferred. If no organism is isolated, ceftazidime and vancomycin should be continued for the remainder of the course.

Netilmicin (and other aminoglycosides) must be used with care by the intraperitoneal route. Systemic absorption from the peritoneum may lead to potentially ototoxic and nephrotoxic serum levels (the latter being relevant for patients who still have some remaining renal function), particularly after an extended course of treatment. Netilmicin, although more expensive, is reported to be the least toxic of the aminoglycosides. A recommended intraperitoneal regimen is netilmicin 7.5 mg/L four times daily for 48 hours, reducing to 7.5 mg/L twice daily (alternating with drug-free bags). A serum netilmicin level should be measured after 96 hours; if the level is greater than 4 mg/L, the dose or frequency should be further reduced.

Aztreonam has a similar potency and spectrum of activity to the aminoglycosides but does not share their systemic toxicity. It has been used successfully by the intraperitoneal route but experience is limited. It is relatively expensive but does not need serum level monitoring.

Other reported regimens for the effective treatment of CAPD peritonitis have included:

(a) For confirmed Gram-positive peritonitis, intravenous administration of vancomycin 1 g on the day of confirmation followed by vancomycin 1 g intravenously seven days later.

(b) Concomitant intraperitoneal use of an aminoglycoside and vancomycin, both in various doses.

(c) Concomitant intraperitonal use of a cephalosporin and an aminoglycoside, both in various doses.

(d) Concomitant intraperitoneal use of other cephalosporins and vancomycin, both in various doses.

(e) Use of two high intraperitoneal doses of

vancomycin (30 mg/kg), one week apart, with the addition of an intraperitoneal aminoglycoside daily if Gram-positive culture is not confirmed.

(f) Use of the broad-spectrum drug ciprofloxacin as a single agent, either by the intraperitoneal route (25 mg/L), or orally (250–500 mg four times daily).

(g) Use of bolus intravenous vancomycin with oral ciprofloxacin.

As yet, none of these alternative regimens has been shown to be therapeutically superior to the one recommended. However, some offer the advantages of simplicity of regimen, which is useful for aiding patient compliance after hospital discharge, and reduced cost. Reports on the successful use of oral ciprofloxacin in CAPD peritonitis are particularly encouraging. Compliance could be a problem with Mr F on discharge and a simpler antibiotic regimen should be considered when that time comes.

3. Yes. Inflammation of the peritoneal membrane, due to peritonitis, causes an increase in its permeability. Glucose absorption becomes more rapid, which results in a faster dissipation of the osmotic gradient that is essential for ultrafiltration.

Peritoneal inflammation has already affected Mr F in two ways: firstly, the loss of ultrafiltration has caused him to become fluid-overloaded, and secondly, the increased glucose absorption has caused his hyperglycaemia. To correct fluid overload, the number of dialysis fluid exchanges should be increased to six daily, and "strong" and "weak" bags should be alternated. This reduces the dwell time of the dialysate in the peritoneum, thereby maintaining the osmotic gradient. Additionally, the more frequent use of the more hypertonic dialysate will remove the excess fluid from Mr F.

To achieve serum glucose control, subcutaneous insulin should be stopped and an infusion of short-acting insulin started using a syringe pump. The insulin dose can be given in accordance with a sliding scale based on blood glucose measurements. As soon as Mr F's peritonitis and fluid overload is controlled, he can revert to subcutaneous insulin therapy and four dialysis exchanges daily. The use of hypertonic dialysate can cause peritoneal discomfort, and Mr F should be warned about this.

4. Subcutaneous administration is not necessarily the route of choice for insulin in CAPD patients, although it is preferable for Mr F.

Many reports suggest that better control of serum glucose can be achieved with intraperitoneal insulin. The total daily insulin requirement via the intraperitoneal route is approximately 50% greater than via the subcutaneous route. This is due to:

(a) adsorption of insulin onto the PVC of CAPD bags and tubing,

(b) incomplete absorption of the dose during the dwell time,

(c) degradation of insulin in the dialysate, and

(d) insulin resistance and antibody formation.

There is considerable interpatient variation in the dosage required to maintain good serum glucose control, and doses must be individualised. Higher doses of insulin are required in dialysate bags containing the higher concentrations of glucose. A suitable initial intraperitoneal dosage regimen using soluble human insulin is as follows. For preprandial daytime exchanges: CAPD bags with 1.36% glucose, add 0.175 units/L/kg; CAPD bags with 3.86% glucose, add 0.25 units/L/kg. For overnight exchanges: CAPD bags with 1.36% glucose, add 0.1 units/L/kg; CAPD bags with 3.86% glucose, add 0.15 units/L/kg. In order to achieve acceptable levels of glycaemia, doses should be adjusted according to four-hourly serum glucose profiles taken over the previous 24 hours.

Reports indicate that loss of glycaemic control during peritonitis is less common in patients treated with intraperitoneal insulin, probably because the permeability of the peritoneum increases for insulin as well as for glucose. Another report has indicated that the incidence of peritonitis in diabetic CAPD patients treated with intraperitoneal insulin is lower than in any other group of CAPD patients, although the reason for this is unclear.

Despite these arguments in favour of intraperitoneal insulin therapy, after taking into account Mr F's social circumstances, visual handicap and the fact that he is trained and familiar with self-administration of subcutaneous insulin, it is better that he continues to use the latter route.

5. Reduced calcitriol (the physiologically active form of vitamin D) synthesis in the failing kidney results in reduced serum calcitriol levels and reduced calcium absorption from the gut. This, together with hyperphosphataemia and reduced bone resorption, causes hypocalcaemia.

Hypocalcaemia and a reduction in the direct suppressive action of calcitriol on the parathyroid gland results in an increased secretion of parathyroid hormone (PTH). Since it is not possible for the failing kidney to increase synthesis of calcitriol in response to the increased serum PTH levels (which would result in a decrease in PTH levels in a patient with normal renal function), the serum PTH levels remain chronically elevated and hyperplasia of the parathyroid glands occur. The resultant secondary hyperparathyroidism is central to the development of renal osteodystrophy.

Mr F's hypocalcaemia should be treated with oral alfacalcidol (metabolised to calcitriol in the liver) at an initial dose of 250 nanograms daily. This dose can be adjusted according to his response. During therapy his serum calcium level should be regularly monitored, particularly if he is changed to a calcium-based phosphate-binder. If Mr F becomes hypercalcaemic, stopping alfacalcidol should quickly result in a reduced serum calcium level. Although not relevant in Mr F's case, significant hyperphosphataemia should always be corrected prior to correcting hypocalcaemia, as elevated phosphate and calcium levels can result in metastatic calcification of soft tissue.

The oral administration of calcitriol or alfacalcidol results in a rise in serum calcitriol and calcium, which suppresses PTH secretion to some extent. To suppress serum PTH to normal levels, large oral doses of calcitriol (or alfacalcidol) would have to be given and hypercalcaemia would quickly ensue. However, it has been demonstrated that intravenous administration of calcitriol to hyperparathyroid chronic haemodialysis patients (1 microgram three times weekly after dialysis) can reduce serum PTH levels to within the normal range without causing hypercalcaemia. The reason for this is not yet fully understood.

Transdermal and subcutaneous calcitriol are alternative routes worthy of investigation. In the future, management of renal osteodystrophy will probably centre around the normalisation of serum PTH by the parenteral administration of calcitriol.

6. Heparin is being added to each bag of CAPD fluid to help break down the fibrin that appears in the peritoneum as a result of peritonitis, and which contributes to the cloudy appearance of the CAPD effluent. The breakdown of the fibrin helps prevent blockage of the CAPD catheter.

Heparin additions should continue until the CAPD effluent becomes clear. The dose of heparin per bag varies considerably between renal units and is somewhat empirical. We find that 200 units per bag (irrespective of volume) is a simple and effective regimen, although some reports recommend as much as 1000 units/L. We use heparin flush (ampoules of 200 units in 2 mL) as a convenient source of the 200 unit dose. This simplifies the regimen for patients making the additions at home. Although not the case with Mr F, a proportion of patients always have a cloudy fibrinous CAPD effluent that is not associated with peritonitis. These patients add heparin to each of their CAPD bags routinely.

7(a) Mr F's aluminium hydroxide therapy should be stopped and calcium carbonate 900 mg three times daily started, using calcium carbonate 300 mg tablets (USP). Following this change in therapy, his serum phosphate and calcium levels should be monitored regularly and the dose adjusted in response to changes in these concentrations. A low-calcium dialysate (Baxter Special Dialysis Solutions) could be considered if hypercalcaemia proves to be a problem.

Serum phosphate levels rise in patients with renal failure, mainly due to the decreased renal excretion of phosphate. The resulting hyperphosphataemia plays a major role in the development of secondary hyperparathyroidism and, consequently, renal osteodystrophy, since excessive PTH release is stimulated by hyperphosphataemia-induced hypocalcaemia and also hypocalcitriolaemia. Management of hyperphosphataemia centres around a combination of dialysis and the binding of orally ingested phosphate in the gut, using a phosphate-binding agent to prevent its systemic absorption. Such an agent is usually the salt of a di- or tri-valent metallic ion.

Aluminium, usually as the hydroxide, has been widely used as a phosphate-binder. However, aluminium that is systemically absorbed from the binding agent is toxic, causing encephalopathy, osteomalacia, proximal myopathy and anaemia. Aluminium salts also cause constipation, which can quickly lead to drainage problems in CAPD patients.

Alternatives to aluminium salts are based on magnesium and/or calcium salts, usually the carbonate. Magnesium carbonate (up to 4.8 g daily) has been used successfully in chronic haemodialysis patients but diarrhoea is a major side-effect. Calcium carbonate has been used with some success in chronic haemodialysis patients. However, calcium has a relatively low phosphate-binding capacity, necessitating the use of impractically large doses (up to 10 g daily), and, in some haemodialysis patients, the concomitant use of another phosphate-binding agent to control serum phosphate adequately. The dose of calcium carbonate required to control serum phosphate in CAPD patients is, however, generally lower (1.2–3.78 g daily), probably due to the continuous removal of serum phosphate by this method of dialysis. However, unpredictable episodes of hypercalcaemia, due to systemic calcium absorption, are a problem in this patient group.

For both haemodialysis and CAPD patients, if

serum phosphate is high and a significant amount of calcium is systemically absorbed from the calcium carbonate (a problem that is more likely if large doses are being used), there is a risk of metastatic calcification of soft tissue. Calcium salts are also constipating.

Dose volumes of existing aluminium, calcium and magnesium phosphate-binders tend to be large and taste unpleasant, factors that decrease patient compliance and, as a consequence, reduce the patient's serum phosphate control. To reduce this problem, a phosphate-binder combining magnesium and calcium carbonates in a pleasant-tasting, chewable tablet form has been developed jointly by pharmacy and renal unit staff and is currently under clinical trial. The product is designed to be non-toxic, have a potent phosphate-binding capacity in a small dose volume (one or two tablets three times daily being adequate for most patients), and be relatively free of side-effects. In addition, the dialysate used for patients treated with this product is formulated to have a lower calcium and magnesium concentration than usual.

Until research reveals a more satisfactory phosphate-binder than those already in use, calcium carbonate is the drug of choice for Mr F.

(b) Co-proxamol therapy should be discontinued and replaced by paracetamol 500 mg, up to two tablets four times daily when necessary. If Mr F's pain is continuous, regular therapy should be recommended.

Co-proxamol (containing paracetamol 325 mg and dextropropoxyphene 32.5 mg), although commonly used, is not the analgesic of choice in renal failure. The active metabolite of dextropropoxyphene, norpropoxyphene, accumulates in renal failure, enhancing side-effects such as constipation and sedation. This has probably contributed to Mr F's feeling of lethargy and his need for laxatives. There is no conclusive evidence that co-proxamol is a stronger analgesic than paracetamol alone. If pain relief is not achieved with paracetamol, a non-steroidal anti-inflammatory drug could be considered, although such a drug may cause gastro-intestinal bleeding and reduce any residual renal function Mr F may have. Sulindac may be the drug of choice from this group as it is reported to have no effect on renal function at normal therapeutic doses, although gastro-intestinal side-effects can still be a problem. Alternatively it may be considered that the benefit of using co-proxamol could outweigh its disadvantages. Co-dydramol could also be considered as an alternative, but sedation and respiratory depression can occur.

(c) Lactulose should be prescribed regularly. Ispaghula husk sachets should be discontinued and paracetamol should be prescribed as analgesia in place of co-proxamol.

Constipation in CAPD patients can lead to obstruction of drainage of the dialysate from the peritoneum. Three factors are probably contributing to Mr F's constipation:
(i) his aluminium phosphate-binder (however, calcium phosphate-binders also cause constipation);
(ii) the use of an analgesic containing dextropropoxyphene, a synthetic narcotic analgesic with morphine-like action; and
(iii) inappropriate "when necessary" use of his prescribed laxatives.

Lactulose acts as both an osmotic and a bulking laxative. Because of its physiological mode of action it is unsuitable for use on a "when necessary" basis and should be prescribed regularly. Lactulose can also produce a significant reduction in colonic pH, which may reduce the formation and systemic absorption of ammonium ions and other nitrogenous toxins, thus aiding the control of uraemia. It is not significantly absorbed and is unlikely to affect Mr F's diabetic control adversely. A dose of 15 mL twice daily is suitable to start, with adjustment according to response. The concomitant use of ispaghula husk sachets is illogical, and, in addition, both brands (Fybogel® and Regulan®) contain between 6 and 7 mmol potassium per sachet. By discontinuing such therapy, an unnecessary intake of potassium in a patient with renal failure can be avoided.

(d) Change Mr F's antihypertensive therapy from propranolol to captopril.

Hypertension in end-stage renal failure is attributed to either increased cardiac output, or increased peripheral vascular resistance, or both. Increased cardiac output reflects volume expansion secondary to sodium and water retention and/or the anaemia of chronic renal failure. Increased peripheral resistance may reflect an increase in circulating renin and angiotensin II or, possibly, decreased levels of vasodilators such as prostaglandins, bradykinin or renal medullary lipids. Hypertension is occasionally controlled by dialysis, but most patients, including Mr F, need antihypertensive medication.

Propranolol and other beta-blockers have the potential to affect diabetics by increasing the frequency of hypoglycaemic attacks and delaying the rate of recovery, and by impairing carbohydrate tolerance. This risk is lessened by the use of the more cardioselective beta-blockers, atenolol or metoprolol. Atenolol is excreted renally and therefore needs dosage adjustment in renal failure. Metoprolol is cleared hepatically and needs no dosage adjustment, although small initial doses are advised in renal failure. Even the more cardioselective beta-blockers can cause some vasoconstriction in both the peritoneum and the periphery by blockade of vascular beta$_2$-adrenoreceptors which allows unopposed alpha-receptor-mediated vasoconstriction. This may reduce the efficiency of dialysis in CAPD patients. Although there is no absolute contra-indication to beta-blocker therapy in Mr F, it is not the treatment of choice. If a beta-blocker is desired, metoprolol therapy would be most appropriate.

A logical antihypertensive for Mr F is an angiotensin-converting enzyme (ACE) inhibitor, which causes vasodilation and reduced sodium retention by reducing the amount of circulating angiotensin II. There is little to choose clinically between captopril, enalapril and lisinopril. Captopril, with a shorter half-life, has acute activity which is useful for testing response to ACE inhibitors prior to initiating routine therapy. ACE inhibitors can cause a profound drop in blood pressure in patients with renal failure. Enalapril and lisinopril offer the benefit of once-daily dosing.

Sudden beta-blocker withdrawal can be dangerous, but Mr F is taking a relatively small dose. Mr F's propranolol can therefore be stopped and a test dose of captopril 6.25 mg be given. His blood pressure should be closely monitored for about four hours. A dose of 12.5 mg twice daily is suitable for Mr F to start, with adjustment according to response. Neutropenia has been reported in patients with renal failure, and fortnightly white cell counts are advised for the first three months of therapy. Other more common side-effects are transient loss of taste, dry cough and rashes. There are reports that ACE inhibitors reduce thirst, which is potentially useful in those dialysis patients who have a tendency to fluid overload as a result of excessive drinking.

Nifedipine would also be a suitable choice for Mr F. Headache, facial flushing and oedema are the main side-effects.

The vasodilators hydralazine, prazosin and minoxidil are not contra-indicated in renal failure but are not the antihypertensives of choice for Mr F. Hydralazine and minoxidil should be used with a beta-blocker to reduce reflex tachycardia. Nausea can be problematic and a syndrome like systemic lupus erythematosus can be induced when high doses of hydralazine are used long term. Postural hypotension, drowsiness and nasal stuffiness can be problems with prazosin. The sensitivity of patients to all these drugs in end-stage renal failure is increased and, if used, therapy should be initiated with small doses.

The use of methyldopa in hypertension has considerably decreased, mainly due to its side-effect profile. If used in renal failure, initial doses should be small, because of the increased sensitivity of such patients to the drug.

8. Mr F should be treated with intravenous recombinant human erythropoietin (rhuEPO), a bioengineered form of the hormone which is immunologically and biologically indistinguishable from native erythropoietin (EPO).

Mr F's anaemia is probably the major contributor to his continuous feeling of lethargy and fatigue. This, combined with other central nervous system and non-central nervous system related disorders primarily caused by the hypoxaemia of anaemia, results in a diminished quality of life. The anaemia of chronic renal failure is probably caused by a deficiency in the renal production of the hormone EPO, which leads to reduced bone marrow erythropoiesis. Other contributing factors include the inhibition of erythropoiesis by uraemic toxins, a shortening of red cell survival, uraemic bleeding, iron deficiency, aluminium toxicity, hyperparathyroidism and hypersplenism.

Red blood cell transfusions have been the cornerstone of management of the anaemia of CRF, but erythroid marrow suppression, HLA antibody induction, and iron overload make this treatment increasingly unpopular. Drug therapy has centred around the use of anabolic steroids or even cobalt; hepatic and cardiac toxicity and virilisation limit their use and, in any case, we have not found them to be particularly efficacious. Iron and/or folic acid are given if the patient is found to be deficient.

A slow rise in haemoglobin should minimise aggravation of Mr F's hypertension and avoid other reported haemodynamically induced side-effects, such as seizures and clotting of vascular accesses. The hypertension sometimes seen during rhuEPO therapy is probably due to a reverse of vasodilation caused by chronic anaemia. Mr F's blood pressure should be regularly monitored and controlled, if necessary, by adjustment of his antihypertensive therapy. Depletion of available iron is common during rhuEPO therapy because of the greatly increased marrow requirements. Mr F's iron status should thus be regularly monitored; if his transferrin saturation falls below 20%, iron supplementation should be given to maintain maximum response to the rhuEPO therapy. Improved appetite on rhuEPO therapy can also increase potassium intake, which can necessitate the institution of some dietary control.

As yet, there is no definitive dose or route recommendation for rhuEPO. An initial intravenous dose of 50 units/kg body weight three times weekly should produce the required slow rise in haemoglobin. A rise of no more than 1 g/dL/month is advised. The target haemoglobin is commonly 9–11 g/dL, with a haematocrit of 0.30–0.35. Once the target has been reached, a dose in the region of 75 units/kg/week in two or three divided doses should maintain the level. RhuEPO has been shown to be equally effective clinically when administered subcutaneously using similar or smaller doses than those used intravenously. The subcutaneous route would be ideal for Mr F, who has no permanent vascular access and is used to subcutaneous drug administration. The current presentations of 2000 and 4000 units/mL in 1 mL ampoules are not convenient for subcutaneous dosing or intravenous dosing in fractions of 1 mL; a presentation of 10,000 units/mL in a "penfill"-type cartridge device would be optimum for this route. When a suitable subcutaneous presentation of rhuEPO becomes available, this route should be considered for Mr F. RhuEPO has also been shown to be effective by the intraperitoneal route. Early studies indicated that much larger doses than those used intravenously are needed for successful intraperitoneal therapy, but it has been suggested that adjustment of the dialysis regimen can increase the intraperitoneal bioavailability of rhuEPO considerably.

9. Mr F, who is blind, can be helped to comply with the remainder of his intraperitoneal vancomycin course in one of two ways.

(a) By making 100 mg vancomycin additions to a further two days' supply of his CAPD bags under aseptic conditions in the pharmacy. The stability (less than 10% loss in potency) of vancomycin in CAPD fluid at room temperature has been demonstrated over this period. Mr F could store the bags in a refrigerator until they are ready for warming just prior to instillation.

(b) By supplying him with reconstituted vancomycin 100 mg in pre-filled syringes assembled under aseptic conditions in the pharmacy. Reconstituted vancomycin has been shown to be stable for at least 14 days at room temperature and at least 60 days if stored in a refrigerator. Refrigeration until use should be recommended.

Under the circumstances, the first option is preferable, as this requires no manipulations by either Mr F or his sister. The bags with vancomycin added must be clearly identifiable to Mr F. His sister could help in this respect by assembling the bags that he is to use during the day, before she goes to work.

An alternative simple therapeutic option would have been to measure Mr F's serum vancomyin level on the day of discharge and then stop his intraperitoneal vancomycin therapy. Using pharmacokinetic principles, an intravenous top-up dose of vancomycin could have been calculated that would have increased his serum level to a peak of around 30 mg/L. Owing to the long half-life of vancomycin in impaired renal function, his serum concentration would then have remained above the minimum recommended therapeutic concentration (10 mg/L) for at least two days. This regimen is based on the report that intravenous vancomycin can be used successfully to treat Gram-positive CAPD peritonitis (see answer 2).

Although the remainder of Mr F's drug regimen is relatively simple, it is advantageous to counsel him, and his sister if possible, before discharge. If necessary a time-designated, compartmentalised compliance aid (such as the Dosette®), could be supplied. This would allow oral solid doses to be assembled by his sister in advance. Alternatively, the different drugs can be dispensed in different-sized bottles which Mr F can clearly identify. He should be informed that the calcium carbonate tablets can be chewed before swallowing if preferred, and that the "sweet-tasting" lactulose liquid should now be taken regularly. He is proficient at subcutaneous insulin dosing and his sister monitors his blood glucose levels. The district nurse will administer the intravenous rhuEPO. Mr F should also be reminded not to take any other drugs, either purchased or prescribed, without first checking with the Unit.

Acknowledgements

I should like to acknowledge the assistance of Stephen Smith, Senior Registrar in Nephrology, St Helier Hospital, and the support of my fellow pharmacists, David Roberts, Janet Zimmerman, Douglas McLean, and Sandra Briant, during the preparation of this case study.

References and Further Reading

Beardsworth S.F. *et al.*, Intraperitoneal insulin: a protocol for administration during CAPD and a review of published protocols, *Peritoneal Dialysis Int.*, 1988, **8**, 145–151.

British Society for Antimicrobial Chemotherapy Report, Diagnosis and management of peritonitis in continuous ambulatory peritoneal dialysis, *Lancet*, 1987, **1**, 845–849.

Nephrology forum, The anaemia of chronic renal failure: pathophysiology and the effects of recombinant erythropoietin, *Kidney Int.*, 1989, **35**, 134–148.

Scott D.K. and Roberts DE., Drugs and continuous ambulatory peritoneal dialysis (part 1), *Pharm. J.*, 1985, **234**, 592–593.

Scott D.K. and Roberts D.E., Drugs and continuous ambulatory peritoneal dialysis (part 2), *ibid.* 621–624.

RENAL TRANSPLANTATION

Sharron K. Marshment

Principal Pharmacist (Clinical Services Manager), Royal Free Hospital, London

Day 1 Thirty-eight-year-old Mr O was urgently admitted from home for a cadaveric renal transplant. He had a six-year history of renal impairment. He had first presented to his general practitioner with persistent headaches, which had resulted in an increased plasma urea being detected. Two years later he had presented with weakness, fatigue and generally "not feeling well" and was diagnosed as having chronic renal failure. Since then he had received continuous ambulatory peritoneal dialysis, and for the past three months had been in end-stage renal failure, awaiting a transplant.

His drug therapy on admission was:

Titralac® (calcium carbonate 420 mg + glycine 180 mg), one tablet three times daily
Alfacalcidol 250 nanograms daily
Folic acid 5 mg daily
Ferrous sulphate 200 mg daily
Ketovite®, one tablet daily.

Mr O was noted to be allergic to penicillin.

Mr O was a non-smoker who rarely drank alcohol. He was married with a five-year-old daughter, and worked as a draughtsman. He had recently been having difficulty maintaining his job, owing to a constant lack of energy.

On examination, Mr O was noted to be pale, but generally quite well. He was normotensive (blood pressure 120/90 mmHg), had a pulse of 70 beats per minute, and had no oedema or signs of cardiac failure. He had no haematuria, but his urine output was less than 250 mL/day. He weighed 55 kg.

His serum biochemistry and haematology results were:

Sodium 140 mmol/L (reference range 135–146)
Potassium 4.0 mmol/L (3.5–5.0)
Urea 17.4 mmol/L (3.0–6.5)
Creatinine 1074 micromol/L (60–120)
Phosphate 1.66 mmol/L (0.8–1.4)
Haemoglobin 9.0 g/dL (13.5–18.0)
White blood cells (WBC) 8.0×10^9/L $(4.0–10.0 \times 10^9)$
Liver function tests within normal limits

Day 2 (p.m.) Mr O was prepared for transplant. One hour prior to the operation he was given cyclosporin 150 mg intravenously, azathioprine 50 mg intravenously, and netilmicin 100 mg intravenously. The latter was given to cover the introduction of a subclavian line.

During the procedure, at the release of the vascular clamps, he was given methylprednisolone 1 g intravenously.

1. How should these injections be administered?

2. What are the therapeutic aims on return from theatre?

3. Which immunosuppressant(s) would you recommend be prescribed subsequently and why?

On return to the renal unit later that evening, Mr O was started on:

Cyclosporin 150 mg intravenously, to be repeated every 12 hours
Azathioprine 50 mg intravenously, to be repeated once each day
Methylprednisolone 15 mg intravenously, to be repeated once each day.

4. How should the cyclosporin therapy be monitored?

5. Which parameters should be monitored when azathioprine is prescribed?

Accurate fluid balance charts and intensive temperature, blood pressure and respiration rate monitoring were started. Initially Mr O had a renal output of 40 mL/hr. He was given Hemofiltrasol 22® (an electrolyte replacement solution containing calcium, sodium, magnesium, chloride and lactate ions) intravenously in a volume to replace the urine output over the first 24 hours plus an additional 2 L, using the central venous pressure as a guide to fluid replacement needs. Additional electrolytes were supplemented as appropriate, based on laboratory results. To improve renal perfusion, a dopamine infusion of 3 microgram/kg/min was started.

Mr O's blood pressure was noted to be 125/95 mmHg and it was decided that antihypertensive therapy was not necessary. He was, however, started on ranitidine to prevent stress ulceration.

Serum biochemistry and haematology results were:

Sodium 139 mmol/L (135–146)
Potassium 3.6 mmol/L (3.5–5.0)
Urea 16.8 mmol/L (3.0–6.5)
Creatinine 615 micromol/L (60–120)
Haemoglobin 9.0 g/dL (13.5–18.0)
WBC 7.8×10^9/L (4.0–10.0×10^9)

6. What dosage of ranitidine is appropriate for this indication?

Day 3 Mr O was well, apyrexial, and his urine output was good (approximately 150 mL/hr). The dopamine infusion was stopped and it was decided to give his remaining intravenous medications by the oral route.

Serum biochemistry and haematology results were:

Creatinine 459 micromol/L (60–120)
WBC 10.5×10^9/L (4.0–10.0×10^9)
Cyclosporin 184 nanogram/mL (100–120)

7. What oral doses of immunosuppressants would you recommend?

Nifedipine 10 mg sublingually when required was prescribed as an antihypertensive, to be used if Mr O's diastolic blood pressure was greater than 110 mmHg. Mr O complained about the taste of the cyclosporin liquid.

8. Would you have recommended nifedipine as an antihypertensive for Mr O?

9. How can the palatability of cyclosporin be improved?

Day 4 Serum biochemistry and haematology results were:

Creatinine 383 micromol/L (60–120)
WBC 8.1×10^9/L (4.0–10.0×10^9)

Day 5 Mr O became pyrexial, with a temperature of 37.5°C, and his kidney site was slightly tender. His blood pressure was 130/100 mmHg.

Serum biochemistry and haematology results were:

Creatinine 420 micromol/L (60–120)
WBC 7.4×10^9/L (4.0–10.0×10^9)
Cyclosporin 130 nanogram/mL (100–120)

An indium-labelled diethylenetriamine penta-acetic acid (DTPA) scan showed reduced perfusion of the kidney, and it was decided that Mr O was suffering from a rejection episode.

10. How should Mr O's acute rejection episode be managed?

Day 8 Mr O was looking better. His serum creatinine level had fallen to 280 micromol/L and the graft site was no longer tender. His cyclosporin level (trough) was 150 nanogram/mL.

Day 11 Mr O became pyrexial again, but this time the transplant site was not tender. He had developed a dry cough, complained of a sore throat, and had white patches in his mouth. He had some shortness of breath and looked ashen, but was alert and lucid.

His serum biochemistry and haematology results were:

Creatinine 274 micromol/L (60–120)
WBC 18.9×10^9/L (4.0–10.0×10^9)
Cyclosporin 121 nanogram/mL (100–120)

Blood samples and mid-stream urine samples were sent for microscopy, culture and sensitivity, and a chest x-ray was performed, which showed diffuse shadowing in both lung fields. There was marked deterioration in Mr O's blood gases, particularly after exercise.

11. What has pre-disposed Mr O to infection?

12. What types of infection is Mr O susceptible to?

Mr O was diagnosed as having a pneumonitis and was given a bronchial lavage to obtain "washings" that could be sent for microscopy, culture and sensitivity. *Pneumocystis carinii* infection was subsequently confirmed, and "high dose" oral co-trimoxazole therapy was started. *Listeria* was also cultured, and oral erythromycin 1 g four times daily was co-prescribed. Amphotericin lozenges were prescribed to treat oral candidiasis.

13. What dosage regimen of co-trimoxazole would you recommend?

Over the next seven days Mr O's temperature returned to normal and he appeared to be progressing well. His urine output was approximately 4 L/24 hrs and his blood gases were improving.

Day 20 The antibiotics were stopped and Mr O remained apyrexial. His urine output had fallen to 1250 mL in the last 24 hours and he had become oedematous. He was given frusemide 40 mg intravenously over 10 minutes, and was fluid-restricted to 500 mL per 24 hours. A DTPA scan showed deterioration of renal perfusion but a biopsy of the transplant showed no evidence of rejection. The possible diagnosis was cyclosporin toxicity.

Serum biochemistry and haematology results were:

Creatinine 380 micromol/L (60–120)
WBC 5.3×10^9/L (4.0–10.0×10^9)
Cyclosporin 258 nanogram/mL (100–120)

14. What could have potentiated cyclosporin toxicity?

15. Which drugs interact with cyclosporin?

16. How can cyclosporin nephrotoxicity be differentiated from rejection?

17. How should Mr O's cyclosporin dose be adjusted?

Mr O's cyclosporin dose was adjusted as recommended.

Day 22 Mr O again became pyrexial and the transplant had become tender and had increased in size. There was no obvious infection.

Serum biochemistry and haematology results were:

Creatinine 450 micromol (60–120)
WBC 4.6×10^9/L (4.0–10.0×10^9)
Cyclosporin 175 nanogram/mL (100–120)

As the cyclosporin level was still high, the next dose of cyclosporin was omitted and Mr O's dose was reduced to 150 mg twice daily.

This episode was considered to be a rejection episode and this was later confirmed by biopsy. It was treated as before.

Day 24 The graft was not functioning well, despite the immunosuppression with cyclosporin, azathioprine and corticosteroids.

Serum biochemistry and haematology results were:

Creatinine 560 micromol/L (60–120)
WBC 4.2×10^9/L (4.0–10.0×10^9)
Cyclosporin 95 nanogram/mL (100–120)

It was decided that Mr O required further immunosuppression with anti-thymocyte immunoglobulin (ATG).

18. What precautions should be taken when starting ATG?

19. How should the dose be calculated?

20. How should ATG be administered?

21. How does ATG differ from anti-lymphocyte immunoglobulin (ALG)?

22. Should the doses of his other immunosuppressants be adjusted during ATG therapy?

Day 25 A subclavian line was inserted and a ten-day course of ATG started. Initially 10×25 mg vials were administered.

Day 26 WBC 4.2×10^9/L 10 vials ATG given
Day 27 WBC 1.2×10^9/L dose omitted
Day 28 WBC 2.5×10^9/L 2 vials ATG given
Day 29 WBC 2.2×10^9/L 2 vials ATG given
Day 30 WBC 2.6×10^9/L 2 vials ATG given
Day 31 WBC 3.3×10^9/L 4 vials ATG given
Day 32 WBC 3.0×10^9/L 6 vials ATG given
Day 33 WBC 2.2×10^9/L 2 vials ATG given
Day 34 WBC 2.7×10^9/L 4 vials ATG given

Day 35 Mr O had markedly improved and a DTPA scan showed increased renal perfusion.

His serum biochemistry and haematology results were

Creatinine 268 micromol/L (60–120)
WBC 3.1×10^9/L (4.0–10.0×10^9)
Cyclosporin 73 nanogram/mL (100–120)

The cyclosporin dose was increased and azathioprine therapy was restarted at a dose of 25 mg each day. Mr O continued to improve over the next week.

Day 42 Mr O was discharged on the following medication:

Cyclosporin 200 mg orally twice daily
Azathioprine 25 mg orally daily
Prednisolone 17.5 mg orally each morning
Ranitidine 150 mg orally twice daily
Amphotericin lozenges, one to be sucked four times
 each day.

23. How long should Mr O remain on immunosuppressants?

24. How long is Mr O likely to require ranitidine and amphotericin therapy?

25. What points would you cover when counselling Mr O about his medication?

Answers

1. (a) Cyclosporin 150 mg: in 250 mL dextrose 5% over 30 minutes.

Cyclosporin for injection should be diluted at least one in 20, i.e. the minimum volume for 150 mg (3 mL) is 60 mL. An alternative diluent is 0.9% sodium chloride, but dextrose 5% is preferable in a renal patient such as Mr O because sodium intake is usually restricted to minimise sodium and fluid overload. The manufacturer's data sheet recommends administration over two to six hours, but there is rarely sufficient time for this with cadaveric transplants. Faster infusion rates are associated with a higher incidence of nausea and vomiting. Mr O should be observed throughout the infusion as cyclosporin contains polyethoxylated castor oil, which has been reported to cause anaphylactoid reactions.

(b) Azathioprine 50 mg: as a slow bolus over at least one minute.

Injectable azathioprine is a very alkaline and irritant solution, and therefore the line should be flushed with 50 mL 0.9% sodium chloride or dextrose/saline after administration.

(c) Netilmicin 100 mg: as a slow bolus over three to five minutes.

(d) Methylprednisolone 1 g: in 100 mL dextrose 5% infused over at least 30 minutes.

The reconstituted solution may also be diluted with 0.9% sodium chloride or dextrose/saline. It must be given slowly to minimise the cardiac arrhythmias, circulatory collapse and cardiac arrests associated with rapid infusions.

2. (a) Maintain good renal perfusion, by using dopamine if the urine output is less than 50 mL/hr, and ensure Mr O is volume-replete.
(b) Control any post-operative hypertension. This will reduce the risk of fitting and/or renal damage.
(c) Treat any systemic vasoconstriction using vasodilators.
(d) Maintain adequate immunosuppression to prevent rejection.
(e) Avoid infection.

3. Mr O should receive combined immunosuppressive therapy with azathioprine, corticosteroids and cyclosporin.

Rejection occurs when Mr O's grafted kidney is recognised as "foreign" and is attacked by his immune system. On recognition of the "foreign" tissue, the T-lymphocytes differentiate in his lymph nodes into T-helpers (lymphocytes that provide information to B-lymphocytes about the antigens), T-killers (cytotoxic lymphocytes that cause direct damage to "foreign" cells), and T-suppressors (which suppress B-lymphocytes and prevent multiplication and antibody formation). Sensitised lymphocytes return to the graft site in large numbers, reacting with the antigenic material and releasing lymphokines ("messenger" substances), which attract macrophages to the site. These, together with T-killer cells, destroy the grafted kidney.

Immunosuppression either reduces to ineffective numbers the number of cells reacting against the transplanted organ, or inhibits their normal function. Prophylactic regimens against rejection vary between transplant centres. The main immunosuppressants used are azathioprine, prednisolone, cyclosporin, polyclonal antibodies (such as ATG), and monoclonal antibodies (such as OKT3). They can be used alone, but are usually prescribed in combination.

(a) Azathioprine. This is metabolised to 6-mercaptopurine, which disrupts purine metabolism and consequently interferes with DNA synthesis and cell proliferation, thereby reducing lymphocyte function.

(b) Corticosteroids. These have several possible mechanisms of action, for example, anti-inflammatory activity, blocking production of interleukins 1 and 2 (lymphokines), and causing sequestration of circulating lymphocytes and monocytes in lymphoid tissue, particularly the bone marrow. Adverse effects are commonly encountered, and include Cushingoid appearance, hypertension, hyperglycaemia, weight gain, increased susceptibility to infection, and personality changes.

(c) Cyclosporin. This appears to act primarily by blocking, in T-lymphocytes, the production of interleukin 2 through inhibition of its messenger RNA. It also inhibits T-lymphocyte activity (mainly of T-helpers). Unlike azathioprine it is not myelosuppressive. Cyclosporin has been used as a single agent at oral doses of 14–18 mg/kg/day for one to two weeks, and then tapered to 6–8 mg/kg/day over several months. Some workers advocate lower starting doses (approximately 10 mg/kg/day) to minimise the potential for nephrotoxicity. Individual patient handling of cyclosporin is very variable and doses must be tailored, based on measured serum levels.

(d) Monoclonal antibodies. Numerous types are

becoming available, each with differing specificities to dendritic cells (cells that activate T-helpers).

(e) Polyclonal antibodies. These remove circulating T-lymphocytes and block their formation and proliferation in response to antigenic stimuli.

Monoclonals and polyclonals are very expensive, and their use tends to be reserved for prophylaxis from day 1 in sensitised recipients or in second or subsequent transplants.

Combining immunosuppressants provides a synergistic effect, allows lower doses of each agent, and a lower incidence of toxicity and rejection. The traditional combination is azathioprine and prednisolone. When used as single therapy, each agent rarely provides sufficient immunosuppression. In combination with corticosteroids, azathioprine may be used in an initial pre-transplantation dose of 3–5 mg/kg/day and then a maintenance dose of 1–2 mg/kg/day. Maintenance doses must be sharply reduced or discontinued in the presence of severe infection, malignancy or WBC counts less than 4×10^9/L. Methylprednisolone 1 g is usually given on the cadaveric transplant day; oral prednisolone (or the equivalent as intravenous methylprednisolone) is then started, initially at 0.5–2 mg/kg/day, and then tapered over several months to a maintenance dose of 100–200 microgram/kg/day.

The addition of cyclosporin to this combination has provided encouraging results, with reduced incidence of infection; although one small controlled study using cyclosporin 8 mg/kg, azathioprine 1.5 mg/kg and prednisolone 300 microgram/kg daily demonstrated increased mortality due to infection. This study was, however, criticised for using an azathioprine dose that was too high.

The manufacturer's data sheet cautions against the use of cyclosporin with other immunosuppressants, with the exception of corticosteroids, as this strategy is thought to increase the risk of oversuppression, possibly by increasing the risk of lymphoma development. In practice, "triple therapy" is frequently used for the reasons outlined above, and is recommended for Mr O. Post-operatively, our centre currently uses cyclosporin 5 mg/kg/day intravenously (10 mg/kg/day orally), azathioprine 1 mg/kg/day intravenously, and methylprednisolone 250 microgram/kg/day intravenously. Some transplant centres avoid cyclosporin until post-operative diuresis has begun, whereas others start pre-operatively.

4. By regular monitoring of cyclosporin serum levels, serum glucose levels and liver function tests, and by regular blood pressure measurement.

(a) Cyclosporin serum level monitoring.

(i) Trough levels should be taken before the morning dose every two to three days until therapy is stabilised, then monthly. A diurnal variation in cyclosporin clearance occurs, and therefore sampling should be at a fixed time each day. Times to achieve peak levels are variable (one to eight hours after oral dosing); trough levels provide more consistent results.

The risk of rejection is greatest shortly after transplant and pathophysiological changes occur rapidly. The half-life of cyclosporin has been reported to be six to 40 hours, and hence two to three days is the time normally required to achieve steady-state concentrations. Monitoring is required initially every two to three days until therapy is stabilised, and two to three days after any dosing change.

(ii) Whole blood, plasma or serum samples may be used but quoted therapeutic ranges differ, depending on the sample type and the assay method. Cyclosporin in blood distributes between erythrocytes (50%) leucocytes (10%) and plasma (40%). Concentrations measured in whole blood may be up to twice that in plasma. Distribution is temperature-dependent, increased temperature resulting in increased plasma concentrations. If plasma samples are used, the temperature must be kept at 37°C during separation from the blood.

Two main assay methods are available. Radioimmunoassay (RIA) uses an antibody that cross-reacts with a number of cyclosporin metabolites, and therefore tends to overestimate cyclosporin levels. High-performance liquid chromatography (HPLC) tends to be more laborious, requiring extractions, but gives more accurate measurements of the parent compound. Levels determined by RIA are usually two to three times those determined by HPLC.

(iii) Samples should be drawn from a separate line from that used for cyclosporin administration. Cyclosporin may bind to the catheter material despite flushing with standard intravenous fluids. Studies have demonstrated that it can be easily displaced when blood is drawn back up the catheter.

(b) Liver function tests.

Reversible dose-related hepatotoxicity may be induced by cyclosporin therapy. This may result in increases in serum bilirubin and liver enzymes.

(c) Serum glucose levels.

Hyperglycaemia may develop as a result of cyclosporin therapy or concomitant corticosteroid therapy.

(d) Blood pressure monitoring.

Hypertension is frequently observed and has been associated with seizures. It is not generally dose-related.

5. Haematology and liver function.

Full blood counts, including platelets, should be carried out at least weekly for the first two months, and then less frequently. Azathioprine causes dose-related, reversible bone marrow suppression, which is usually seen early in therapy, but can develop on long-term treatment.

Liver function tests should also be performed, as cholestatic and/or reversible dose-related hepatotoxicity can develop.

6. Initially, ranitidine 50 mg intravenously three times daily, changing to 150 mg orally twice daily when Mr O is able to take oral medication.

Ranitidine is excreted via the kidneys and the dosage is usually halved if the glomerular filtration rate (GFR) is less than 10 mL/min. Mr O has a high serum creatinine, but it is lower than pre-transplant. Most of the equations available to estimate the creatinine clearance from the serum creatinine are inaccurate if there are acute changes in renal function. Accepting these inaccuracies, an estimated GFR for Mr O is between 10 and 15 mL/min. Future serum creatinine results should be monitored to check renal function is continuing to improve.

7. Prednisolone 17.5 mg orally each morning, azathioprine 50 mg orally each morning, and cyclosporin 300 mg orally twice daily.

Oral absorption of prednisolone is "normal" in renal transplant patients. Methylprednisolone and prednisolone differ in anti-inflammatory potency: 5 mg prednisolone is equivalent to 4 mg methylprednisolone, therefore 18.75 mg prednisolone is equivalent to 15 mg methylprednisolone.

Azathioprine oral absorption is variable in renal transplant patients, but generally the same dose is given orally as intravenously.

Oral absorption of cyclosporin is slow, variable and incomplete. One study of adult renal transplant patients demonstrated a mean bioavailability of $28\% \pm 20\%$. Therefore the oral dose of cyclosporin is two to three times the intravenous dose. Mr O's last measured cyclosporin level was high and therefore he should be given twice the intravenous dose orally, and levels measured after two days.

8. Yes.

Renal patients often have high renin profiles resulting in systemic vasoconstriction and hypertension. Vasoconstriction may also be catecholamine-mediated. Vasodilators are probably the most appropriate method of reducing the blood pressure acutely.

Nifedipine is a vasodilator and does not require dosage adjustment in renal failure. For a quicker onset of action, it can be taken sublingually by biting the capsule and holding the liquid contents in the mouth.

Intravenous antihypertensives such as hydralazine and labetolol are usually reserved for more severe hypertension. Overzealous treatment of hypertension could produce further renal impairment by reducing renal perfusion.

9. To mask the taste, Mr O could dilute the oral cyclosporin solution with milk, chocolate drink or fruit juice immediately before taking the dose. Cyclosporin is also marketed in 25 mg and 100 mg capsules, which may be a convenient, but more expensive, alternative to the liquid.

10. Methylprednisolone 1 g intravenously in 100 mL 5% dextrose administered over 60 minutes each day for three days.

Acute rejection is most often seen 5–10 days post transplant.

The four agents most commonly used to treat acute rejection are: Methylprednisolone, monoclonal antibodies, polyclonal antibodies, and radiotherapy.

(a) Methylprednisolone. This is the cheapest alternative and has been demonstrated to reverse 72–83% of first allograft rejections.

(b) Monoclonal and polyclonal antibodies. These are very expensive and their use tends to be reserved for:

(i) Second or subsequent rejection episodes

(ii) Severe acute rejection not responsive to intravenous methylprednisolone.

(c) Radiotherapy. This is indicated if the kidney is hard and severely swollen, or possibly on third and subsequent rejection episodes.

Methylprednisolone 1 g/day for one to five days (usually three days) is thus the preferred option for Mr O.'s first rejection episode.

11. Corticosteroid, azathioprine and cyclosporin therapy all increase Mr O.'s susceptibility to infection.

12. Any infection.

Mr O. could develop fungal (eg. opportunistic infections with *Candida, Aspergillus*), protozoal, viral (eg. cytomegalovirus, herpes) or common or uncommon bacterial infections.

13. Co-trimoxazole seven 480 mg tablets twice each day for three days, then four 480 mg tablets twice each day.

For *Pneumocystis carinii* infection the dose is 120 mg co-trimoxazole (20 mg trimethoprim and 100 mg sulphamethoxazole)/kg/day intravenously or orally. This dosage regimen must be reduced in renal impairment.

Estimating Mr O's creatinine clearance accurately is beset by the same problems as before, although his serum creatinine results appear more stable (i.e., on day 8 his serum creatinine level was 280 micromol/L, while on day 11 it was 274 micromol/L).

Using the Cockcroft and Gault formula, Mr O's creatinine clearance is estimated to be 25 mL/min. For patients with this level of renal function, the manufacturer's data sheet recommends using a standard co-trimoxazole dosage for three days, and then half the standard dosage. If required, the adult suspension can be used to allow the standard dosage to be halved more accurately.

14. Erythromycin and co-trimoxazole co-administration.

Acute reversible nephrotoxicity has been associated with cyclosporin levels greater than 200 nanogram/mL. Mr O's cyclosporin levels may have been increased by concurrent erythromycin therapy. Studies in healthy adults suggest that erythromycin can substantially reduce the plasma clearance of cyclosporin, possibly by inhibiting drug metabolism, although the exact mechanism remains to be determined. The trimethoprim component of co-trimoxazole is also potentially nephrotoxic, and concurrent use of trimethoprim and cyclosporin can accentuate cyclosporin nephrotoxicity.

It is also worth noting that it is most unlikely that the administration of intravenous frusemide 40 mg worsened Mr O's established cyclosporin nephrotoxicity. Only diuretic doses large enough to cause a marked hypovolaemia would be likely to have such an adverse effect.

15. (a) Drugs reported to increase the nephrotoxicity of cyclosporin include: acyclovir, aminoglycosides, amphotericin (systemically), co-trimoxazole, melphalan, frusemide (and other potent diuretics), cephalosporins, and indomethacin.

(b) Drugs reported to *increase* cyclosporin levels, possibly by inhibition of metabolism, include: erythromycin, ketoconazole, methylprednisolone, oral contraceptives, and diltiazem.

(c) Drugs reported to *decrease* cyclosporin levels, possibly by induction of metabolism, include phenytoin, phenobarbitone, rifampicin, co-trimoxazole, and isoniazid.

16. Cyclosporin nephrotoxicity is difficult to differentiate from organ rejection. Differentiation is necessary to determine whether an increased dose of immunosuppressants or a decreased cyclosporin dose is appropriate.

Rejection is usually associated with fever, low urine output, a rapidly rising serum creatinine level, graft tenderness or enlargement, and DTPA scans that show reduced renal perfusion. Cyclosporin levels are usually low (less than 100 nanogram/mL), and on further reduction of the dose there is either no change or a worsening of renal function.

Cyclosporin toxicity is usually associated with an afebrile patient, low urine output, slowly or rapidly increasing serum creatinine levels, non-tender grafts, and DTPA scans that show reduced renal perfusion. Cyclosporin levels are usually high (greater than 200 nanogram/mL) and reduction of the cyclosporin dose improves renal function.

The differentiation of the two is, however, often unclear, and histological examination is often required. This may reveal renal tubular atrophy in the case of cyclosporin toxicity. The mechanism of cyclosporin nephrotoxicity is unclear, but it has been proposed that the drug reduces renal perfusion by interfering with renal prostaglandin release. Animal studies have suggested that co-administered synthetic prostaglandins, such as misoprostol, may protect against cyclosporin nephrotoxicity, although this has still to be substantiated in man.

17. Omit the next dose, then reduce the cyclosporin to 200 mg orally twice daily.

Cyclosporin kinetics are complex. The drug has numerous (at least 25) metabolites, and little is known about their contribution to cyclosporin's activity or its adverse effects. Additionally, rapid physiological changes in the patient may hinder calculation of his pharmacokinetic parameters. Therefore, dosage adjustment tends to be empirical rather than a result of calculation, with the aim of achieving a trough concentration within the therapeutic range.

In a case of cyclosporin toxicity such as Mr O's, doses of cyclosporin would ideally be withheld until levels were back within the therapeutic range, and the maintenance dose would then be reduced. During this time, additional immunosuppression (such as increased doses of prednisolone or azathioprine) may be required. However, in practice (because of delays in obtaining cyclosporin level results), the next dose is usually omitted, and a new maintenance dose initiated, which is subsequently adjusted on the basis of reported serum levels.

18. (a) Carry out a scratch skin test with ATG (not intra- or sub-dermal) to check Mr O's tolerance, as ATG has been associated with anaphylaxis.

(b) Ensure adrenaline, hydrocortisone and chlorpheniramine are available during administration of the first dose, and ready for use if required urgently.

(c) Administer ATG via a large vein, such as a central line, to avoid thrombophlebitis.

19. At the time of writing the initial treatment dosage regimen is one to two 25 mg vials per 10 kg of body weight per day. The usual course length is ten days. Each subsequent day's dosage is determined by monitoring the WBC count and aiming to maintain the count in the range 2.0–4.0×10^9/L.

Platelets should also be monitored, and any thrombocytopenia below 50,000/mm^3 will require interruption of treatment.

20. Each 25 mg vial should be diluted in 50 mL 0.9% sodium chloride; but, in practice, on the prescriber's responsibility, a higher concentration (e.g. 1 mg/mL) is administered, so that the sodium and fluid load is not too great for the patient. The infusion is usually administered over 8–12 hours via a large vein. Any associated fever or shivering may be relieved by administering chlorpheniramine or hydrocortisone intravenously, one hour prior to the infusion.

21. ALG and ATG primarily differ in the animal used for their production. The name ATG is usually reserved for the substance produced in rabbits, and ALG for that produced in horses.

Both are prepared by hyperimmunisation of the respective animals with human T-cell lymphocytes. The immunoglobulins produced are purified and concentrated. The choice of agent depends on the patient's ability to tolerate horse or rabbit proteins. Generally, there is a higher incidence of adverse reactions to horse-derived products. Extreme caution should be taken if the patient has had ALG or any other horse serum on a previous occasion.

22. Mr O's azathioprine therapy should be stopped whilst the ATG course is in progress. Both drugs are myelosuppressive, and concurrent use may cause a marked leucopenia necessitating the withdrawal of the ATG. The prednisolone and cyclosporin doses should initially be unchanged; however, three days before the end of the ATG course, the prednisolone dose should be doubled, as practice has shown episodes of rapid rejection can occur on stopping ATG.

Immediately the ATG course finishes, the azathioprine should be re-started at the pre-ATG dose, and the prednisolone therapy reduced over three or four days to the maintenance dose of 17.5 mg each morning. The cyclosporin should remain at the same dose, provided serum level monitoring indicates that this is still appropriate.

23. Immunosuppressive therapy can rarely be stopped completely after transplant. Even the briefest cessation may precipitate rejection. Intensive immunosuppression is, however, usually only required for the first few weeks post-transplant, or during a rejection crisis. Subsequently, the graft may often be maintained on relatively small doses of immunosuppressive drugs, and hence fewer adverse drug effects are experienced.

Some authors favour switching from "triple therapy" to azathioprine plus corticosteroids. This usually results in lower serum creatinine levels, but may also result in a higher incidence of acute rejection episodes or infection.

The dosage of Mr O's immunosuppressants should be reduced as follows:

(a) Prednisolone. Mr O should be maintained on approximately 300 microgram/kg/day for the first six months, then gradually reduced to 150 micrograms/kg/day.

(b) Azathioprine. The dosage should usually be modified in the light of the WBC count, which should not be allowed to fall below 4×10^9/L.

(c) Cyclosporin. Serum levels of 50–75 nanogram/mL should be aimed for within the first year, and levels of 50 nanogram/mL after one year (an approximate dose of 2–4 mg/kg/day).

24. Ranitidine therapy is likely to continue while Mr O remains on prednisolone, but can probably be reduced to a maintenance dose of 150 mg at night as his condition stabilises. Amphotericin may be required as long as Mr O receives immunosuppressive therapy, but in practice is likely to be stopped shortly after discharge, and restarted only if his oral candidiasis recurs.

25. (a) Azathioprine:

(i) Take after food to minimise gastro-intestinal adverse effects.

(ii) Report any unusual bleeding or bruising, as this could indicate bone marrow depression.

(b) Cyclosporin:

(i) If possible, take before meals or on an empty stomach, as food has been shown to have variable effects on absorption, both increasing and decreasing it. The effect observed may depend on the diet composition, as cyclosporin is a lipid-soluble drug.
(ii) Maintain good oral hygiene, removing plaque, as cyclosporin may cause gum hyperplasia. Good oral hygiene will also help prevent opportunistic oral infections such as *Candida*.

(c) Prednisolone:

(i) Take the dose at approximately the same time each day, preferably in the morning in order to mimic diurnal production of endogenous steroids.
(ii) Always carry a steroid card. It must also be ensured that Mr O understands the written instructions on the card.

(d) Ranitidine:

(i) Take one dose in the morning and the second dose at night, with food if supper is eaten.

(e) Amphotericin lozenges:

(i) Take at regular intervals throughout the day.
(ii) Suck the lozenges slowly.
(iii) If taken near to meal times, suck after meals rather than before.

(f) General:

(i) Do not discontinue any of the medication unless advised so by the doctor.
(ii) Keep all medication out of the reach of children.

(iii) Report to the doctor any signs of infection, including sore throats.

Acknowledgement

I am grateful to Dr J. E. Scoble, Senior Registrar, Renal Unit, Royal Free Hospital, for his assistance in the preparation of this case study.

References and Further Reading

Anon., Cyclosporin for ever?, *Lancet*, 1986, **1**, 419–420.

Bryson S.M., Monitoring cyclosporin therapy, *Pharm. J.*, 1988, **241**, 42–43.

Calne R.Y., Cyclosporin in cadaveric renal transplantation: 5-year follow-up of a multicentre trial, *Lancet*, 1987, **2**, 506–507.

Canafax D.M. and Draxler C.A., Renal transplantation, in *Applied Therapeutics—the Clinical Use of Drugs*, 4th edn, Young L.Y. and Koda-Kimble M.A. (eds), Vancouver, WA, Applied Therapeutics, 1988, 529–544.

Hiesse C. *et al.*, Safety of triple immunosuppressive treatment (cyclosporin, azathioprine and prednisolone), *Lancet*, 1985, **2**, 1355.

Morris P.J. *et al.*, Cyclosporin conversion versus conventional immunosuppression; long-term follow-up and histological evaluation, *ibid.* 1987, **1**, 586–591.

Ptachcinski R.J. *et al.*, Clinical pharmacokinetics of cyclosporin, *Clin. Pharmacokinet.*, 1986, **11**, 107–132.

Rodighiero V., Therapeutic drug monitoring of cyclosporin—practical applications and limitations, *ibid.*, 1989, **16**, 27–37.

Salaman J.R. and Griffin P.J.A., Immunosuppression with a combination of cyclosporin, azathioprine, and prednisolone may be unsafe, *Lancet*, 1985, **2**, 1066–1067.

Slapak M. and Digard N., Safety of triple immunosuppressive treatment (cyclosporin, azathioprine, and prednisolone), *ibid.*, 1355.

Taube D.H. *et al.*, Differentiation between allograft rejection and cyclosporin nephrotoxicity in renal-transplant recipients, *ibid.*, 171–174.

Venkataramanan R. *et al.*, Clinical pharmacokinetics in organ transplant patients, *Clin. Pharmacokinet.*, 1989, **16**, 134–161

DUODENAL ULCER

Linda J. Dodds

Principal Pharmacist (Clinical Trainer), Kent and Canterbury Hospital, Canterbury

Day 1 Fifty-three-year-old Mr T was admitted from casualty. He had a three-day history of stomach pains and nausea. During the past few hours his symptoms had worsened considerably and he had vomited material that resembled coffee grounds. He had also passed several loose, black and tarry stools but he had not had frank diarrhoea or seen fresh blood.

He described his pain as gnawing and generalised over his abdomen, but said it did not appear to relate to food ingestion. He added that he had had similar, but less severe, bouts of stomach pain several times in the past few months, but all had resolved spontaneously. He had thought his symptoms on this occasion were the result of food poisoning and he had been taking kaolin and morphine mixture.

His regular drug therapy was atenolol 50 mg, which he had been taking once daily for three years to control hypertension, and temazepam 10 mg at night when required. He had also recently been prescribed a course of "painkillers" by his general practitioner for a sprained knee.

Mr T admitted to smoking about 20 cigarettes a day and drinking about 20 units of alcohol a week, mostly in connection with his job as a sales representative.

On examination he was found to be pale, sweating, shocked and hypotensive (blood pressure 120/60 mmHg) with a pulse rate of 105 beats per minute. His stools were positive for occult blood and his abdomen was tender. An emergency endoscopy revealed a duodenal ulcer adjacent to the antral mucosa. The ulcer was no longer bleeding and had not perforated.

His serum biochemistry and haematology results were:

Sodium 135 mmol/L (reference range 137–150)
Potassium 3.8 mmol/L (3.5–5.0)
Urea 7.2 mmol/L (2.5–6.6)
Creatinine 93 micromol/L (80–150)

Haemoglobin 9.7 g/dL (14–18)
Haematocrit 0.31 (0.36–0.46)
Liver function tests within normal limits

Three units of whole blood were ordered, and an intravenous line was set up with one litre of normal saline to run until cross-matching was complete. Mr T was designated "nil by mouth" and half-hourly observations were started. He was written up for ranitidine 50 mg intravenously three times daily; and metoclopramide 10 mg intravenously at once, then 10 mg every eight hours if required.

1. What are the therapeutic aims for Mr T?

2. Does the therapy ordered meet these aims satisfactorily?

3. Would you recommend concurrent antibiotic therapy?

4. Should analgesia be written up for Mr T?

5. What factors may have contributed to Mr T suffering from a duodenal ulcer?

6. What information will you be particularly interested in when you take a medication history from Mr T?

Day 2 Mr T was no longer vomiting. His haemoglobin was 12.2 g/dL and he was feeling and looking much better. There was no evidence of rebleeding. His intravenous line was kept open with dextrose/saline and one further unit of whole blood was ordered.

Serum biochemistry results were:

Sodium 130 mmol/L (135–150)
Potassium 4.8 mmol/L (3.5–5.0)
Urea 6.5 mmol/L (2.5–6.6)
Creatinine 110 micromol/L (80–150)

The medication history taken by the pharmacist established that the "painkillers" prescribed for Mr T were ibuprofen 400 mg three times daily. He had taken them regularly for one week, but for the past ten days had been taking them only when necessary (usually at night). He had not been taking any other over-the-counter drugs that may have contributed to his admission, although he did admit to suffering from frequent headaches, which he usually treated with 1.0–1.5 g paracetamol.

The team treating Mr T decided to prescribe a course of oral H_2-receptor blocker therapy.

7. Which H_2-receptor blocker do you recommend and at what dose?

8. Do you agree that an H_2-receptor blocker is the ulcer-healing agent of choice for Mr T?

9. How long should H_2-receptor blocker therapy be continued?

10. Does Mr T need any other therapy written up?

11. What do Mr T's serum biochemistry results indicate?

12. What action should be taken in the light of these results?

13. Could Mr T's short history of ibuprofen ingestion have contributed to his admission?

Day 3 Mr T continued to improve. His intravenous line was discontinued and his fluid input was limited to output plus 300 mL.

Serum biochemistry results were:

Sodium 131 mmol/L (135–150)
Potassium 4.5 mmol/L (3.5–5.0)
Urea 3.2 mmol/L (2.5–6.6)
Creatinine 98 micromol/L (80–150)

Day 4 Mr T continued to improve. His urea and electrolyte results were all within normal limits and he was allowed free fluids and a semi-liquid diet.

Day 6 Mr T was ready for discharge. His blood pressure was 150/105 mmHg and it was decided to re-start antihypertensive therapy. His haemoglobin was 13.5 g/dL. In view of his history, it was also decided to prescribe a course of iron therapy.

14. Can his previous antihypertensive therapy be re-prescribed?

15. Which iron preparation do you recommend, and at what dose? For how long should treatment continue?

Day 8 Mr T was discharged with seven days' supply of the following:

Cimetidine 800 mg at night
Maalox® 15 mL when required
Atenolol 50 mg each morning
Ferrous sulphate 200 mg twice daily

16. What points would you cover when counselling Mr T on his discharge medications?

Month 4 Mr T had re-presented to his general practitioner complaining of symptoms of pain between meals and at night, two months after completing an eight-week course of cimetidine. Endoscopy revealed a new ulcer crater. This time the biopsy findings on a sample of his gastric mucosa reported histological signs of chronic active gastritis. On questioning, Mr T admitted he was still smoking about 20 cigarettes daily and drinking 10–20 units of alcohol per week. He was, however, avoiding foods that caused indigestion.

17. Is such rapid relapse common?

18. Is there any difference in relapse rates following healing with the different ulcer-healing agents?

19. Which ulcer-healing regimen would you recommend this time?

Month 6 Ulcer healing was confirmed endoscopically and a biopsy of Mr T's gastric mucosa showed no signs of chronic gastritis. In view of his history it was decided to prescribe maintenance anti-ulcer therapy.

20. Which agent do you recommend and for how long should it be prescribed?

Answers

1. (a) Treat shock;
   (b) relieve nausea and vomiting;
   (c) prevent ulcer rebleeding; and
   (d) initiate ulcer healing.

2. Yes.

(a) Shock. Mr T urgently requires plasma expanders, preferably whole blood, as he has lost a lot of blood. His low haemoglobin with haemodilution not yet complete, and low haematocrit, indicate probable chronic blood loss. Sodium chloride 0.9% is an appropriate interim intravenous fluid as vomiting depletes sodium and chloride ions. Additions of potassium are not advisable, as the whole blood ordered may contain large amounts of this ion from lysed cells.

(b) Nausea and vomiting. Furthur vomiting must be avoided, both to ensure Mr T's comfort and to prevent furthur fluid loss. Persistent vomiting may also precipitate rebleeding. Metoclopramide is an effective anti-emetic for this indication; it increases gastric emptying and also acts centrally at the chemoreceptor trigger zone to relieve vomiting.

(c) Ulcer rebleeding. No agent has been shown conclusively to prevent ulcer rebleeding. The evidence for ranitidine's effectiveness is equivocal from small studies. Large multicentre studies have indicated that cimetidine does not have this property. Tranexamic acid has been evaluated and may reduce mortality in the elderly, but again does not appear to actually prevent rebleeding episodes, when compared with placebo and cimetidine.

(d) Ulcer healing. As Mr T has been vomiting, intravenous therapy is preferable. Only cimetidine and ranitidine are available as intravenous formulations at present. Ulcer-healing rates are similar for both drugs, but as ranitidine has the advantage discussed in (c) it is an appropriate choice for Mr T. Each dose should be diluted to 20 mL with normal saline and administered as a slow intravenous bolus over two minutes.

3. No. On present data, antibiotic therapy is warranted:

   (a) if the ulcer perforates,
   (b) in response to clear signs of infection, or
   (c) (controversial) to eradicate the Gram-negative spiral bacterium *Helicobacter pylori*.

Mr T's ulcer has not perforated and he does not have clinical signs of infection, therefore (c) would be the only reason to initiate antibiotic therapy.

Helicobacter pylori colonises the mucus-secreting epithelial cells of the stomach, and, although non-invasive, produces the characteristic cytopathic changes that constitute the lesion of "chronic active gastritis" (CAG). The aetiological role of the organism in peptic ulcer disease is still open to speculation. Some studies have shown that about 90% of patients with duodenal ulcer (DU) have CAG. It has been hypothesised that the organism may colonise the islands of metaplastic gastric epithelium that are found in the duodenum, and somehow weaken the mechanisms that usually protect the duodenal cells. More recently, it has been proposed that the presence of *H. pylori* in the gastric antrum increases the release of gastrin and is responsible for hypergastrinaemia in patients with DU.

Eradication of the organism with antibiotics has, in small trials, resulted in ulcer healing, although reinfection and relapse appear common. Concurrent antibiotic and ulcer-healing agent therapy is strongly advocated by some clinicians, but others have had less success with using antibiotics, either alone or in combination with ulcer-healing agents, and these strategies are thus still controversial in the absence of proven CAG. Furthermore, it is not yet clear what constitutes an appropriate regimen to eradicate *H. pylori*. The organism appears able to develop resistance *in vivo* to antibiotics that are highly toxic *in vitro*, although it may be that the organism "hides" in the gastric mucosa, thus evading the antibiotic.

As Mr T does not have proven CAG and as there is no clearly effective antibiotic regimen for the eradication of *H. pylori* at the time of writing, antibiotic therapy is not recommended at this stage of his disease.

4. Once Mr T's condition has stabilised he is unlikely to require analgesia, but if he is very restless or anxious an anxiolytic (e.g. lorazepam 1 mg sublingually) is preferable to an opiate, which could induce vomiting and hypotension.

5. (a) Smoking,
   (b) ingestion of agents known to predispose to ulcer formation,
   (c) genetic factors, and
   (d) stress (controversial).

6. (a) The identity of the "painkillers" he has been taking.
   (b) Whether he has a history of ingestion of over-the-counter non-steroidal anti-inflammatory drugs (NSAIDs), or has recently been pres-

cribed corticosteroids or any other drugs known to cause gastro-intestinal ulceration.

(c) Whether he has been taking over-the-counter antacids.

7. Cimetidine 800 mg at 9 p.m. There are four H_2-receptor blockers marketed at present: cimetidine, ranitidine, nizatidine and famotidine. Factors to be taken into account when choosing the most appropriate agent for Mr T are: clinical efficacy (i.e. healing rate, symptom relief, relapse rate), dosage regimen, side-effect profile, the fact that he smokes and takes antihypertensive therapy, and the cost.

(a) Clinical efficacy. There is little to choose between the four agents in terms of clinical efficacy. Symptom relief may be slightly faster with the more potent agents but healing rates appear similar. Recent meta-analysis of pooled data comparing cimetidine (800–1000 mg per day) with ranitidine (200–300 mg per day) concluded that ranitidine had healed significantly more ulcers at four weeks than cimetidine; however, the six-week healing rates of all four H_2-receptor blockers are similar. Relapse rates following healing also appear to be similar.

(b) Dosage regimen. Each of the four agents can be taken as a single evening dose, which may encourage compliance.

(c) Side-effect profile. Cimetidine has anti-androgenic effects, and impotence, gynaecomastia and breast tenderness have been reported to occur as a result of treatment. These side-effects are, however, very rare, and do not usually preclude the agent from being prescribed. Although the other three agents do not have specific anti-androgenic effects, each has been reported to cause reversible impotence.

Histamine exerts positive inotropic effects, mainly via H_2-receptors; thus H_2-receptor blockers may theoretically exert negative inotropic effects. Studies in healthy volunteers have concluded that H_2-receptor blockers can decrease heart rate, and possibly blood pressure at rest and during exercise, in a small segment of the population, although not in the general population. The only agent for which it has been postulated that this property may be clinically relevant is famotidine. Although this effect may actually be beneficial to a hypertensive patient like Mr T, it is probably prudent to avoid famotidine as it is likely that he will need to be restabilised on antihypertensive therapy in the near future.

(d) Interactions with concurrent therapy. There would be no clinically relevant interactions between Mr T's admission medications and any of the H_2-receptor blockers. Cimetidine inhibits the cytochrome P448/450 system and therefore inhibits the metabolism of drugs requiring oxidative pathways, but this would not be relevant to Mr T at present.

(e) Smoking. It has been suggested that, as smoking appears to stimulate nocturnal acid secretion and enhance the rate of relapse, then the more potent H_2-receptor blockers may be preferable for smokers. However, a carefully controlled crossover trial failed to show that smoking interfered with the inhibitory effects of H_2-receptor blockers on gastric secretion, suggesting that smoking primarily affects mucosal defence mechanisms. Thus, Mr T must be advised to stop smoking, but the fact that he smokes does not influence the choice of H_2-receptor blocker at present, although his chance of rapid relapse will increase if he continues to smoke.

From the criteria considered it can be seen that there is little to choose between the four H_2-receptor blockers available, so the final choice of agent can be based on the cost of treatment. At present, cimetidine therapy represents the most cost-effective H_2-receptor blocker available, both to this hospital and to patients in the community. It is therefore appropriate that Mr T is prescribed cimetidine as a single dose, which should be taken in the early evening, after the last food of the day, as studies have shown that administration at this time promotes faster healing.

8. Yes. On present evidence H_2-receptor blocker therapy is the best first-line therapy for Mr T's DU, as the dosage regimen is easy to follow and the healing rates for H_2-receptor blockers are as high or higher than for other ulcer-healing agents.

Bismuth chelate does have some advantages over the H_2-receptor blockers in that:

(a) Relapse rates are approximately 25% lower in the first year after healing with bismuth chelate than with an H_2-receptor blocker. This is true whether the patient is a smoker or a non-smoker.

(b) Bismuth chelate is bactericidal to *H. pylori* and can eradicate proven infection in up to one-third of treated patients. This property has been used to explain the difference in relapse rates after healing with bismuth chelate compared with other agents.

However, bismuth chelate also has disadvantages for Mr T. Firstly, it has a more difficult-to-follow dosage regimen (two tablets twice daily, half-an-hour before meals, with antacids and dairy products to be avoided within half-an-hour of a dose to ensure the chelate does not adhere to these products preferentially over the ulcer crater). It is also recommended that the ingestion of dairy products is kept to the minimum throughout the course of treatment. Secondly, bismuth chelate may cause blackening of the mouth and tongue. Although this is avoidable if the product is not held in the mouth, it would prove an embarrassment to Mr T, who is a salesman, if it did occur. In addition, the advantage of the lower relapse rate does not appear to be maintained beyond one year.

Other options for Mr T are sucralfate, pirenzepine, carbenoxolone, misoprostol and omeprazole. Sucralfate, a mucosal protective, also has a more difficult-to-follow dosage regimen (two tablets twice a day, half-an-hour before meals, with antacids to be avoided within half-an-hour of a dose). Pirenzepine (an anti-muscarinic) has a side-effect profile that is likely to make it unacceptable to Mr T, who has to drive as part of his job – dry mouth [15%], blurred vision and central nervous system effects [5%]. Carbenoxolone (cytoprotective) has a steroid-like structure, and mineralocorticoid effects are noted in up to 66% of patients (sodium and water retention, potassium excretion). It is therefore unacceptable for a patient who requires antihypertensive therapy. Misoprostol, a synthetic analogue of prostaglandin E_1, can cause hypotension. In addition, its principal side-effect of diarrhoea can be troublesome, even when the total dose is given in four aliquots. Finally, clinical trials have demonstrated that omeprazole, a proton pump inhibitor, is at least as effective as the H_2-receptor blockers for treatment of DU, and may in fact induce faster healing; however, lack of clinical experience with the drug, and the concern surrounding the observation that high-dose treatment in rats has induced reversible gastric hypertrophy and, after long-term use, gastric tumours, mean that it cannot be considered as a first-line agent for Mr T.

9. Until ulcer healing is demonstrated endoscopically.

Sixty to ninety per cent of duodenal ulcers are healed by H_2-receptor blockers in four to eight weeks. If Mr T cannot be re-endoscoped, then a treatment length of eight weeks is most appropriate.

10. Antacid therapy.

Although symptomatic relief is good with cimetidine, some patients may require antacids on an "as required" basis for seven to ten days. Mr T should thus be prescribed a low-sodium, balanced antacid (e.g. Maalox® or Mucogel®) to avoid aggravating his hypertension or causing bowel disturbances.

11. Low serum sodium plus rising potassium and

creatinine can signal the onset of acute renal failure. Alternatively, Mr T's low sodium may reflect over-hydration with salt-poor fluids, his rising potassium the effect of whole blood transfusions, and his raised creatinine value (compared with his admission level) merely the ten per cent error that is intrinsic to such measurements. His high normal urea may still reflect the presence of blood in his gastro-intestinal tract.

12. (a) Monitor fluid balance and take appropriate action on the results (e.g. consider fluid restriction if there is evidence of over-hydration, consider prescribing diuretics if he is oliguric).

(b) Monitor urea, creatinine and electrolyte levels regularly. It should, however, be remembered when interpreting future serum creatinine levels that cimetidine therapy can cause a slight rise in serum creatinine. This is probably due to competition between cimetidine and creatinine for excretion at the renal tubule and is of no clinical significance.

(c) Carry out a 24-hour urine collection if acute renal failure appears to be the most likely explanation for the changes noted.

13. Yes. Ibuprofen may have contributed to the development of his ulcer. NSAID use has also been postulated to mask ulcer pain and delay diagnosis.

NSAIDs are postulated to be ulcerogenic by two mechanisms: local irritation, and inhibition of the enzyme cyclo-oxygenase. The latter effect results in the inhibition of prostaglandin production from arachidonic acid. Until recently there was no convincing *in-vivo* evidence that non-aspirin NSAIDs predisposed to peptic ulcer disease; however, a case-control study of patients over 60 years of age admitted with bleeding peptic ulcer showed that the risk of admission for bleeding peptic ulcer was substantially increased for users of non-aspirin NSAIDs. Ibuprofen appears less toxic to the gastric mucosa than other NSAIDs, but between 1969 and 1985, 218 cases of gastro-intestinal haemorrhage or perforation were reported following its use.

14. Yes.

Although an interaction has been reported between cimetidine and beta-blocker therapy, it appears to be confined to beta-blockers that are hepatically metabolised and have a large first-pass effect. For example, elevated propranolol levels and reduced resting pulse rates have been noted after concurrent propranol and cimetidine therapy, although such effects appear to be of little or no clinical significance. The postulated mechanism of the interaction is that the cimetidine reduces hepatic blood flow, probably as a result of an effect on vascular histamine H_2-receptors, and that this results in an increase in the bioavailability of drugs that undergo significant first-pass metabolism. Atenolol is a beta-blocker that is renally excreted. It is not subject to first-pass metabolism and can be re-prescribed for Mr T.

15. Ferrous sulphate 200 mg twice daily for one month.

Before prescribing iron supplements it is essential to confirm that Mr T's low haemoglobin does reflect iron deficiency. This would be confirmed by the findings of a reduced mean cell volume and mean cell haemoglobin, reduced serum iron levels, and increased total iron-binding capacity.

Although Mr T's haemoglobin result is now only just below the normal range for an adult male, his admission haematology indicated that he had probably been bleeding chronically, and his iron stores may now be depleted. A normal adult absorbs about 1 mg (10%) of the elemental iron presented in an average diet, but an anaemic patient will absorb much more. It is usually appropriate to prescribe approximately 120 mg daily of elemental iron as a simple ferrous salt (e.g. ferrous sulphate 200 mg, containing 65 mg elemental iron per tablet) to ensure adequate iron absorption. The dose should be divided to ensure optimal absorption, as iron is actively absorbed in the upper small intestine only. Sustained-release products are not warranted. They are about ten times more expensive than plain ferrous salts, and the fact that they are less likely to cause gastro-intestinal toxicity is related to the fact that they release less iron at the absorbing site, and hence may result in less iron uptake. Iron's gastro-intestinal toxicity is due to a mild astringent effect and appears to be directly proportional to the iron concentration. If ferrous sulphate tablets cause gastro-intestinal discomfort to Mr T, ferrous gluconate (35 mg elemental iron per tablet) may prove to be an acceptable alternative. Therapy for one month should replenish iron stores adequately, provided he has no further bleeds. Longer therapy may incur iron overload, with deposition of the element in the liver.

16.(a) Cimetidine.

(i) This is a course of tablets, which must not be discontinued until told to do so, even if there is total pain relief.

(ii) Take at about 9 p.m., with food if supper is eaten. Do not eat again after the dose is taken.

(b) Maalox®.

(i) May need to be taken until cimetidine is fully effective (usually seven to ten days).

(ii) If buying an alternative over-the-counter product, tell the pharmacist you are taking tablets for hypertension (to ensure that a low-sodium product is recommended).

(c) Atenolol.

(i) Take at the same time each day, preferably after breakfast.

(ii) Do not discontinue unless advised so by the doctor.

(d) Ferrous sulphate.

(i) Take after food.

(ii) This is a month's course of tablets only.

(iii) May make stools look black.

(iv) May alter bowel habits (constipation or diarrhoea). If severe, discuss with your general practitioner and get an alternative preparation prescribed.

(e) General.

(i) Try to stop smoking. This can delay ulcer healing and predispose to relapse.

(ii) Avoid over-the-counter aspirin and aspirin-like drugs for pain relief. Use paracetamol, or check suitability with a pharmacist if an alternative product is desired.

(iii) When buying any over-the-counter product (e.g. for coughs or colds) at a pharmacy, tell the pharmacist that you are taking atenolol and have had a peptic ulcer.

(iv) Avoid foods that cause discomfort, and minimise alcohol consumption as that also can delay ulcer healing.

17. Yes. H_2-receptor blockers can heal ulcers but do not appear to alter the natural history of DU disease, which may last up to 20 years, although it more commonly "burns out" after five to ten years.

Studies have shown that after healing with an H_2-receptor blocker, symptomatic relapse in the first year occurs in about 65% of patients, while asymptomatic relapse occurs in a further 15–20%. Unfortunately, the rate and frequency of relapse in an individual cannot be predicted. Smoking has been clearly demonstrated to enhance the rate of DU recurrence, as well as to slow the rate of healing during treatment, and Mr T must be advised again to stop smoking.

18. Yes. Relapse rates after healing with bismuth chelate are approximately 60% in the first year, compared with about 85% after healing with an H_2-receptor blocker. Relapse rates may also be lower for the other ulcer-healing agents than for the H_2-receptor blockers, but the evidence is less clear.

Suggested mechanisms for the difference in relapse rates after treatment with an H_2-receptor blocker and bismuth chelate include:

(a) Cessation of treatment with an H_2-receptor blocker induces rebound hypersecretion secondary to previous acid suppression, which leads to hypergastrinaemia and an increase in parietal cell mass.

(b) Failure (by mechanism/s unknown) of the duodenal mucosal cell to return to normal after H_2-receptor blocker therapy but not after bismuth chelate therapy.

(c) Bismuth accumulates in the body and continues to be excreted after treatment with bismuth chelate stops. This implies a systemic, and not just a local, effect of bismuth. It also raises the possibility that bismuth encephalopathy could be a consequence of long-term bismuth chelate use. As yet, no cases of encephalopathy have been associated with bismuth chelate.

(d) The fact that bismuth chelate is bactericidal to *H. pylori* and H_2-receptor blockers are not. In one study, *H. pylori* status was found to be a significant predictor of endoscopic relapse. Patients found to be free of the organism after healing with bismuth chelate had only a 27% relapse rate in the first year, compared with 79% in those who were still infected with the organism. These findings have since been reproduced in a prospective double-blind trial of DU relapse after eradication of *H. pylori*. The explanation for these findings may be related to the observation reported in a further study that a fall in post-prandial plasma gastrin response occurs after eradication of *H. pylori*. This, the authors speculated, may eventually lead to a reduction in the number of parietal cells.

19. Bismuth chelate, two tablets twice daily, half-an-hour before food, for 28 days; plus metronidazole 400 mg three times daily for the first two weeks of the course. If re-examination by endoscopy reveals that the ulcer has not healed, and there is still evidence of *H. pylori* infection, repeat the course of bismuth chelate, with the addition of amoxycillin 500 mg four times daily for seven days in the middle of the course.

As Mr T now has proven CAG, and hence *H. pylori* infection, it is appropriate to try and eradicate the organism as well as heal the ulcer, in order to reduce his chance of a further rapid relapse (see answer 18). Bismuth chelate alone will eradicate infection in up to one-third of treated patients. Metronidazole has been demonstrated to be bactericidal *in vivo* to *H. pylori*, and is used in the UK as a cost-effective alternative to tinidazole, the antibiotic used in the early Australian studies to eradicate the organism. As discussed earlier, *H. pylori* can be difficult to eradicate, and amoxycillin therapy has been proposed for patients resistant to tinidazole. Other antibiotics found to eradicate *H. pylori in vivo* include penicillin, erythromycin, tetracycline and furazolidone.

At the time of writing, there is controversy not only over which is the most effective antibiotic to eradicate *H. pylori*, but also over the period over which antibiotics should be prescribed in relation to the ulcer-healing agent. Some clinicians favour prescribing the antibiotic therapy in the middle or at the end of the course of ulcer-healing agent, rather than at the beginning. Further clinical trials are needed to establish the optimal therapy to eradicate *H. pylori* and heal the DU concurrently.

20. Cimetidine 400 mg at 9 p.m. for six months, then review.

Bismuth chelate is not licenced for long-term maintenance treatment because its long-term safety is in doubt. Sucralfate and pirenzepine also do not have product licences for this indication at the time of writing, although both have been used with as much success as the H_2-receptor blockers in clinical trials.

Maintenance treatment with an H_2-receptor blocker can however be offered to Mr T. Most experience has been with cimetidine and ranitidine. In trials, treatment with these drugs, at a dose of half the therapeutic dose (taken at night), reduced cumulative rates of symptomatic relapse to approximately 20% and 50% respectively at one and two years post-healing, compared with about 50% and 80% respectively for those taking placebo. It is, however, worth noting that, in a trial that followed up patients like Mr T whose ulcers had been healed and *H. pylori* eradicated by bismuth chelate and antibiotic therapy, the relapse rate in the 12-month follow-up period was only 21% without any maintenance treatment. It is not yet clear whether H_2-receptor blocker maintenance therapy in such patients will lower this relapse rate furthur. If relapse does occur during maintenance treatment, remission can usually be induced by doubling the dose of drug.

The time to continue maintenance treatment is controversial. There is little good evidence that maintenance treatment alters the natural course of DU disease, and many trials have indicated that a period of maintenance therapy does not influence relapse rate once such treatment is stopped. As maintenance treatment is costly, many clinicians prefer to treat relapses as they occur ("intermittent" treatment), and offer maintenance therapy only while the patient attempts to eradicate ulcerogenic factors in their life-style (e.g. smoking or alcohol consumption). As Mr T is still smoking and drinking to excess, this strategy could be of value to him. Once he has controlled these factors it may be more cost-effective to offer him intermittent treatment. However, if it is decided that maintenance therapy is appropriate for a longer period, studies have indicated that cimetidine 400 mg at night for up to six years is both effective and safe.

Acknowledgement

I would like to thank Dr Andrew Carmichael, Medical Registrar, Kent and Canterbury Hospital, for reviewing this article.

References and Further Reading

Anon., The influence of relapse rate on the choice of duodenal ulcer therapy, *Drug Ther. Bull.*, 1987, **25**, 77–80.

Anon., New H_2 blockers: does more choice help?, *ibid.*, 1988, **26**, 65–66.

Axon A.T.R., *Campylobacter pylori*: what role in gastritis and peptic ulcer?, *Br. med. J.*, 1986, **293**, 772–773.

Coghlan J.G. *et al.*, *Campylobacter pylori* and recurrence of duodenal ulcers – a 12-month follow-up study, *Lancet*, 1987, **2**, 1109–1111.

Crean G.P. and Sherman D.J.C., Diseases of the alimentary tract and pancreas, in *Davidson's Principles and Practice of Medicine*, 15th edn, Macleod J., Edward C. and Bouchier I. (eds), Edinburgh, Churchill Livingstone, 1987, 283–292.

Culshaw M., Peptic ulceration, *Pharm. J.*, 1988, **240**, 821–824.

Hazell S.L. and Lee A., *Campylobacter pylori*, urease, hydrogen ion back diffusion and gastric ulcers, *Lancet*, 1986, **2**, 15–17.

Levi S. *et al.*, Antral *Helicobacter pylori*, hypergastrinaemia, and duodenal ulcers: effect of eradicating the organism. *Br. med. J.*, 1989, **299**, 1504–1505.

Marshall B.J. *et al.*, Prospective double-blind trial of duodenal ulcer relapse after eradication of *Campylobacter pylori*, *Lancet*, 1988, **2**, 1437–1442.

Miller J.P. and Faragher E.B., Relapse of duodenal ulcer: does it matter which drug is used in initial treatment?, *Br. med. J.*, 1986, **293**, 1117–1118.

Stewart Goodwin C., Duodenal ulcer, *Campylobacter pylori* and the "leaking roof" concept, *Lancet*, 1988, **2**, 1467–1469.

Weir D.G., Peptic ulceration, *Br. med. J.*, 1988, **296**, 195–200.

CROHN'S DISEASE

Sandra Ross

Staff Pharmacist (Clinical Education), City Hospital, Nottingham

Day 1 Mr J, a 23-year-old man, presented with a six-month history of diarrhoea, abdominal pain, and anorexia. He had suffered a weight loss of 13 lb during this period. Over the past week he had noticed bright red blood in his stools.

On examination he was found to have left-sided abdominal tenderness and a temperature of 38.5°C. Two fleshy anal skin tags were noted.

Stool cultures were negative. Sigmoidoscopy and rectal biopsy revealed discontinuous inflammatory changes of the mucosa, and aphthous ulceration. Small bowel enema showed no evidence of ileal involvement. A diagnosis of Crohn's disease of the colon and rectum was made.

His serum biochemistry and haematology results were:

Haematocrit 0.32 (reference range 0.36–0.46)
Haemoglobin 9 g/dL (14–18)
Albumin 24 g/L (35–50)
Erythrocyte sedimentation rate (ESR) 70 mm/hour (0–20)
Potassium 3.0 mmol/L (3.5–5.3)
Sodium 136 mmol/L (137–145)
Urea 8.3 mmol/L (2.5–6.6)
Creatinine 88 micromol/L (80–150)

Blood was sent for cross-matching, and intravenous saline with potassium was started. An elemental diet was ordered and Mr J was written up for intravenous hydrocortisone 100 mg three times daily.

1. What are the therapeutic aims for Mr J?

2. What subjective and objective parameters will give an indication that these aims are being met?

3. Has appropriate intravenous therapy been prescribed? Which other serum electrolyte would it be advisable to monitor at this point?

4. What is the rationale for the use of intravenous steroid therapy? Is hydrocortisone the most appropriate steroid for Mr J?

5. What biochemical monitoring should be carried out while Mr J is receiving hydrocortisone?

6. Should an antidiarrhoeal agent such as codeine phosphate be prescribed for Mr J?

7. Why is it important to provide nutritional support?

8. What role does an elemental diet play in remission induction?

9. Would total parenteral nutrition (TPN) be a more effective alternative to the elemental diet?

10. How should Mr J's anaemia be treated?

Day 6 Mr J had shown improvement over the intervening days, and thus after five days' intravenous therapy he was written up for oral steroids (prednisolone 40 mg daily). It was decided on the ward round to prescribe sulphasalazine therapy.

11. What is sulphasalazine's postulated mode of action in inflammatory bowel disease?

12. What factors limit its usefulness in Crohn's disease?

13. Do you agree with the addition of sulphasalazine to Mr J's regimen?

14. What starting dose of sulphasalazine do you recommend for Mr J and why?

15. How should his treatment be monitored biochemically?

16. If he is unable to tolerate sulphasalazine, what alternatives could you recommend?

17. Would you have recommended one of these agents as first-line treatment in preference to sulphasalazine for Mr J?

18. Is there a place for antibiotic therapy in acute Crohn's disease? If so, should an antibiotic be prescribed for Mr J?

Day 14 Mr J was ready for discharge on:

Prednisolone 40 mg daily
Sulphasalazine 1 g twice daily
Ferrous sulphate 200 mg daily.

19. *What points would you cover when counselling Mr J on his discharge medication?*

20. *Will Mr J need dietary advice?*

Day 42 Mr J was seen in the out-patient department with very few signs and symptoms of Crohn's disease remaining.

21. *Should sulphasalazine and/or prednisolone be continued to maintain disease remission?*

Month 44 Mr J had remained in remission for several years, but had now been admitted to hospital with a history of abdominal distension and vomiting. A plain abdominal x-ray revealed extensive dilatation of the colon. Surgical opinion was sought, and subsequently Mr J underwent panproctocolectomy with an ileostomy.

22. *What medical problems might Mr J's ileostomy present him with, and how can these be treated?*

23. *What drugs should be avoided or prescribed with caution in patients with ileostomies and why?*

Month 80 Mr J had again remained reasonably well for several years, although he had had several admissions to hospital with increased output from his ileostomy, which had left him dehydrated. On each occasion, he was given intravenous fluids and settled quickly.

On this admission, Mr J complained of abdominal pain and general malaise in addition to increased ileostomy output. A small bowel enema revealed three short stretches in the ileum of recurrent Crohn's disease.

He was prescribed prednisolone 30 mg daily. He improved over the next few weeks, and so his prednisolone dose was gradually reduced to 2 mg daily; however, he was then readmitted with a three-day history of abdominal pain. His prednisolone dose was thus increased to 40 mg daily, and azathioprine 100 mg daily was added to his regimen.

24. *What is the rationale for prescribing azathioprine?*

25. *What maximum dose of azathioprine would you recommend and why? How should azathioprine therapy be monitored?*

26. *Can azathioprine be used as sole therapy in Crohn's disease?*

Month 85 Mr J had improved on the regimen of prednisolone and azathioprine and so it was decided to reduce his prednisolone by 5 mg every two weeks. However, it proved impossible to drop below a dose of 15 mg prednisolone daily; if the dose was reduced further, the recurrence of symptoms necessitated the re-introduction of full steroid doses to induce remission. This situation occurred several times, so it was decided to try Mr J on cyclosporin therapy.

27. *What is the rationale behind prescribing cyclosporin for Mr J?*

28. *What should be checked before starting cyclosporin therapy?*

Mr J was prescribed cyclosporin 350 mg daily. His azathioprine therapy was stopped and the prednisolone dose reduced.

29. *Were the dosage adjustments made to his other therapies appropriate?*

30. *How should cyclosporin therapy be monitored biochemically?*

31. *What side-effects should be monitored for?*

32. *If Mr J suffers an exacerbation of his disease, how would you recommend his cyclosporin therapy be administered?*

Answers

1. (a) Induce remission of active disease,
   (b) correct fluid and electrolyte imbalances,
   (c) treat anaemia, and
   (d) give nutritional support.

2. (a) Reduction in diarrhoea and abdominal pain,
   (b) weight gain,
   (c) rising serum albumin,
   (d) no rectal blood loss,
   (e) absence of fever,
   (f) reduction in ESR and levels of acute phase proteins, such as C-reactive peptide and orosomucoid (thus indicating a reduction in the inflammatory process),
   (g) rising haemoglobin, and
   (h) normalisation of serum electrolytes.

3. Mr J's intravenous therapy is appropriate, provided it is monitored closely. In addition, it is advisable to monitor his serum magnesium level prior to initiating this therapy.

Blood transfusion is appropriate to compensate for Mr J's prolonged colonic blood loss (low haemoglobin plus low haematocrit). Acute or chronic diarrhoea can cause depletion of sodium, potassium, and chloride, as well as water. The ensuing dehydration will result in a raised blood urea, as in Mr J, but the serum sodium may remain in the normal range because of mixed depletion of sodium and water. Appropriate therapy is isotonic sodium chloride solution: administration of water in the form of glucose 5% solution will further aggravate the reduction in extracellular fluid volume. Potassium should be replaced conservatively, with careful monitoring of serum potassium levels, as Mr J is to receive whole blood (which can contain large amounts of potassium).

Prolonged diarrhoea can also deplete the body of magnesium. A potential added complication in the replacement of potassium is the requirement for the body to be magnesium-replete before this is possible (magnesium being necessary for the functioning of the sodium-potassium pump which maintains the potassium concentration intracellularly). If Mr J is found to be magnesium-deficient, replacement by oral magnesium compounds such as magnesium hydroxide may be inappropriate, as these tend to cause diarrhoea, which would be undesirable for Mr J. Magnesium infusion is the preferred route (e.g. 35–50 mmol of magnesium per litre of normal saline or dextrose over 12–24 hours).

4. Intravenous corticosteroids are the drugs of choice for remission induction in severe attacks of Crohn's disease. Methylprednisolone may have been more appropriate than hydrocortisone for Mr J.

It is standard practice to give five days' intravenous therapy and then to switch to oral prednisolone. Failure to respond after the initial five days may be taken as an indication for surgery.

The glucocorticoid properties of corticosteroids, namely immunosuppression and reduction of inflammation, are important in the therapy of Crohn's disease. The aetiology of the disease is as yet unknown, but there are theories that centre on a role for immunological mechanisms, as well as a role for diet and infective agents.

Studies have shown that absorption of oral corticosteroids is impaired in acutely ill patients like Mr J, so intravenous therapy is appropriate initially, although a corticosteroid with less mineralocorticoid activity than hydrocortisone, such as methylprednisolone, might have been more appropriate. However, the intravenous course he is to receive is short, and any electrolyte problems that may occur should be picked up early by monitoring.

5. Serum sodium and potassium levels, and blood sugar measurements.

The mineralocorticoid properties of hydrocortisone may cause sodium and water retention and potassium depletion. In view of Mr J's diarrhoea-induced hypokalaemia, it is particularly important to monitor his serum potassium level. The glucocorticoid property of hydrocortisone may produce a rise in blood sugar; this parameter should thus be monitored on a four-hourly basis.

6. No. The reduction in gut motility induced by drugs such as codeine phosphate may precipitate a state of toxic megacolon in a patient like Mr J.

Toxic megacolon is a life-threatening complication of Crohn's disease, in which the colon is very dilated. This carries the risk of gut perforation and haemorrhage. Other drugs reducing gut motility, such as anticholinergics, should also be avoided.

7. Nutritional support is required because patients like Mr J are generally malnourished, owing to anorexia and malabsorption.

Mr J's low serum albumin is indicative of malnutrition, although it may also be the result of a protein-losing enteropathy induced by the disease. Both an elemental diet and TPN would provide the high-protein, high-calorie intake (e.g. 0.2–0.3 grams of nitrogen per kg body weight per day, 200 kcal per gram of nitrogen) required to replace nutritional stores.

Anthropometric measurements, such as triceps skinfold thickness, are better indicators of improving nutritional status than serum albumin, which has a long half-life.

8. It rests the large bowel.

An elemental diet is a nutritionally complete liquid enteral feed in which the nitrogen is present as simple amino acids. Some studies claim it is as effective as oral prednisolone in inducing remission in patients with active Crohn's disease. This may be due to the inflamed gut being rested, as the components of the diet are absorbed mainly in the upper small bowel. Another postulated mechanism is that Crohn's patients have an immunological reaction to the passage of large amounts of foreign protein through the damaged gut wall, and the diet would treat this aspect of the disease.

One patient factor worth noting is the unpalatability of these elemental diets: patients find it difficult to persevere with them over the four to six weeks generally required for remission induction. This problem can be circumvented by passing a soft fine-bore nasogastric tube and feeding the patient through this.

9. Not on present evidence.

Bowel rest is again the reason for a possible role for TPN in acute Crohn's disease. It has been suggested that the inflamed intestine might heal more quickly without the passage of food, which causes mechanical trauma and the release of digestive enzymes. However, to date, controlled trials have not produced evidence that TPN can influence the outcome in active Crohn's colitis. TPN is very expensive, invasive and has many potential complications. Further controlled trials are awaited.

10. By further clinical investigations, then ferrous sulphate 200 mg twice daily, if appropriate.

It is most likely that Mr J has iron-deficiency anaemia due to prolonged colonic blood loss (low haemoglobin plus low haematocrit); however, this must be confirmed by a blood film result that gives a microcytic, hypochromic picture with a low serum iron concentration, before treatment is commenced. A macrocytic picture might be produced if there was ileal involvement, owing to malabsorption of vitamin B_{12}. However, Mr J has no evidence of ileal disease.

Mr J has already received blood transfusions. If appropriate these should be followed by iron supplementation on resumption of oral intake. Ferrous

sulphate 200 mg twice daily, for three months after normalisation of the haemoglobin level, is sufficient to replace iron stores in the body. There is no advantage to using a thrice daily dose and this may even increase the gastric intolerance experienced by some patients. Crohn's patients can be particularly intolerant of oral iron and a total dose infusion may be necessary. Slow-release preparations of iron are generally released past the site of absorption of iron in the jejunum and are therefore to be avoided.

11. Sulphasalazine is a conjugate of 5-aminosalicylic acid (5-ASA) and sulphapyridine, linked by an azo bond. The current theory is that the active moiety in inflammatory bowel disease is 5-ASA, an anti-inflammatory salicylate, with the sulphonamide moiety being a carrier to ensure the drug reaches the colon intact.

Sulphasalazine is in fact absorbed in the ileum but is secreted unchanged in the bile to reach the colon intact; the normal gut flora then release enzymes which split the azo bond and release 5-ASA to exert a topical anti-inflammatory action. The sulphapyridine moiety is absorbed in the colon, metabolised, and then excreted in the urine.

In addition, some recent study results suggest that sulphasalazine may possess intrinsic therapeutic activity, i.e. that it may be a drug as well as a pro-drug.

12. The anatomical site of the disease and the drug's adverse effects.

Crohn's disease can affect any part of the gastro-intestinal tract from the mouth to the anus. However, from the previous answer it is obvious that sulphasalazine can only be effective in colonic and, possibly, terminal ileal disease. An exception to this may be in patients with a blind loop and bacterial overgrowth, as sulphasalazine is then split in the small intestine.

The usefulness of sulphasalazine is also limited by its dose-related side-effects and occasional adverse reactions. Dose-related side-effects include headache, nausea, anorexia and haemolysis. Adverse reactions which are not dose-related include fever, rash, hepatic dysfunction, toxic epidermal necrolysis, and the blood dyscrasias, agranulocytosis and thrombocytopenia. Infertility can be produced in males through a decrease in the sperm count and sperm motility, although this resolves completely two months after withdrawal of therapy.

13. Yes.

The combination of sulphasalazine and prednisolone has been shown in a large controlled study to be more effective than either drug alone in remission induction in two groups of patients: those who were previously untreated, and those with colonic disease alone. Mr J fits into both these categories.

14. 500 mg daily, increasing every two to three days until maximum benefit and minimal adverse effects are seen.

The dose usually arrived at is a compromise between effectiveness and minimisation of side-effects, and is generally in the range 2–4 g per day. It is wise to start with smaller doses, such as 500 mg–1 g per day and increase gradually to avoid the dose-related side-effects discussed in answer 12. If these side-effects appear, the drug should be stopped and re-started at a lower dose.

Desensitisation to some of the less serious adverse reactions, such as rash, can be attempted by starting with a very small dose, for example 1 mg, and increasing very gradually. In the event of more serious adverse reactions, such as blood dyscrasias, sulphasalazine therapy should be withdrawn.

15. Liver function tests and full blood counts should be carried out on a regular basis.

16. Mesalazine or olsalazine.

Mesalazine (5-ASA) alone, coated with a resin that remains intact below pH 7 (marketed as Asacol®) allows delivery of 5-ASA to the colon and terminal ileum. This avoids the side-effects attributed to the sulphonamide moiety of sulphasalazine, but some side-effects do occur, mainly gastrointestinal ones, such as abdominal pain, nausea and diarrhoea.

Mesalazine is also available as a slow-release preparation (Pentasa®) on a named-patient basis at the time of writing. Pentasa® comprises granulated 5-ASA, where each granule is coated with a semipermeable membrane of ethylcellulose. The release is only partly pH-dependent; claims that effective treatment is possible throughout the small bowel have not been substantiated to date in controlled trials.

Olsalazine consists of two molecules of 5-ASA linked by an azo bond which requires colonic bacteria to cleave it. Olsalazine is not effective in the terminal ileum, although this would not affect Mr J.

Topical formulations of sulphasalazine and mesalazine are available as enemas, but these can only be of benefit in rectal and distal colonic disease.

17. It would have been more appropriate to start Mr J on mesalazine therapy to avoid any of the serious adverse reactions that may result from sulphasalazine therapy. Also, Mr J may wish to avoid the problem of infertility, which is often caused by sulphasalazine.

As regards the choice between mesalazine and olsalazine, there is little to choose between them in terms of efficacy and side-effects, although as yet unknown side-effects of olsalazine may emerge with its wider use. Mesalazine would therefore seem to be an appropriate first-line treatment for Mr J. An appropriate starting dose is 400 mg three times daily. It should, however, be noted that mesalazine treatment is approximately three times more expensive than sulphasalazine therapy.

18. Antibiotic therapy is not warranted for Mr J at present.

To date, there is no substantial evidence of the presence of an infective agent in Crohn's disease, although there is continuing interest in this area, particularly regarding the role of atypical mycobacteria. It is thought that bacteria might exacerbate inflammation by:

(a) getting through to the gut wall in diseased areas, or

(b) presenting an antigenic load to the lymphatic system in the gut.

Despite the lack of evidence of an infective agent, metronidazole has been shown to compare favourably with sulphasalazine in remission induction of colonic disease (controlled trial), and has been widely used in peri-anal disease (controlled trials awaited). Its use is limited by the incidence of peripheral neuropathy, which can occur after only two weeks of therapy.

Other antibiotics used with some success in the treatment of chronic, symptomatic Crohn's disease include tetracycline, erythromycin, and ampicillin, but these studies were uncontrolled. It should also be remembered that parenteral broad-spectrum antibiotics have a clear role in the treatment of local perforation of the disease.

Should Mr J fail the trial of sulphasalazine (or of mesalazine should he prove intolerant to sulphasalazine), metronidazole might be an appropriate alternative therapy, with careful monitoring to detect emergence of peripheral neuropathy.

19. (a) Sulphasalazine induces orange colouration of urine (also contact lenses, if appropriate).

(b) Take prednisolone and iron with food to lessen gastric irritation.

(c) To avoid the possibility of sulphasalazine binding with ferrous sulphate, take the two drugs at least two hours apart.

(d) Continue with all therapies until advised otherwise.

(e) Advise every doctor or pharmacist (if purchasing over-the-counter drugs) that you are taking steroid therapy. Carry the steroid card at all times.

20. Yes. Mr J should be advised to maintain a well-balanced diet, with a high protein and calorie intake. If necessary, liquid supplements can help achieve the latter.

More controversial is the area of elimination diets. One school of thought believes that Crohn's disease is caused by a food intolerance, and that patients might be able to discover which, if any, foods are implicated by gradually re-introducing foods individually. Obviously this is a very slow process and patients need to be highly motivated.

21. No.

Only one study has shown any significant difference in numbers of patients maintaining remission on steroids, as compared to placebo. In contrast, several studies have shown no difference, with both sulphasalazine and prednisolone being no more effective than placebo in preventing recurrence of Crohn's disease.

Prednisolone therapy should, however, be tailed off gradually over the next four to six weeks, to allow recovery of normal adrenocortical function.

22. Nutritional, fluid and electrolyte disturbances may occur, depending on the extent of ileal resection.

Initially, TPN may be necessary to maintain adequate nutrition. Fluid balance should be checked daily and electrolytes monitored, particularly calcium and magnesium. Vitamin B_{12} may have to be given parenterally for life every three months, as its site of absorption in the ileum may have been removed.

A longer-term problem is diarrhoea, which may arise for several reasons:

(a) Reduced transit time, owing to the shortened gut. This can be controlled with loperamide or codeine phosphate, although the former is preferred for long-term use, to avoid dependence.

(b) Unabsorbed bile acids. This problem can be controlled with cholestyramine.

(c) Steatorrhoea. This is due to malabsorption of fats and should be controlled by a reduction in dietary fats.

(d) Small bowel contamination. This should be treated with appropriate antibiotics, such as metronidazole or tetracycline.

23. Laxatives, drugs affecting fluid balance, and iron. Enteric-coated and sustained-release preparations should not be used, as there may not be sufficient release of the active ingredient.

Laxatives should not be prescribed for patients with ileostomies. Problems will arise from drugs that increase the fluid content of the effluent, as this will lead to dehydration without the regulatory control of the colon. An example is antacids with an osmotic effect, such as magnesium-containing compounds; a mixed antacid, or perhaps even an aluminium-containing one, would be preferred.

Diuretics may produce excessive dehydration and potassium depletion may occur. Iron preparations may cause loose stools and sore skin around the ileostomy site.

24. To reduce the side-effects associated with high-dose, long-term steroid therapy.

Mr J is suffering a relapse on reduction of his steroid dose, a frequent occurrence after remission induction. It seems likely that to reduce his symptoms Mr J may have to remain on prednisolone long-term. The immunosuppressant azathioprine has a steroid-sparing effect, allowing the dose of prednisolone to be reduced, and thereby reducing the incidence of side-effects (such as moon face, bruising, hirsutism, impaired glucose tolerance, hypertension, acne, weight gain, osteoporosis, predisposition to infection, and striae).

25. The dose should not exceed 2 mg/kg/day, as larger doses greatly increase the risk of bone marrow suppression.

Other adverse effects which can occur include cholestatic jaundice, pancreatitis, fever with arthralgia, and malignancy. Liver function tests and full blood counts should thus be carried out regularly.

26. Azathioprine as sole therapy for Crohn's disease has been studied both in remission induction and as maintenance therapy, but the results are conflicting.

One study did show a relapse rate (after six months' remission) of only 5% on azathioprine (at a dose of 2 mg/kg daily) compared to 41% on placebo. However, because of the increased incidence of lymphoma with long-term use, it is mainly used in patients refractory to other treatment. It must be given for at least six months before any benefit is noted.

27. For its immunosuppressant activity.

Although the aetiology of Crohn's disease is unknown, there is a hypothesis (discussed in answer

4) that it is partially auto-immune in origin, and so may respond to immunosuppressive therapy.

28. Serum creatinine, urea, bilirubin, and liver enzymes should be monitored before therapy, as cyclosporin may affect liver and kidney function.

29. Yes.

There is only limited information available on the adjustment of existing therapy after the addition of cyclosporin to the regimen. Cyclosporin has been used in combination with azathioprine and steroid therapy, but the potential benefit of using azathioprine and cyclosporin together has to be weighed against the risk of enhanced toxicity. Azathioprine has been stopped abruptly in some patients, and phased out in others. A recent report suggests the response to cyclosporin plus steroid therapy is good.

30. Mr J's cyclosporin levels should be monitored regularly, and his liver and kidney function, and potassium levels, should be checked at regular intervals.

Serum biochemistry should be checked weekly, initially. Any changes noted (e.g. an increase in serum creatinine) are dose-dependent and reversible.

Cyclosporin blood levels should be checked twice weekly, initially. After about two weeks' therapy, patients should have achieved 80% of their final level, with stabilisation by three or four weeks. Some Crohn's patients show impaired absorption of cyclosporin, and it is important to remember that as the disease improves, cyclosporin absorption may increase.

It is important to use the reference range for cyclosporin levels corresponding to the assay type employed. Also, only whole blood should be used for analysis, plasma assays being difficult to interpret, owing to the reversible binding of cyclosporin to red blood cells. Samples should be taken just before a dose is given.

31. Hypertension has been reported in transplant patients taking cyclosporin, and therefore Mr J's blood pressure should be monitored regularly.

In addition to the effects on liver and kidney function, and blood pressure already discussed, hirsutism, tremor, gingival hypertrophy, anorexia, nausea and vomiting, and hyperkalaemia have been noted. A burning sensation in hands and feet may also occur, usually in the first week of therapy.

32. Oral absorption may be impaired, so intravenous cyclosporin at one-third of the oral dose should be used. After suitable dilution, the infusion should be given over two to six hours.

References and Further Reading

Allan R., Crohn's disease, *Med. Int.*, 1986, **26**, 1049–1055.

Baker P., Inflammatory bowel disease, *Pharm. J.*, 1988, **241**, 180–182.

Piper D.W. *et al.*, Gastrointestinal and hepatic diseases, in *Avery's Drug Treatment – principles and practice of clinical pharmacology and therapeutics*, 3rd edn, Speight T.M. (ed.), Edinburgh, Churchill Livingstone, 1987, 770–772.

Sack D.M. and Peppercorn M.A., Drug therapy of inflammatory bowel disease, *Pharmacotherapy*, 1983, **3**, 158–176.

Truelove S.C., Crohn's disease, in *Oxford Textbook of Medicine*, 2nd edn, Weatherall D.J., Ledingham J.G.G. and Warrell D.A. (eds), Oxford, Oxford University Press, 1987, 12.127–12.133.

Ursing B. *et al.*, A comparative study of metronidazole and sulphasalazine for active Crohn's disease, *Gastroenterology*, 1982, **83**, 550–562.

HEPATO-BILIARY DISEASE WITH JAUNDICE

Elizabeth G. Kennedy

Staff Pharmacist (Clinical), Ninewells Hospital, Dundee

Day 1 (1979) Twenty-year-old Mrs R was referred to the gastro-enterology out-patients' clinic by her general practitioner. She was jaundiced. Four-and-a-half months earlier she had given birth to a normal baby after an uncomplicated pregnancy with no hepatic problems. For one-and-a-half years prior to conception she had taken the oral contraceptive Eugynon 30® (ethinyloestradiol 30 micrograms, levonorgestrol 250 micrograms) and ten weeks ago she had re-commenced Eugynon 30®. Two weeks later she had started to feel tired and listless, and her next two menstrual periods had been very heavy. For the last five or six weeks she had been passing frequent pale yellow loose stools, both during the day and the night, and these bowel motions had been associated with epigastric or generalised abdominal pain, and flatus. In addition, she had experienced occasional episodes of vomiting, anorexia, nocturia and increased urinary frequency with dark urine, and marked generalised itching. She also complained of lethargy, weakness, and occasional headaches. Mrs R had no other relevant medical history. She rarely drank alcohol and did not smoke.

Her present medication was Lomotil® (diphenoxylate 2.5 mg, atropine 25 micrograms) two tablets every six hours, and cholestyramine 4 g, eight sachets daily.

On examination she was noted to be jaundiced, with scratch marks on her skin, spider naevi on her face and back, and bruising on her shins, but there were no clinical features of anaemia. Her liver was just palpable but there was no evidence of splenomegaly or ascites.

Her serum biochemistry and haematology results were:

Alkaline phosphatase (Alk phos) 600 iu/L (reference range 20–120)
Aspartate transaminase (AST) 51 iu/L (0–35)

Bilirubin (total) 124 micromol/L (0–17)
Gamma-glutamyl transferase (GGT) 350 iu/L (5–42)
Albumin 32 g/L (36–50)
Protein 66 g/L (65–80)
Calcium (corrected) 2.4 mmol/L (2.2–2.6)
Chloride 99 mmol/L (96–108)
Creatinine 80 micromol/L (44–150)
Glucose (fasting) 6.7 mmol/L (3.3–5.8)
Potassium 3.4 mmol/L (3.5–5.0)
Sodium 141 mmol/L (135–147)
Urea 4 mmol/L (3.3–6.6)
Haemoglobin 12.8 g/dL (12–16)
White blood cells (WBC) 6.5×10^9/L ($4–11 \times 10^9$)
Prothrombin time 20 s (control 14 s)
KCCT (Kaolin Cephalin Clotting Time) 43 s (control 43 s)
Hbs Ag (Hepatitis B Surface Antigen) negative
Anti-HBc (Hepatitis B Core Antibody) negative
Anti-nuclear factor negative
Anti-mitochondrial antibody strongly positive
Anti-smooth muscle antibody negative

Bilirubinuria was present, but urobilinogen was not detected in the urine. Nothing abnormal was detected from a stool culture, and abdominal ultrasound revealed normal liver texture, and normal bile ducts with no dilation. No gall stones were seen.

The initial diagnosis was of cholestatic jaundice, possibly induced by the oral contraceptive pill, which was discontinued. Intravenous Vitamin K (10 mg) was prescribed for three days and this brought the prothrombin time towards normal. Mrs R's cholestyramine dose was reduced to one sachet four times daily.

1. What symptoms and signs of hepato-biliary disease does Mrs R exhibit?

2. What are the main mechanisms of drug-induced liver disease?

3. *Can the oral contraceptive cause cholestatic jaundice? Do you think Eugynon 30 therapy caused Mrs R's problems?*

4. *How would you recommend that drug-induced liver disease be treated? Is there a place for corticosteroid therapy?*

5. *Why has cholestyramine been prescribed for Mrs R and what symptoms may it aggravate? Is the dose appropriate and how should she be counselled to take it?*

6. *What other drugs could be prescribed for the same purpose as cholestyramine?*

7. *Why has Vitamin K been prescribed? Is the route of administration appropriate?*

8. *Would you recommend that Mrs R be prescribed any other nutritional supplements?*

9. *If liver failure developed and Mrs R required total parenteral nutrition (TPN), what formulation considerations would you make?*

Month 9 A liver biopsy was performed and this confirmed a diagnosis of primary biliary cirrhosis.

Month 18 (1980) Mrs R was still tired and listless and she had gained 2 kg in weight. After large meals she experienced immediate urgency to open her bowels. Her stools were sometimes difficult to flush away and were foul-smelling. She had no rectal bleeding or melaena.

She complained of heavy menstrual periods and she was jaundiced, especially during menstruation. She was also suffering from frequent headaches.

Serum biochemistry and haematology were:

Alk phos 710 iu/L (20–120)
AST 71 iu/L (0–35)
Bilirubin 150 micromol/L (0–17)
GGT 450 iu/L (0–17)
Albumin 33 g/L (35–50)
Protein 72 g/L (65–80)
Haemoglobin 9.9 g/dL (12–16)
WBC 7.0×10^9/L ($4–11 \times 10^9$)
Platelets 431×10^9/L ($100–400 \times 10^9$)
Prothrombin time 19 s (control 13.5 s)
KCCT 50 s (control 40 s)

Because of her low haemoglobin, Mrs R had a gastroscopy performed. This revealed oesophageal varices and linear oesophagitis. Iron therapy was commenced with oral ferrous sulphate at a dose of 200 mg three times daily.

10. *Why might Mrs R have developed anaemia? Is iron therapy appropriate?*

Month 45 (1982) Mrs R had been experiencing increasing pruritus. Ultrasound had excluded gallstones as a cause of her jaundice. She had developed xanthelasma (flat or slightly raised yellow patchy deposits on the skin which develop in proportion to the total serum lipid level) over the previous two months, but no longer had any diarrhoea. She was entered into a double-blind randomised trial to investigate the value of propranolol (80 mg long-acting daily) in the management of chronic liver disease.

11. *Why might propranolol benefit Mrs R?*

Month 75 (1985) Mrs R was admitted to hospital following three days of epigastric pain, vomiting, and diarrhoea, which had been associated with episodes of melaena and a small haematemesis. She stated she had been suffering epigastric discomfort for several months. Her past medical history of primary biliary cirrhosis and oesophagitis were noted. Her pulse was 96 beats per minute and regular.

Endoscopy revealed that Mrs R had bleeding oesophageal varices, and terlipressin (2 mg) was administered intravenously.

12. *How does terlipressin decrease bleeding? What side-effects would you warn ward staff about?*

13. *What alternative treatments are available for bleeding oesophageal varices?*

It was noted that Mrs R had gained 8 kg in weight since her first presentation and that she had developed ascites.

A Warren shunt operation was performed surgically two days later. This distal splenorenal shunt decompresses the varices, while preserving much of the portal blood flow to the liver. Encephalopathy thus ensues much less frequently than with non-selective portal-systemic shunt surgery.

Serum biochemistry results were:

Alk phos 693 iu/L (20–120)
Bilirubin 160 micromol/L (0–17)
Protein 57 g/L (65–80)
Albumin 25 g/L (36–50)

14. *What drug therapy would you recommend for treating Mrs R's ascites?*

Month 96 (1987) Mrs R's medication was:

Ferrous sulphate 200 mg orally three times daily
Spironolactone 300 mg orally daily
Frusemide 40 mg orally daily
Ranitidine 150 mg orally twice daily
Gaviscon® 10 mL orally, as required for indigestion
Diazepam 2 mg orally at night
Menadiol sodium phosphate 10 mg orally daily

15. *Why is diazepam an inappropriate sedative for Mrs R, and what would you recommend instead?*

16. *What other alterations to Mrs R's therapy might be appropriate?*

Month 99 Mrs R was experiencing painful joints. Piroxicam 10 mg orally twice daily was prescribed.

17. *What might be the reason for Mrs R developing painful joints?*

18. *Would you have recommended a non-steroidal anti-inflammatory drug (NSAID)?*

Month 120 (1989) Mrs R was placed on the waiting list for a liver transplant, ten years after first presentation.

Month 125 Mrs R received a liver transplant and splenectomy. She experienced rejection in the early days post-transplant, but this was controlled effectively with prednisolone and azathioprine therapy.

Her serum biochemistry results were:

Alk phos 116 iu/L (20–120)
AST 47 iu/L (0–35)
Bilirubin 17 micromol/L (0–17)
Albumin 41 g/L (36–50)
Protein 66 g/L (65–80)

Mrs R's current medication is:

Azathioprine 100 mg orally daily
Cyclosporin 800 mg orally daily
Prednisolone 15 mg orally daily
Penicillin V 250 mg orally twice daily
Nystatin suspension 5 mL orally four times daily
Ranitidine 150 mg orally at night

Mrs R feels better now than at any time over the last ten years.

19. *What points would you cover when counselling Mrs R about her medication?*

Answers

1. Mrs R's clinical symptoms and signs indicating hepato-biliary disease are:

   (a) jaundice, itching, and scratch marks, with pale stools and dark urine (due to abnormal bilirubin metabolism);

   (b) diarrhoea with pale yellow stools (due to fat malabsorption);

   (c) spider naevi (dilated spider-shaped blood vessels which occur in liver disease and with the contraceptive pill);

   (d) hepatomegaly; and

   (e) bruising (coagulation defects may occur either from impaired liver cell function or reduced vitamin K absorption in association with cholestasis).

Other features of severe liver disease, not present in Mrs R, are ascites, ankle oedema, and hepatic encephalopathy.

Mrs R's laboratory results clearly indicate underlying hepato-biliary disease; however, they do not yet enable a firm diagnosis to be made, although some possible causes (such as hepatitis B) have been excluded. Most of the biochemical investigations carried out on Mrs R are not actual tests of liver "function" per se. In the presence of hepato-biliary disease these tests are usually abnormal, but normal values do not exclude severe disease. It must be remembered that these tests are not specific to the liver.

Bilirubin is normally removed from blood only by the liver, and therefore its serum level can be used as a true test of liver function, provided there is no bile duct obstruction.

Aminotransferases (or transaminases) are enzymes that are present in hepatocytes and leak into the blood when liver cells are damaged. They are therefore tests of liver cell integrity. The enzymes are not specific to the liver, but are of value in differentiating hepato-cellular from obstructive jaundice. Alkaline phosphatase is an enzyme which is present in the canalicular and sinusoidal membranes of the liver, but it is also present in many other tissues (e.g. bone, intestine, placenta). The enzyme is raised in cholestasis from any cause, whether intra- or extra-hepatic disease. The highest levels are seen with hepatic metastases and primary biliary cirrhosis. Gamma-glutamyl transferase is a microsomal enzyme. In cholestasis the serum level rises in parallel with that of alkaline phosphatase.

Serum albumin is a sensitive marker of hepatic synthetic function, as albumin is synthesised entirely in the liver. Albumin has a half-life of about 20 days, and low levels may thus be an indication of chronic disease of the liver.

2. The main mechanisms are intrinsic and idiosyncratic hepatotoxicity.

Intrinsic damage is caused by drugs that are direct or indirect hepatoxins, inducing cytotoxic, cholestatic, or mixed hepatotoxicity. Idiosyncratic damage results from a hypersensitivity reaction, an individual's auto-immune predisposition to the drug, or as a result of a metabolic abnormality in a susceptible patient. These reactions are dose-independent. Chronic active hepatitis can also be drug-induced.

3. Oral contraceptive therapy may cause a number of adverse effects on the liver, including cholestasis; however, it is unlikely that Eugynon 30® has caused Mrs R's problems.

Cholestasis is a rare complication in the millions of women worldwide who take sex hormones. The reaction is dose-dependent, and the incidence associated with oral contraceptive use has declined as the dose of hormones contained in the oral contraceptive has been reduced.

The oral contraceptive is particularly likely to cause jaundice in women with a history of cholestasis of pregnancy, and vice versa. The common basis for these conditions is that oestrogens appear to reduce hepatic excretion of bile in those patients who are generally susceptible. This is in accord with the known familial tendency to this adverse effect, and the finding of a higher incidence of its occurrence in Scandinavia, Northern Europe, and Chile.

Oral contraceptive-induced jaundice usually occurs in the first three cycles of treatment and resolves on drug discontinuation. The serum bilirubin level is usually less than 150 micromol/L, with a high alkaline phosphatase level, indicative of cholestasis.

It is unlikely that Mrs R's liver disease was caused by Eugynon 30®, as she had no jaundice during her first course of oral contraceptives, nor during pregnancy. Instead, the combination of jaundice and pruritus with a strongly positive anti-mitochondrial antibody is very suggestive of primary biliary cirrhosis.

4. The suspected drug must be withdrawn and, in most cases, its future use must be cautioned against. Otherwise, management of drug-induced liver disease is generally supportive, with any complications receiving appropriate treatment. The value of corticosteroid therapy is

controversial and depends on the nature of the liver damage.

Bed rest and dietary restriction are only necessary if the patient is severely ill. Patients who feel well should be encouraged to take a normal diet; however, if they feel nauseated, a light diet supplemented with fruit drinks and glucose may be better tolerated. If the patient vomits, then intravenous fluids and glucose should be administered.

Corticosteroids should not be given to patients with drug-induced liver disease in whom there is no liver failure, and even in patients with established liver failure they are of doubtful value. In fulminant hepatic failure, controlled trials have failed to show benefit from large doses of corticosteroids, and such therapy may even have a deleterious effect, predisposing to infection, gastric erosions, and pancreatitis.

Although corticosteroid therapy can produce a feeling of well-being and improved appetite in patients with viral hepatitis, most trials show no improvement in outcome. Indeed, corticosteroid use is associated with more frequent relapse, and it may worsen liver damage from hepatitis B infection, as well as inducing a carrier state. Corticosteroids are also contra-indicated in most cases of primary biliary cirrhosis because they increase the risk of bone fractures. However, corticosteroids can be life-saving in the auto-immune variety of chronic active hepatitis.

5. Cholestyramine has been prescribed to reduce Mrs R's pruritus, although a dose of one or two sachets daily is more appropriate for this indication. Cholestyramine therapy may aggravate Mrs R's diarrhoea, and reduce her absorption of fat-soluble vitamins.

High systemic concentrations of bile acids, and their consequent deposition in tissues, cause the itch experienced by jaundiced patients. Cholestyramine is a strongly basic anionic-exchange resin. The 9 g sachet contains 4 g anhydrous resin. It decreases bile acid concentrations by binding bile salts in the intestine, and thus increases their excretion in the faeces. It will normally stop itching in four to seven days in patients with partial biliary obstruction.

Cholestyramine can also reduce the diarrhoea experienced by some patients with terminal ileal disease or bowel resection, in whom unabsorbed bile salts stimulate secretion from the colon; however, it may worsen the diarrhoea in patients like Mrs R, because by binding bile salts it may reduce fat absorption further. Cholestyramine can also bind fat-soluble vitamins and make any deficiency state worse.

Mrs R's cholestyramine dose is inappropriate, as the dose to relieve pruritus is usually one or two sachets daily (4–8 g). Two formulations of cholestyramine are available: Questran Classic® and Questran A®. Questran Classic contains 3.5 g of sugar per sachet. Questran A contains less than 0.3 g of sugar, but also contains aspartame. Although Questran A is not as soluble as Questran Classic, it requires less water for reconstitution (75 mL) because it contains less bulking agent, and the resin is finer. As Mrs R is not diabetic, Questran Classic should be prescribed for her.

Before counselling Mrs R on her cholestyramine therapy, it should be ascertained whether she is breast-feeding, as it is recommended that cholestyramine should not be taken by breast-feeding mothers. If she is, advice on this matter will be required from appropriate experts.

Mrs R should be counselled to take the main dose of cholestyramine before breakfast, to ensure that arrival of the drug in the duodenum coincides with gall bladder contraction and maximum duodenal bile acid concentration. If more than one sachet is required, the additional doses should be taken before the mid-day and evening meals. The contents of the sachet should be mixed with 150 mL of water, or other drinks, *immediately* before being taken. It may also be incorporated into food (a cookery book is available).

Cholestyramine, as well as binding bile salts, will bind drugs. It is known to reduce absorption of digitalis and its alkaloids, tetracyclines, chlorothiazide, penicillin G, warfarin and thyroxine. Therefore, Mrs R should be told not to take cholestyramine at the same time as any other drugs she may be prescribed in the future. Other drugs should be taken at least one hour before cholestyramine, or four to six hours afterwards.

It should be explained to Mrs R that cholestyramine can cause nausea and constipation, but that she should discuss any such side-effects with her doctor before stopping treatment, as it is important that she takes this drug.

6. Alternative therapies to control pruritus induced by high bile acid concentrations include other anionic-binding agents, hormonal therapy, antihistamines, and topical measures.

Colestipol (5 g twice daily) is as effective as cholestyramine, and can be tried if a patient cannot tolerate cholestyramine. If a patient has complete biliary obstruction, then anionic-binding resins are of no help.

Methyltestosterone therapy (25 mg sublingually daily) can relieve itching within seven days. Norethandrolone (10 mg twice or thrice daily) or stanozolol (5 mg twice daily) are less virilising and are therefore more appropriate for females. However, these agents greatly increase jaundice, can cause intra-hepatic cholestasis in normal patients, and cause bone thinning, especially in post-menopausal women. The smallest effective dose should be given, and such therapy should be reserved for intractable (usually malignant) pruritus. However, hormonal therapy is of use in total biliary obstruction where cholestyramine is ineffective.

Antihistamines can be tried, as their sedating effect may alleviate itch, but they should be prescribed with caution where impaired hepatic metabolism is present, as encephalopathy may ensue. The non-sedating agents (e.g. terfenadine 60 mg twice daily) may also be of benefit.

Ursodeoxycholic acid (10–15 mg/kg/day) has been shown to reduce pruritus in patients with primary biliary cirrhosis. It becomes the predominant bile acid.

Topical measures can also help. Skin dryness can be treated with aqueous cream, and soap replaced by Oilatum Emollient®. Topical phenolated calamine lotion is also of use. Non-drug measures advocated for the treatment of pruritus are the use of ultra-violet radiation (at a specific wavelength) and plasmapheresis. Both are of questionable benefit in the majority of patients, but may be useful in some patients.

Finally, it should be ensured that Mrs R is not prescribed any drugs that may increase her pruritus, such as clofibrate, which increases biliary cholesterol excretion.

7. Vitamin K has been prescribed to ensure adequate production of clotting factors and thus prevent haemorrhage. Parenteral therapy is appropriate for Mrs R.

In patients with hepato-biliary disease, the synthesis of certain coagulation factors may be reduced, either because the liver cells are damaged, or because cholestasis impairs intestinal absorption of vitamin K, which is needed to synthesise coagulation factors II (prothrombin), VII, IX and X. As the half-lives of some of these factors are very short, coagulation abnormalities can develop rapidly after liver cell damage. In patients with severe liver cell damage, vitamin K may not increase synthesis of coagulation factors, but if cholestasis predominates, parenteral vitamin K usually corrects coagulation defects. Parenteral vitamin K should thus be given to all patients with a prolonged prothrombin time. In addition it can be given prophylactically in the early stages of liver disease, and it should always

be given to patients with conjugated hyperbilirubinaemia.

Vitamin K should be given by a slow intravenous injection (over ten minutes) when coagulation is severely impaired. It can also be given intramuscularly. Injections should be repeated once daily until coagulation normalises; if this has not occurred within five days, then significant liver cell damage is likely.

In the presence of cholestasis, oral phytomenadione therapy is inappropriate, as the lack of bile salts will impair absorption of this fat-soluble vitamin. A water-soluble vitamin K analogue (menadiol sodium phosphate) is available for oral use, but its value in chronic cholestatic disorders, such as primary biliary cirrhosis, is questionable. In these disorders, minor coagulation abnormalities need not be corrected unless frank bleeding occurs, or invasive procedures such as liver biopsy are planned.

8. Vitamin A and D supplements should be considered to correct any deficiencies, and also because Mrs R is currently taking cholestyramine.

Vitamin A deficiency is uncommon but can cause night-blindness. If supplementation is required, 100,000 units may be administered intramuscularly once each month. Vitamin D deficiency may be due to inadequate dietary intake, reduced absorption due to steatorrhoea, reduced exposure to sun (as itching may be worse in the sun), or impaired entero-hepatic circulation of bile salts. Vitamin D deficiency causes peripheral bone pain and muscle weakness. Prophylactic therapy may be given to Mrs R as parenteral calciferol (vitamin D_2) 100,000 units monthly, or as oral calcitriol (1,25-dihydroxycholecalciferol). Therapy should be monitored by assaying her 25-hydroxycholecalciferol levels.

9. A number of factors need to be taken into account when formulating a feed for a patient in liver failure.

Patients with acute liver failure are more prone to hypoglycaemia, while those with chronic liver failure are more prone to hyperglycaemia. Therefore, blood glucose levels must be measured regularly, especially as levels can fluctuate, and undetected hypoglycaemia can exacerbate hepatic encephalopathy. If a patient has a low blood sugar, glucose infusions should be administered; whereas if there is hyperglycaemia, insulin should also be administered, although insulin resistance can occur in acute hepatitis. If hypertonic glucose solutions are required as a calorie source they must be administered through a central line to reduce the risk of thrombosis.

Intravenous lipids (e.g. Intralipid®) should be used with caution. They are poorly utilised by patients in liver failure and will also exacerbate an increase in plasma levels of free fatty acids, which are a result of the disease state itself. The patient's ability to clear lipid from the circulation should be checked. The administration of lipids once weekly could be considered.

A daily nitrogen supply of 9–11 g is usually appropriate, provided no encephalopathy is present. Nitrogen can be provided as an amino acid solution, but for adequate nitrogen utilisation, a ratio of 200 kcal of glucose per gram of nitrogen is necessary.

Amino acids derived from the diet and muscle breakdown arrive in the liver for metabolism. Some of these are transaminated or deaminated to keto-acids, while others are metabolised to ammonia and urea. The maximal rate of urea synthesis in chronic liver disease is markedly reduced, and a generalised or selective amino aciduria is a feature of hepato-cellular disease. In patients with severe liver disease, there is usually a picture of raised plasma concentrations of aromatic amino acids, and reduced levels of branched chain amino acids. These changes are due to impaired hepatic function, portal-systemic shunting of blood, hyperinsulinaemia, and hyper-glucagonaemia.

From the above facts, it can be seen that an amino acid solution containing a higher proportion of the branched chain amino acids (leucine, isoleucine, and valine) and smaller amounts of the aromatic amino acids (phenylalanine, tyrosine, tryptophan, and methionine) should be beneficial; however, although branched chain amino acid solutions are available, their clinical value remains controversial.

Serum electrolyte levels must be carefully monitored and supplemented accordingly. Hypokalaemia can be life-threatening. Sodium intake should be greatly reduced (to 20 mmol/day) as there is usually an inappropriately high renal retention of sodium and water. Calcium and phosphate supplementation may also be required. Appropriate and regular vitamin and mineral supplementation must be given if long-term TPN is planned.

10. A number of factors may have contributed to Mrs R's anaemia, but it is not yet clear whether ferrous sulphate therapy is appropriate.

Mrs R's anaemia may have developed as a result of her known menorrhagia, occult internal haemorrhage, or reduced iron intake secondary to the anorexia which is common in such patients. However, iron supplements are only appropriate if the anaemia is proven to be a result of iron deficiency, and further investigations are thus required.

11. Propranolol therapy may reduce her portal hypertension, thereby reducing the risk of bleeding from oesophageal varices.

In patients with liver cirrhosis, scar tissue obstructs the intra-hepatic venous system, thereby raising the portal venous pressure above the upper normal limit of 5 mmHg. Once the pressure exceeds 15 mmHg, clinical sequelae are likely, and although portal hypertension contributes to the development of ascites and hepatic encephalopathy, bleeding from oesophageal varices is the most important complication. The raised portal venous pressure distends adjoining collateral vessels, which results in varicose veins within the distal oesophagus and proximal stomach, and sometimes within the distal rectum and anal canal. Eventually the raised pressure may rupture the oesophageal varices, causing a severe intestinal bleed which may be aggravated by the reduced clotting factors. Portal hypertension can also cause the spleen to enlarge, which results in more rapid removal of platelets from the circulation, and this further accentuates the bleeding problems.

These complications can be treated, but unless portal pressure is reduced, bleeding will recur. Unfortunately, surgical decompensation may precipitate irreversible hepatic encephalopathy. Oral propranolol, in a dosage sufficient to reduce the resting heart rate by 25%, has been shown to reduce portal pressure and to lower significantly the incidence of rebleeding from varices. However, it is not yet known if propranolol will benefit those patients who have not bled. Its long-term safety and efficacy, optimal duration of treatment, and consequences of stopping therapy, are not yet known. In addition, there may be difficulties in resuscitating patients treated with beta-blockers.

12. Terlipressin decreases bleeding by constricting splanchnic arterioles and reducing vascular resistance.

Terlipressin (triglycyl-lysine-vasopressin) is a synthetic analogue of vasopressin. It has a more prolonged action, fewer side-effects, and may be more effective than the parent compound. It is not active itself but is metabolised to vasopressin, which is slowly released over several hours in amounts sufficient to reduce portal pressure without producing the same degree of systemic and cardiac effects as accompany vasopressin administration. Initially terlipressin was thought to act solely by constricting splanchnic arterioles, which decreased portal venous flow, but recent studies show that it has the unique property of reducing portal vascular resistance. An appropriate dose is 2 mg every six hours until bleeding stops; this should be followed by 1–2 mg every six hours for a further 24–72 hours.

The ward staff should be aware of the potential side-effects of terlipressin, but it must be noted that the absence of these effects indicates an inadequate therapeutic effect. Colicky abdominal pain, facial pallor, and bowel evacuation are all predictable effects. Myocardial ischaemia and angina can be seen in some patients, and the administration of sublingual glyceryl trinitrate may minimise such a reaction.

13. Alternative measures to stop bleeding from oesophageal varices are intravenous somatostatin (which is very expensive), or balloon tamponade.

Somatostatin is given as a bolus of 50–250 micrograms, then infused at 250 micrograms per hour. Once the immediate bleeding from the varices has stopped, recurrent bleeding is usually prevented by the use of fibre optic endoscopic injection sclerotherapy with sodium tetradecyl sulphate, ethanolamine oleate, or alcohol. Alternative prophylactic measures are propranolol (see answer 11) or portal-systemic shunt surgery.

14. Diuretic therapy, with the aldosterone antagonist spironolactone, is the treatment of choice.

A dose of 100–200 mg spironolactone per day is used initially, but because of the drug's long half-life, the maximal effect will not be seen for three to four days. The dose may then be increased slowly by 100 mg every two to four days. However, hyperkalaemia may be a dose-limiting factor.

Triamterene or amiloride are alternative potassium-sparing diuretics that can be considered if Mrs R suffers intolerable side-effects of spironolactone, but they are generally not as effective as spironolactone. Frusemide (40–120 mg daily) may be added to the diuretic regimen if there is inadequate response to spironolactone, or if Mrs R experiences adverse effects. Frusemide reduces the more proximal reabsorption of sodium. It is not the first-line treatment for this indication and must be used with care, as too rapid a diuresis can induce renal failure and hepatic encephalopathy. During diuretic therapy, a weight, and therefore fluid, loss of 0.5 kg daily should be aimed for, although this can be higher if peripheral oedema is present.

If ascites is resistant to diuretic treatment it is important to establish whether the reason for treatment failure is ascitic infection or inappropriate ingestion of salt. In severe ascites, especially if it is impairing respiration, paracentesis may be performed. However, because this can precipitate renal failure, it is wise to remove no more than five litres of ascitic fluid at a time, and to administer salt-poor albumin intravenously. The latter prevents intravascular fluid leaking back into the abdomen.

15. Diazepam may predispose Mrs R to encephalopathy for a variety of reasons. If a benzodiazepine is deemed essential, a small dose of oxazepam or lorazepam would be a safer choice.

In patients with liver disease there is an increased pharmacological sensitivity in the brain to benzodiazepines. They are highly plasma protein-bound, and therefore an increased amount of free drug is available initially (see case study 11). Diazepam has a half-life of 20–50 hours and is hepatically demethylated to an active metabolite (desmethyldiazepam) which has a half-life of 36–200 hours. Where there is hepatic impairment, both compounds will accumulate.

If itching is keeping Mrs R awake at night, then appropriate treatment for the itching should be given. If it is true insomnia, Mrs R could be prescribed a small dose of oxazepam or lorazepam. These drugs, which have half-lives of 5–20 and 10–20 hours, respectively, are the safest choices if a benzodiazepine is required. They are not hepatically metabolised to active compounds, but are glucuronidated.

16. Mrs R should be prescribed a low sodium alternative to Gaviscon®, and a medication history should be taken to ascertain whether changes to her iron or spironolactone therapy are appropriate. The need for menadiol sodium phosphate therapy should be questioned.

Gaviscon has a sodium content of 6 mmol/10 mL. Sodium is retained avidly by the cirrhotic patient, by complex renal mechanisms; water excretion is also defective and additional sodium intake would accentuate this situation. Thus, after ascertaining whether Mrs R needs an antacid or a "raft" preparation, a low-sodium alternative should be recommended, (e.g. Mucogel® or Algicon®, respectively). A further consideration in the selection of an antacid would be the effect it would have on Mrs R's bowels. One with a more constipating effect could be chosen.

Because iron salts are astringent, gastro-intestinal irritation may occur. Nausea and epigastric pain are directly associated with the amount of elemental iron in the preparation prescribed. If Mrs R was experiencing such side-effects, an alternative preparation with a lower elemental iron content could be selected; however, her total daily intake of elemental iron should be 100–200 mg. If Mrs R does feel nauseated, a further strategy would be to split her dose of spironolactone, as high plasma levels of this drug are associated with an increased incidence of gastro-intestinal side-effects.

The therapeutic benefit of long-term menadiol sodium phosphate therapy in patients like Mrs R was discussed in answer 7.

Finally, the sodium content of other drugs must be borne in mind when future therapy is prescribed. In particular, effervescent tablets and injectable drugs can have a high sodium content.

17. Underlying bone disease.

Underlying bone disease can complicate all forms of chronic cholestasis and chronic hepato-cellular disease, and bone pain is common. Serum biochemistry may reveal normal or low calcium and phosphate levels. Osteomalacia and osteoporosis are slow to develop but their progress can be hastened by the inappropriate use of corticosteroids. Osteomalacia (softening of bone) is primarily due to a deficiency of vitamin D, and to a lesser extent calcium, or both. Osteoporosis (atrophy of bone) is believed to be due to predominance of resorption over formation of the cellular matrix of the bone, leading to a reduction in the total mass of bone.

18. No. Correction of the underlying problem is preferable.

NSAIDs, while reducing pain and inflammation, are generally contra-indicated in patients with liver disease as they cause excess fluid retention and lead to an increased risk of gastro-intestinal bleeding. The latter complication can have fatal consequences. The co-prescribing of an H_2-receptor blocker has been advocated, but this may not prevent gastro-intestinal bleeding from occurring.

Simple analgesia could be tried but may not be adequate. Aspirin is contra-indicated where varices are present. Paracetamol may be used with caution. Nefopam may be effective. Corticosteroids can exacerbate the underlying disease state. Thus, correction of the underlying cause is thus the most appropriate treatment.

Mrs R should be given vitamin D in the form of calciferol (vitamin D_2) injections or calcitriol (1,25-dihydroxycholecalciferol) orally. Oral calcium and phosphate supplements may be required, depending on Mrs R's serum levels. Severe bone pain may be controlled by parenteral calcium therapy.

19. (a) General.

The importance of compliance must be stressed to Mrs R. She will probably be taking most of these drugs for life. The indication for each drug should thus be clearly explained. Mrs R should also be warned of potential drug interactions with additional prescribed or over-the-counter medications. She should be told to inform the pharmacist of the prescribed drugs she is taking before purchasing any over-the-counter medicines.

(b) Azathioprine.

This is an immunosuppressant. It is given to reduce the risk of rejection in the initial phase post-transplant and may be stopped in due course.

(c) Cyclosporin.

This drug is also an immunosuppressant and given to prevent rejection. Mrs R should be told that she will need to have blood samples taken regularly to check that she is receiving the correct dose of cyclosporin. This drug is available as a liquid, or as liquid-filled capsules, which are more palatable but large. The former must be measured accurately with the syringe provided and may then be mixed, immediately before taking, with milk, chocolate drink or strongly flavoured fruit juice, to disguise the unpleasant taste. The liquid preparation should not be stored in the refrigerator.

(d) Prednisolone.

Prednisolone is also given as an immunosuppressant, and in some patients it may be possible to withdraw it at a later date. It should be taken on a full stomach, that is, after food. The precautions on the steroid card should be discussed.

(e) Penicillin V.

This is an antibiotic which has been given to prevent Mrs R developing infections, to which she is predisposed as a consequence of undergoing splenectomy. Penicillin V should be taken on an empty stomach, that is half to one hour before a meal, at 12-hourly intervals.

(f) Nystatin.

Nystatin therapy is to prevent Mrs R from acquiring fungal infections of the gastro-intestinal tract. The solution should be taken after meals. It should be rinsed around the mouth, then retained in the mouth for as long as possible before swallowing. Food and drink should be avoided for half-an-hour after each dose.

(g) Ranitidine.

Ranitidine therapy is to protect Mrs R from gastric and duodenal ulcers, and because she has experienced gastritis and oesophageal varices in the past. The dose should be taken at 9 p.m., after the last meal of the day.

Acknowledgement

I would like to acknowledge the help of Dr Grahame Barclay, Senior Registrar, Gastro-enterology, Ninewells Hospital and Medical School.

References and Further Reading

Finlayson N.D.C. and Richmond J., Diseases of the liver and biliary tract, in *Davidson's Principles and Practice of Medicine*, 15th edn, Macleod J., Edward C. and Bouchier I. (eds), Edinburgh, Churchill Livingstone, 1987, 326–369.

Jim L.K., Hepatic disorders, part I: adverse effects of drugs on the liver, in *Applied Therapeutics – the Clinical Use of Drugs*, 4th edn, Young L.Y. and Koda-Kimble M.A. (eds), Vancouver, WA, Applied Therapeutics, 1988, 485–500.

Kiire C.R., Controlled trial of propranolol to prevent recurrent variceal bleeding in patients with non-cirrhotic portal fibrosis, *Br. med. J.*, 1989, **298**, 1363–1365.

Shearman D.J. and Finlayson N.D.C., *Diseases of the Gastrointestinal Tract and Liver*, 2nd edn, Oxford, Churchill Livingstone, 1989.

Sherlock S., *Diseases of the Liver and Biliary System*, 7th edn, Oxford, Blackwell Scientific, 1985.

Stricker B.H. and Spoelstra P., *Drug-induced Hepatic Injury, Drug-induced Disorders Vol. 1*, Amsterdam, Elsevier, 1985.

ALCOHOLIC LIVER DISEASE

Gillian F. Cavell

Teacher/Practitioner (Clinical Services), Dulwich Hospital, London

Day 1 Mr N, a 53-year-old gentleman with known alcoholic liver disease (ALD) and cirrhosis was admitted to the ward from the medical out-patient clinic, where he had been referred by his general practitioner.

He was complaining of weakness in both legs and an unstable balance. He had a three-week history of swelling of the ankles and shortness of breath on exertion, which had become increasingly worse over the last week.

His drug history on admission was frusemide 40 mg once daily, and amiloride 5 mg once daily. Both diuretics had been prescribed two months previously by his general practitioner.

Mr N had been a pub landlord for 20 years and used to drink approximately six pints of beer, in addition to several measures of spirits, daily. At the time of his admission he was unemployed. He admitted to smoking 10–20 cigarettes a day and to indulging in "the odd pint".

On examination Mr N was noted to smell of alcohol. He appeared jaundiced and was found to have several stigmata of chronic liver disease, including spider naevi on his face and abdomen, and palmar erythema. Pitting oedema was present in both ankles. His abdomen was grossly enlarged with shifting dullness and a fluid thrill due to the presence of ascites. Distended veins were visible on the abdominal wall and he had a small umbilical hernia.

His serum biochemistry results were:

Sodium 133 mmol/L (reference range 130–145)
Potassium 3.7 mmol/L (3.5–5.3)
Urea 3.7 mmol/L (2.5–6.5)
Creatinine 69 micromol/L (50–120)
Bilirubin (total) 144 micromol/L (5–17)
Alkaline phosphatase 413 iu/L (30–85)
Aspartate transaminase 201 iu/L (10–50)
Gamma-glutamyl transferase 337 iu/L (5–55)
Albumin 24 g/L (35–50)
Prothrombin time 23 s (control 15 s)

1. What are the main therapeutic aims for Mr N on this admission?

2. What drug therapy would you recommend to meet these aims?

3. What general pharmacokinetic and pharmacodynamic considerations need to be taken into account when prescribing for Mr N?

That night, Mr N complained of being unable to sleep and of feeling sick. The nursing staff had noted that he had developed a tremor and that his blood pressure had increased from 110/80 mm Hg to 140/100 mm Hg. He was seen by the doctor who attributed these symptoms to the development of acute alcohol withdrawal syndrome.

4. What therapy would you recommend to suppress Mr N's symptoms of alcohol withdrawal?

Mr N was prescribed chlormethiazole. The nursing staff were requested to inform the doctor if the patient appeared over-sedated or if he remained agitated.

Day 2 Mr N's regimen of chlormethiazole was:

Day 2, two capsules four times daily
Day 3, two capsules three times daily
Day 4, one capsule four times daily
Day 5, one capsule three times daily
Day 6, one capsule twice daily
Day 7, one capsule once daily

His other medications were spironolactone 100 mg once daily, and Parentrovite® Intravenous High Potency, one pair of ampoules daily.

5. How should his diuretic therapy be monitored?

Day 3 Mr N's weight had not reduced significantly from his admission weight of 75.5 kg, and he was still complaining of some breathlessness on exertion, although his peripheral oedema had improved.

The dose of spironolactone was therefore increased to 200 mg once daily.

Laboratory results were as follows:

Serum   sodium 135 mmol/L (130–145)
potassium 3.6 mmol/L (3.5–5.3)
urea 3.4 mmol/L (2.5–6.5)
creatinine 75 micromol/L (50–120)
Urinary sodium 46 mOsmol/kg
potassium 30 mOsmol/kg

Day 5 Mr N's weight had increased to 76.8 kg, so it was decided to increase his spironolactone dose to 200 mg twice daily. This dose effected a rapid diuresis and weight loss of 3.5 kg over the following six days with the result that his breathlessness improved greatly.

Day 11 Serum biochemistry indicated that Mr N was suffering from hyponatraemia (serum sodium of 129 mmol/L) and hyperkalaemia (serum potassium of 6.0 mmol/L). His plasma urea and creatinine were both still within normal limits thereby indicating that the hyperkalaemia was not due to dehydration or acute renal failure. Diuretic therapy was thus reviewed.

6. What changes would you recommend be made to his diuretic therapy?

Days 12–25 Diuresis continued over the following ten days, with a satisfactory urinary sodium output. On day 25 his weight had reduced to 67 kg, and clinically his ascites was much reduced. The spironolactone was reduced to a maintenance dose of 100 mg once daily, and the frusemide dose was reduced to 20 mg once daily for three days and then discontinued.

Mr N remained well on this maintenance dose of spironolactone and, having been given advice regarding dietary sodium restriction, was discharged home.

Day 40 Mr N was readmitted as an emergency through the casualty department of the same hospital.

On examination, in addition to the signs of chronic liver disease he displayed on his previous admission, he was drowsy and disorientated with slurred speech and asterixis. Fetor hepaticus was also noted. He was still taking his prescribed maintenance dose of spironolactone, and his ascites was well controlled. His present condition was attributed to hepatic encephalopathy.

The results of Mr N's serum biochemistry were all normal. He was written up for a protein-free diet and the following drug therapy:

Spironolactone 100 mg once daily
Lactulose 50 mL three times daily
Magnesium sulphate enema, one to be administered immediately

7. What factors can precipitate hepatic encephalopathy in a cirrhotic patient?

8. What are the broad aims of the treatment written up for Mr N's present condition?

9. Why has lactulose been prescribed?

10. What other drugs might be prescribed to produce a similar effect?

11. Why has a protein-free diet been requested?

12. What alternative therapies have been used in the treatment of hepatic encephalopathy?

Day 43 Mr N's mental state had begun to improve. He was less drowsy and the asterixis was less marked. The lactulose had begun to take effect and the frequency and consistency of his bowel motions were being recorded on a stool chart by the nursing staff.

Day 45 Mr N was no longer displaying any signs of encephalopathy. A low-protein diet of 20 g per day was introduced. The dose of lactulose was reduced to 30 mL three times daily, as Mr N was complaining of flatulence.

Day 48 Mr N's protein intake was increased to 40 g per day and he was counselled by the dietician on the need to restrict his protein intake to this level on a long-term basis. His condition continued to improve, and plans were made for his discharge on the following drug therapy:

Spironolactone 100 mg once daily
Lactulose 15 mL twice daily

13. What points would you cover when counselling Mr N on his take-home drugs?

Answers

1. (a) To relieve Mr N's shortness of breath and general discomfort caused by the presence of ascites;

   (b) to reduce his peripheral oedema;

   (c) to monitor for, and prevent, any symptoms of alcohol withdrawal; and

   (d) to correct any dietary deficiencies Mr N may have.

(a) The presence of tense ascites may be responsible for causing Mr N's shortness of breath by impairing inflation of his lungs. The presence of a pleural effusion, which occurs in approximately ten per cent of patients with cirrhosis and ascites, may also be a cause of shortness of breath and should be excluded by chest x-ray.

Ascites occurs in patients with liver disease because of changes in hepatic and intestinal lymph formation and changes in renal sodium handling. Fluid localises in the peritoneal cavity because of an increase in blood pressure in the portal vein. There are two main theories of ascites formation.

(i) The overflow theory. This suggests that renal retention of sodium and water with expansion of plasma volume is the primary event, and that this results in overflow into the extravascular space

(ii) The underfill theory. This suggests that production of lymph exceeds the rate at which it can be returned to the systemic circulation via the thoracic duct. Lymph then accumulates in the peritoneal cavity and draws out fluid and electrolytes from the plasma compartment. The associated reduction in plasma volume activates the renin-angiotensin-aldosterone system, resulting in renal sodium and water retention.

(b) The osmotic pressure of plasma proteins is an important factor in the retention of fluid in the vascular compartment, and the interchange of fluid between the vascular and tissue compartments depends on a balance between the plasma osmotic pressure and the blood pressure. Peripheral oedema occurs in patients like Mr N with impaired hepatic synthetic function, as this results in reduced synthesis of serum albumin and hence a reduction in plasma albumin and colloid osmotic pressure.

(c) Alcohol has an adverse effect on all tissues and organs of the body, as a result of direct toxicity, concomitant malnutrition, and metabolic derangements induced by the metabolism of ethanol. The extent to which body systems are affected will depend on the duration and volume of alcohol consumption.

(d) Mr N has complained of weakness of the legs and an unstable balance. This could be due to peripheral neuropathy secondary to nutritional deficiencies.

Alcoholics tend to have an inadequate food intake, and a diet that is high in carbohydrate and low in protein, vitamins, and minerals. In addition to a reduced intake, absorption of nutrients such as amino acids, xylose, glucose, vitamins, and minerals may be impaired, owing to alteration of active transport and absorption functions in the intestinal mucosa. Thiamine deficiency may result in the development of Wernicke's syndrome, which is characterised by ocular symptoms, ataxia, and irreversible encephalopathy.

2. Mr N should be prescribed spironolactone, starting at a dose of 100 mg once daily; Parentrovite® Intravenous High Potency, one pair of ampoules once daily for three to seven days; and vitamin K 10 mg intramuscularly, as a single dose.

Diuretic therapy is the treatment of choice for Mr N's ascites. The aim of treatment is to induce a negative sodium and water balance. Some patients may respond to a restriction of dietary sodium intake to 22 mmol per day, but patients like Mr N with moderate or tense ascites should be prescribed a distal tubule potassium-sparing diuretic such as spironolactone, in addition to a restricted sodium intake. Spironolactone is a specific antagonist of aldosterone and should initially be prescribed in a dose of 100 mg per 24 hours, as a single daily dose. Diuresis should occur after three days of therapy. A weight loss of 0.5 kg per day is desirable. The rate of fluid loss from the vascular compartment should not exceed the rate at which fluid can be redistributed from the ascitic compartment. An over-vigorous diuresis will result in hypovolaemia, electrolyte disturbances (including hyponatraemia and uraemia), and a risk of inducing hepatic encephalopathy. Spironolactone may also cause hyperkalaemia.

Mr N's response to spironolactone therapy should be reviewed every two days and, if necessary, the prescribed dose increased by increments of 100 mg to a maximum of 600 mg daily. Spironolactone may be given as a single daily dose unless treatment is limited by gastro-intestinal (GI) side-effects, in which case the daily dose can be divided and administered twice a day. If response to treatment with spironolactone alone is poor, then a loop diuretic may be added to the regimen in the lowest dose to achieve an adequate diuresis. Frusemide, in a starting dose of 40 mg on alternate days, would be appropriate. If combined diuretic therapy does not relieve the ascites, or if Mr N is in pain or in distress because of his shortness of breath, then limited-volume paracentesis may be indicated. This is the removal of a volume of ascites via a cannula inserted into the peritoneal cavity through the abdominal wall.

Supplements of vitamins should be prescribed to replenish Mr N's depleted stores and to reduce the risk of Wernicke's syndrome. High-dose vitamins B and C should be prescribed as Parentrovite Intravenous High Potency, in a dose of one pair of ampoules once a day for three to seven days.

As the Committee on the Safety of Medicines has received reports of adverse effects, including anaphylaxis, following the administration of intravenous and intramuscular Parentrovite, the prescriber and nursing staff should be advised of the risk of potentially serious allergic adverse reactions during or after its administration. For this reason it should be administered by slow intravenous infusion over a period of ten minutes, and facilities for treating anaphylaxis should be available. Nursing staff should be requested to monitor the patient for signs of allergic adverse effects, such as shortness of breath, rashes and flushing.

As Mr N has a prolonged prothrombin time owing to a deficiency in clotting factors produced by the liver, a single 10 mg dose of vitamin K should be administered intramuscularly. However, its usefulness in correcting Mr N's prothrombin time long-term will be limited by the synthetic capacity of his cirrhosed liver.

3. A number of pharmacokinetic and pharmacodynamic factors need to be taken into account when prescribing for Mr N.

It is known that Mr N has cirrhosis of the liver, and this will affect the pharmacokinetics of any drug that is metabolised by that organ. The reduced functional capacity of Mr N's liver is reflected in his low serum albumin level, and prolonged prothrombin time (albumin and clotting factors are produced by the liver).

Although the presence of liver disease will influence pharmacokinetic parameters such as absorption, clearance, volume of distribution, and the extent of hepatic extraction of a drug, it is not possible to predict quantitatively the extent to which these variables will be affected in any one individual.

In cirrhosis of the liver a reduction in hepatic blood flow, and the development of portal-systemic shunts (which divert blood from the liver to the systemic circulation), result in an increased bioavailability of drugs that are highly extracted on first pass through the liver (flow-limited drugs). Peak plasma concentrations of such drugs will thus be increased and half-life will be prolonged. This may necessitate a reduction in dose, and/or lengthening of the dosage interval.

In cirrhosis, where necrosis or fibrosis has resulted in disruption of the normal cellular structure of the liver, there is a reduction in hepatic cell mass and a corresponding reduction in the functional capacity of the liver. The consequence of this is again an increase in the bioavailability of drugs with a high extraction ratio, owing to a reduction in first-pass metabolism. Reduced functional capacity, and therefore delayed elimination from the systemic circulation, will also prolong the half-life of drugs with low hepatic extraction (capacity-limited drugs), which are dependent on the functional capacity of the liver for their clearance. In such cases adjustment of the dosing interval will be necessary to avoid toxicity on repeated dosing.

Mr N's low plasma albumin will also result in reduced plasma protein binding of drugs, which in turn will increase the concentration of free, active drug. In the presence of reduced hepatic blood flow, the bioavailability of drugs with a high hepatic extraction will be increased. For drugs that are poorly extracted by the liver at first pass, bioavailability will depend on the capacity of the liver to metabolise that drug. If liver function is not impaired, the increase in free drug concentration due to reduced protein binding will only be temporary, as a new equilibrium will develop.

In addition to pharmacokinetic variations there are also pharmacodynamic variations in drug handling in patients with liver disease, which result in an increase in the patient's cerebral sensitivity to drugs with sedative and hypnotic effects. Because of this, drugs with cerebral depressant activity should only be prescribed with caution to patients with severe liver disease, as there is a risk of precipitating hepatic encephalopathy.

4. Chlormethiazole is the drug of choice for Mr N.

The alcohol withdrawal syndrome occurs after abrupt cessation of heavy alcohol intake. If untreated it may progress from the mild symptoms of tremulousness, anorexia, nausea, vomiting, increased heart rate, increased blood pressure, and raised respiratory rate, through to hyperactivity, insomnia, auditory and visual hallucinations, and then to seizures and delirium tremens. Delirium tremens is a dangerous state of disorientation characterised by marked tremor, extreme agitation requiring restraint, confusion, hallucinations, paranoia, and extreme autonomic hyperactivity (tachycardia, fever, sweating, tachypnoea). Death due to shock, hyperpyrexia, arrhythmias, infection or injury may ultimately ensue.

Not all patients will develop symptoms of alcohol withdrawal, and in many the symptoms will be mild and will resolve within a few days. Although Mr N only admitted to drinking "the odd pint", it was noted on his admission that he did smell of alcohol, which suggests that his consumption was higher than this. The possibility of Mr N developing full-blown alcohol withdrawal syndrome must thus be considered and treatment with a sedative drug should be initiated.

Either chlormethiazole or a benzodiazepine could be prescribed for Mr N. Both drugs are sedative and have anticonvulsant properties. However, in the presence of cirrhosis, chlormethiazole is preferable to a benzodiazepine for the suppression of the symptoms of alcohol withdrawal. Benzodiazepines are capacity-limited drugs and are protein-bound to a greater extent than chlormethiazole. Diazepam and chlordiazepoxide both have half-lives greater than 24 hours, so the risks of accumulation of the drug, and hence over-sedation in Mr N, need to be considered. Chlormethiazole is a flow-limited drug which is extensively cleared on first pass through the liver. Peak plasma concentrations of the drug will be higher in patients with cirrhosis, and there is a risk of accumulation on repeated dosing; however, the half-life of this drug (3–4 hours) is shorter than the benzodiazepines, which means that the dose can be more easily adjusted according to the patient's response. The ideal dose of chlormethiazole will suppress the symptoms of alcohol withdrawal by keeping Mr N lightly sedated and easily rousable.

Chlormethiazole should be prescribed in a reducing dose over a short time period, in order to reduce the risk of Mr N switching from an alcohol-dependent state to a sedative-dependent one. The regimen outlined in the manufacturer's data sheet should be followed, with close monitoring of Mr N's response, and dosage adjustments made accordingly. Chlormethiazole may be administered by intravenous infusion if oral therapy is inappropriate. Intravenous administration of the drug will bypass the first-pass elimination by the liver, so lower doses will be required. The rate of administration should be titrated according to the patient's response.

5. Mr N's diuretic therapy should be monitored both clinically and biochemically.

Clinical monitoring parameters include daily weights, fluid balance, and girth measurements, in addition to the routine monitoring of temperature, pulse, and respiration. The aim of the diuretic therapy is to induce a negative fluid balance, which will be reflected in weight loss.

Serum biochemistry should be monitored closely for electrolyte abnormalities, such as hyperkalaemia and hyponatraemia, and for signs of acute renal failure, such as raised serum creatinine and urea.

Baseline urinary sodium and potassium levels should be measured and then repeated twice a week, to confirm that the prescribed dose of diuretic has increased the urinary sodium output. In secondary hyperaldosteronism, sodium reabsorption from the distal tubule of the kidney is high, and potassium reabsorption is low. In the presence of an aldosterone antagonist, urinary sodium levels should increase if this exchange is being effectively inhibited, so the urinary sodium to potassium ratio should increase. If the ratio does not increase, the dose of potassium-sparing diuretic should be increased with continued monitoring of Mr N's serum electrolyte status.

6. Reduce the dose of spironolactone to 200 mg once daily, and add frusemide 40 mg on alternate days.

Although Mr N is showing a satisfactory weight loss and reduction in ascitic fluid volume, the high dose of spironolactone is inducing electrolyte abnormalities. The diuretic regimen needs to be adjusted to maintain a satisfactory rate of fluid loss without causing hypovolaemia and the associated electrolyte disturbances. Although loop diuretics are not suitable for the first-line treatment of ascites, owing to their tendency to cause electrolyte disturbances, it is appropriate at this time to reduce the dose of spironolactone, as this is probably causing Mr N's elevated serum potassium level, and to add a small dose of frusemide, which is a potassium-losing loop diuretic.

7. Factors that might precipitate hepatic encephalopathy in cirrhotic patients include hypokalaemia (which may be secondary to over-diuresis or diarrhoea and vomiting), GI haemorrhage, infection, inappropriate use of sedatives, alcohol excess, and increased dietary protein intake.

In the presence of a normal serum biochemistry, Mr N's present condition was probably precipitated by an alcoholic binge.

8. (a) To reduce the nitrogen load on the GI tract, and

(b) to correct any metabolic or electrolyte disturbance that may arise.

Hepatic encephalopathy is a metabolic disorder of the central nervous system which occurs in patients with acute or chronic liver disease in the presence or absence of portal-systemic shunting of blood. It is characterized by disturbed consciousness, personality changes, intellectual deterioration, slow speech, asterixis (a flapping tremor of the hands which can be induced by the patient fully extending his arms and flexing his wrists upwards), and fetor hepaticus (a sweet, musty odour on the breath).

The disorder is due to cerebral intoxication by nitrogenous compounds produced by bacteria in the GI tract. In the presence of poor hepato-cellular function, nitrogenous compounds in the portal venous blood pass into the systemic circulation without being metabolised by the liver, and cross the blood-brain barrier. In the early stages the changes in mental function are reversible, suggesting that the disorder is due to biochemical rather than organic disturbances. Several nitrogenous compounds have been implicated as causes of hepatic encephalopathy: they include ammonia, mercaptans, false neurotransmitters, and fatty acids.

9. Lactulose has been prescribed to reduce the nitrogen load on the GI tract.

GI bleeding, dietary protein intake, and constipation all contribute to the nitrogen load on the GI tract. In the absence of any clinical signs of GI bleeding, which should be treated, nitrogen production by the intestinal flora should be reduced. This can be achieved by prescribing drugs that alter the gut flora and decrease GI transit time.

Lactulose is the drug of choice. It is a disaccharide which is converted to lactic, acetic, and formic acids by the intestinal bacteria, thus changing the pH of the intestinal contents from 7 to 5. This acidic pH reduces the absorption of non-ionised ammonia and creates an environment more suitable for the growth of weak ammonia-producing organisms, such as *Lactobacillus acidophilus*, rather than proteolytic ammonia-producing organisms such as *Escherichia coli*. The osmotic laxative effect of lactulose also speeds intestinal transit and so prevents constipation, thereby reducing the time available for the absorption of potentially toxic nitrogenous compounds.

The dose of lactulose should be 30–50 mL three times a day, titrated such that frequent soft motions are produced without diarrhoea. Diarrhoea may result in excessive water and potassium loss from the gut and should be avoided, as dehydration and hypokalaemia may exacerbate Mr N's clinical condition. Lactulose, administered orally, takes two to three days to become effective. Thus, before it exerts its laxative effect, the bowel should be cleared of nitrogen-containing material by the administration of a magnesium sulphate enema.

10. Neomycin may also be prescribed to alter the gut flora in patients with hepatic encephalopathy.

Neomycin may be prescribed as sole therapy, or as an alternative to lactulose (if lactulose is ineffective or not tolerated by Mr N), or in addition to lactulose (when it exerts an additive effect).

Neomycin is a more toxic agent than lactulose. It is absorbed to a small extent. One to three per cent of an orally administered dose is absorbed and may accumulate in patients with compromised renal function. This may result in oto- and nephrotoxicity. Serum creatinine and creatinine clearance should thus be monitored in patients receiving neomycin. Neomycin also decreases the absorption of oral digoxin, penicillin and vitamin K; the latter may be significant in a patient like Mr N who has prolonged clotting times due to reduced hepatocellular function.

Lactulose is the drug of choice for altering the gut flora, but if Mr N's mental function does not improve on lactulose alone then neomycin, in a dose of 1 g four times a day, may be added to the regimen with close monitoring of his renal function.

11. A protein-free diet has been requested because dietary protein contributes to the nitrogen load in the GI tract.

In hepatic encephalopathy all dietary protein should be stopped. When Mr N's clinical condition improves, dietary protein can be re-introduced gradually in increments of 20 g per day, with close monitoring of mental function until a limit of tolerance is reached.

Since Mr N's condition of alcoholic cirrhosis is a chronic one, his dietary protein intake will need to be restricted in the long term to prevent a relapse into an encephalopathic state.

12. Bromocriptine.

Studies have been undertaken to try to demonstrate the effectiveness of bromocriptine and levodopa in the treatment of hepatic encephalopathy. The rationale behind this is the theory that false neurotransmitters accumulate in the brain of patients with cirrhosis and portal-systemic shunting of blood, and displace the active neurotransmitters, dopamine and noradrenaline. Thus, administration of dopamine or dopamine agonists could theoretically reverse this process. Levodopa therapy, limited by side-effects of GI irritation and nausea, has been demonstrated to be ineffective in the treatment of hepatic encephalopathy. Bromocriptine has been shown to be effective in a small number of patients, but its side-effects of sedation, altered liver function tests, constipation, and GI irritation limit its application in this condition. Bromocriptine could be reserved for the treatment of patients unresponsive to other therapies.

13. (a) Spironolactone.

Mr N should be counselled on the importance of continuing his spironolactone therapy and of ensuring that he always has a supply of tablets. He should be advised to take his single daily dose at the same time each day, preferably in the morning, with breakfast, or if he forgets this, at lunchtime. He should be advised against doubling his dose if he forgets to take the tablet for a whole day.

(b) Lactulose.

Although Mr N should continue with a maintenance dose of lactulose to avoid constipation, it could be explained that the dose may be varied to suit his needs, such that he passes regular soft motions. If he has diarrhoea for any reason, he should discontinue the lactulose and contact his doctor.

(c) General.

Mr N should be advised not to take aspirin, or any preparations containing aspirin, because these "irritate the stomach". He may take paracetamol as a simple analgesic occasionally. If regular analgesia is required he should be advised to consult his doctor.

Although Mr N is not on a low-sodium diet, he should be limiting his sodium intake. He should be made aware that over-the-counter indigestion remedies contain a lot of "salt", and that he should ask his pharmacist to recommend a "salt-free" preparation if necessary.

References and Further Reading

Dodds L., Alcoholic liver disease 1: control of acute alcohol withdrawal, *Pharm. J.*, 1986, **237**, 296–298.

Dodds L., Alcoholic liver disease 2: treatment of hepatic encephalopathy, *ibid.*, 549–551.

Gee J.P., Jim L.K. and Kradjan W.A., Hepatic disorders, Part II: Alcoholic cirrhosis, in *Applied Therapeutics – the Clinical Use of Drugs*, 4th edn, Young L.Y. and Koda-Kimble M.A. (eds), Vancouver, WA, Applied Therapeutics, 1988, 501–507.

Panos M. and Williams R., Ascites in cirrhosis: pathophysiology and management, *Br. J. Hosp. Med.*, 1988, **40**, 256–262.

Sherlock S., *Diseases of the Liver and Biliary System*, 7th edn, Oxford, Blackwell Scientific, 1985.

ASTHMA

Mark G. Horsley

Principal Pharmacist (Clinical Services), Kings Mill Hospital, Sutton-in-Ashfield, Nottinghamshire

Day 1 (6 a.m.) Miss V, a 16-year-old schoolgirl, was admitted as an emergency by her general practitioner (GP), with severe shortness of breath. She was accompanied by her anxious parents, with whom she lived. The initial history came from the parents, as Miss V was too breathless to speak.

Miss V had developed both atopic eczema and bronchial asthma in infancy. The eczema had completely subsided; however, the asthma had continued to require regular treatment. Her parents were disappointed by this, and they felt she should have "grown out of it". They stated that the asthma had been quite well controlled over the years, only occasionally causing time off school, and had never required hospital admission.

Miss V had never suffered with hay fever or nasal polyps. The family had owned a cat at one time, but skin-prick testing had confirmed that Miss V may have been allergic to it, and that it could have been worsening the asthma, so they now kept no pets. Miss V had no known drug allergies and never smoked cigarettes. She had no brothers or sisters and neither of her parents had asthma; however, her father suffered from hay fever.

Her usual medication was: sodium cromoglycate 20 mg Spincaps®, inhaled through a Spinhaler® four times a day; and salbutamol inhaler (100 micrograms per inhalation), two puffs when needed. This regimen usually enabled Miss V to lead an active life, although she did need to use the salbutamol for mild wheezing in cold weather and prior to the games period at school. Her parents felt that she had been well in recent weeks and the present attack was "out of the blue". However, on direct questioning they admitted that their daughter had been waking most nights during the previous few weeks with a dry cough, and a tight chest, but that this had always responded promptly to the salbutamol inhaler.

The previous night Miss V's mother had been awakened by her coughing at 2.30 a.m. Miss V had been very wheezy and her chest felt tight. Several doses of inhaled salbutamol and sodium cromoglycate were tried with no effect.

The GP was called at 3.15 a.m. He confirmed that Miss V was suffering from an asthma attack, and administered 5 mg of salbutamol using a nebuliser driven by a foot pump. This seemed to produce some improvement in symptoms but the effects only lasted for 30 minutes. A second dose produced no improvement, so an ambulance was summoned.

On examination in hospital Miss V appeared distressed, with a rapid respiratory rate, and an audible wheeze. She was unable to speak and appeared cyanosed. She had coughed up a small amount of yellow sputum. On auscultation her chest had reduced air entry on both sides with widespread rhonchi. There were no areas of consolidation. Her pulse was 120 beats per minute and regular, and her blood pressure was 140/85 mmHg with 25 mm of paradox. She was apyrexial. Her peak expiratory flow rate (PEFR) was 80 L/min.

An arterial blood sample was sent for urgent blood gas analysis, and an urgent portable chest x-ray was ordered. The resulting chest film showed no evidence of either pneumothorax or pneumonia.

Her blood gases on room air were:

PaO_2 6.1 kPa (reference range 12.0–14.6)
$PaCO_2$ 4.1 kPa (4.5–6.0)
pH 7.45 (7.35–7.45)
HCO_3 21 mmol/L (22–26)

Miss V was promptly started on 35% oxygen. An intravenous line was inserted and a normal saline infusion commenced. The following drug therapy was prescribed:

Hydrocortisone 200 mg intravenously immediately, then 200 mg four times a day (every six hours)
Salbutamol (nebulised), 5 mg six times a day (every four hours)

Ipratropium bromide (nebulised), 500 micrograms
    four times a day
Ampicillin 500 mg intravenously, four times a day

1. What are the important features in assessing the severity of an asthma attack? How bad is this particular attack?

2. Was the therapy administered by Miss V's GP appropriate? What other measures could he have taken?

3. What advice would you have given to Miss V and her parents if they had asked you for help during the acute attack, pending the arrival of the GP?

4. Were the parents right to expect Miss V to grow out of her asthma?

5. What would have been the significance of a history of nasal polyps?

6. Were the treatments written up for Miss V on the ward appropriate? If not, what would you have recommended?

7. What administration parameters should be considered in order to ensure safe, effective delivery of her nebulised drugs?

8. What are the most important parameters to monitor over the first few hours of therapy?

9. How quickly can a response to the prescribed therapy be anticipated?

Day 1 (8.30 a.m.) Miss V was not responding well to initial treatment. Although less cyanosed on the oxygen, her PEFR was now unrecordable.

Repeat blood gases on 35% oxygen showed:

PaO_2 7.7 kPa (12.0–14.6)
$PaCO_2$ 4.5 kPa (4.5–6.0)
pH 7.43 (7.35–7.45)
HCO_3 22 mmol/L (22–26)

It was decided to prescribe intravenous broncho-dilator therapy, and the intensive care unit was alerted in case she became exhausted and needed ventilating.

10. What are the therapeutic options for intra-venous bronchodilator therapy? Which would you recommend, and why? What would be an appropriate dosage regimen for your drug of choice?

Day 2 Miss V was much improved, sitting up in bed, talking, and even asking when she could go home. Her PEFR had climbed to 200 L/min, although it had dropped back to 120 L/min at 6 a.m., prior to the first drug dose from the

nebuliser. She was also complaining of a fine tremor.

During the day, the intravenous bronchodilator was tailed off and her drip was taken down. The hydrocortisone therapy was discontinued, and she was commenced on oral prednisolone 50 mg each morning. The oxygen was also discontinued.

11. Would you have recommended that her intravenous bronchodilator be continued by the oral route?

Day 4 Miss V continued to improve her PEFR, though with wide fluctuations through the day. She now felt "back to normal", apart from a fine tremor, and could not understand why she was being kept in hospital. The prednisolone was reduced to 30 mg each day and the nebulised salbutamol therapy was reduced to four times a day (every six hours).

Miss V asked the ward pharmacist if it would be possible for her to have a nebuliser at home, as she felt that she would not have needed hospital admission if a nebuliser had been available.

12. Would you recommend a home nebuliser for Miss V?

13. Why is it not yet appropriate to discharge Miss V?

Day 5 It was decided to convert Miss V from nebulised to inhaled drug therapy when her PEFR stabilised.

14. What inhaled bronchodilator drug(s) would you recommend, and what dosage regimens would be appropriate?

15. Would you recommend introducing inhaled steroids at this point?

Day 6 The PEFR stabilised at between 300 and 350 L/min. The nebulised drugs were discontinued and Miss V was written up for:

Salbutamol inhaler (100 micrograms per inhalation), two puffs four times a day and when needed
Beclomethasone dipropionate inhaler (100 micrograms per inhalation), two puffs four times a day
Prednisolone 20 mg each morning

Arrangements were made provisionally to dis-charge her on day 7, provided that her peak flow readings remained stable.

16. How can the side-effects from her inhaled steroids be minimised?

17. What would be a suitable "tailing-off" regimen for Miss V's oral steroid therapy?

The ward pharmacist interviewed Miss V to confirm that she would use the medicines appropriately at home. On checking her inhaler technique, this was found to be erratic. She often failed to co-ordinate inhalation with activation of the inhaler, and spray could be seen escaping from her mouth. Despite the pharmacist's best efforts at demonstrating the correct method, her technique remained poor.

18. *How common is poor technique with pressurised aerosol inhalers?*

19. *What alternative devices are available? Which would you recommend for Miss V?*

20. *What general points would you cover when counselling Miss V on her discharge medication?*

Answers

1. Miss V is experiencing an asthma attack of life-threatening severity. This fact is reflected in many features of her presentation.

From the patient's point of view, the most reliable indicator of the severity of an attack is the response to their regular inhaled bronchodilator, in this case salbutamol. For most patients, two puffs provide relief from a mild attack for at least four hours. As the attack progresses, relief may still be complete but the duration of response is reduced. The patient finds themself using the inhaler more frequently. If the attack progresses further, response becomes partial, and transient. In severe acute asthma the response to standard dose bronchodilators is lost completely. This was true in Miss V's case.

From the doctor's point of view, a very good assessment of the severity of the attack can be made clinically without the need for investigations. The degree of dyspnoea can be assessed semi-quantitatively from the ability to speak: so, two-word breathlessness is worse than four-word breathlessness, and so on. Tachycardia and cyanosis are both signs that the patient's arterial oxygen tension is significantly reduced; this only occurs in severe attacks. Paradox is the change in blood pressure between inspiration and expiration. It is due to changes in intra-thoracic pressure and implies severe airflow obstruction. Miss V exhibited all of these clinical features, thus indicating that her asthma attack was of life-threatening severity.

PEFR measurement is the most convenient way of estimating airways calibre. It has been shown to correlate well with symptoms in asthmatics. The predicted normal PEFR for a female of Miss V's age and of average height would be 430 L/min. The minimum recordable flow on most metres is 60 L/min. Miss V's PEFR on admission (80 L/min) demonstrates severe airflow obstruction.

2. The nebulised bronchodilator therapy was appropriate, but Miss V would also have benefited from intravenous corticosteroid therapy.

The nebulised salbutamol administered by the GP was a very appropriate treatment. A nebuliser delivers the drug to the airways reliably and does not require any particular technique from the patient, or even much co-operation. The foot pump means that the GP can give nebulised drugs anywhere, even in the absence of an electricity supply.

The much higher dose of salbutamol delivered by the nebuliser will often produce a response where lower doses from a pressurised aerosol fail. This is because in an asthma attack of moderate severity the dose-response curve to bronchodilators is moved to the right; this means that substantially higher doses are required before bronchodilation occurs.

If the GP had not had a nebuliser available for bronchodilator administration, a reasonable alternative would have been to give terbutaline 500 micrograms subcutaneously. Bolus doses of intravenous aminophylline are still sometimes used by GPs in these circumstances; however, they are inconvenient to administer and relatively toxic. Intravenous aminophylline should be reserved for administration in hospital.

One point where the GP could be criticised is for not giving any corticosteroids to Miss V. While high-dose bronchodilators will reverse an exacerbation of moderate severity, in a severe attack such as that suffered by Miss V, bronchospasm is not the most important component of the airflow obstruction. Inflammation of the airways with oedema, infiltration, and mucus plugging are all involved in the severe attack. None of these factors are reversed by bronchodilators. In addition, delays in the administration of steroids to this group of patients have been implicated as a preventable cause of mortality. It is likely that Miss V would have been easier to treat, and her hospital stay reduced, if she had been given steroid therapy earlier.

3. (a) Take extra doses of inhaled bronchodilator, using a spacer device if available, and

(b) discontinue the use of inhaled sodium cromoglycate.

Miss V and her parents have taken the most important step by realising from the lack of response to the salbutamol inhaler that they are "out of their depth" and that prompt medical assistance is required. Unfortunately, many preventable asthma deaths occur each year because the family either fail to recognise the severity of the attack or believe that they will get over it if they "brave it out". There is a natural reluctance to call out the doctor in the night, but it is a fact that this is when most severe asthma attacks occur.

During such an attack, it is a reasonable idea to give extra doses of any inhaled bronchodilator available. This is perfectly safe: the doses involved are very low when compared, for instance, with nebuliser therapy. Warnings on some inhalers that it is "dangerous to exceed the stated dose" are inappropriate. The main problem with inhaled bronchodilator therapy is that acute breathlessness is likely to interfere with even the most reliable inhaler technique. A ten-second breath hold, for instance, will be completely impossible. Thus the effectiveness of the inhaler is reduced. One way to overcome this is to use large-volume spacer devices. The Nebuhaler® has been shown to be effective in administering terbutaline in these circumstances. A somewhat cruder alternative, which has been reported as being effective in small children, is to use a disposable plastic cup with a hole in the bottom.

By contrast, administration of extra doses of preventative medications, such as inhaled cromoglycate or inhaled steroids, at this late stage is not advisable. They act too slowly to be effective, and the effect of the particles hitting the inflamed airways is to produce paroxysms of coughing.

Finally, is should be noted that, although Miss V is anxious and agitated, this is because acute asthma is a very unpleasant experience. It would be wrong to conclude that "nerves" had brought on the attack. Any attempt to sedate Miss V would be inappropriate and dangerous.

4. No.

Extrinsic or allergic asthma of childhood is at least twice as common in boys as it is in girls. This sex difference is not apparent in adult asthmatics. For boys it can be confidently predicted that their asthma will disappear, or at least improve substantially, at puberty; however, fewer girls grow out of their asthma completely. Those who have mild symptoms not requiring regular treatment have the best chance, but early age of onset and concomitant severe infantile eczema carry a poor prognosis. It is wrong to raise falsely the expectations of girls who have troublesome asthma about improvements at puberty.

5. Miss V may be sensitive to aspirin.

In asthma sufferers, a history of nasal polyps is strongly associated with aspirin sensitivity; however, this is less common in childhood asthmatics than it is in late-onset asthma. In aspirin-sensitive individuals, an asthma attack is typically provoked half to one hour after a dose of aspirin. It would appear to be a pharmacologically mediated adverse reaction, related to the blockade of prostaglandin synthesis. It has been proposed that arachidonic acid metabolism is diverted to produce excess leukotrienes, and that these are responsible for the exacerbation. This view is supported by the fact that similar adverse reactions have been reported with ibuprofen and indomethacin. This adverse reaction should be taken seriously by pharmacists, as deaths have been reported even from over-the-counter products. A history of nasal polyps should always

be sought, by direct questioning, of any asthmatic being considered for therapy with aspirin or other non-steroidal anti-inflammatory drug.

6. Treatment was appropriate, except in the case of the antibiotic therapy.

At partial pressures of oxygen of less than 8 kPa, haemoglobin becomes increasingly unsaturated, cyanosis becomes clinically evident, and oxygen delivery to the tissues is reduced. It is hypoxia that may eventually produce a cardio-respiratory arrest and death in these individuals. It is therefore essential to give Miss V oxygen, preferably at high concentrations.

Owing to her prolonged period of hyperventilation, and being too breathless to drink, Miss V is at risk of dehydration. This is particularly undesirable, as it may thicken bronchial secretions and delay their clearance. The intravenous saline infusion corrects this problem and also allows access for intravenous drugs.

Intravenous steroids are essential, for the reasons outlined in answer 2.

Beta$_2$-adrenoceptor stimulants are the most effective and rapidly acting bronchodilators. The nebulised route is as effective as the intravenous route in most patients, and carries less risk of side-effects.

Nebulised ipratropium bromide is probably less effective than salbutamol as a single agent. However, with its anticholinergic mode of action it appears to offer some additional bronchodilation, when given in combination with salbutamol in severe acute asthma. This is evidenced by a greater rise in PEFRs over the first few hours. In the past, this benefit has had to be weighed against the propensity of nebulised ipratropium to produce paradoxical bronchospasm in a small number of patients. This problem appears to have been eliminated since the manufacturer reformulated the solution for nebulisation to make it isotonic and preservative-free.

There is no evidence that Miss V's asthma attack was caused by an infection. She is apyrexial and there is no sign of consolidation, either clinically or on the chest x-ray. The yellow sputum she expectorated is likely to be due to sputum eosinophilia rather than infection. There is no value in the routine administration of antibiotics to asthmatics unless there is other evidence of infection. The prescription of ampicillin for Miss V is therefore inappropriate and should be challenged.

7. Two factors need to be considered when using a jet nebuliser: firstly, the driving gas and its flow rate must be chosen; secondly, the drug must be

diluted to the correct fill volume using an appropriate diluent.

The choice of driving gas for a jet nebuliser lies between compressed air from an electrical compressor, or oxygen, either from a cylinder or piped onto the ward. As Miss V is hypoxic and there is no evidence of respiratory depression it makes sense to use oxygen to drive the nebuliser.

The flow rate of the driving gas affects the droplet size of the mist produced, and the time taken to nebulise a particular volume of solution. As a rule of thumb, doubling the flow rate halves the droplet size. The bulk of the droplets must be below 5 μm in diameter in order to be deposited in the conducting airways. For most brands of nebuliser in clinical use, an oxygen flow rate of at least 6 L/min is necessary to produce an optimum droplet size. A high flow rate also has the advantage of minimising the time taken to nebulise the dose.

Nebuliser administration is usually continued "to dryness", that is, when no more mist is produced. In fact some drug solution is left behind, trapped on the plastic of the nebuliser. This dead volume (between 0.6 and 1.0 mL, depending on the brand of nebuliser) is not available to the patient. Therefore, if an attempt is made to nebulise a low volume of solution (for example, 1 mL), an unacceptably low fraction of the dose will reach the patient. Thus it is necessary to dilute the solution to increase the fill volume and maximise the fraction of drug reaching the patient. In the hospital setting, a fill volume of 4–5 mL is optimal; this releases approximately 80% of the dose, without producing an excessively long administration time.

When necessary, dilution of the solution should always be with normal saline rather than water. This is because nebulisation of hypotonic solutions may provoke bronchospasm in asthmatics. Although not specifically recommended by the manufacturers, it is acceptable to mix salbutamol and ipratropium in the same nebuliser, provided they are then administered immediately. This reduces the need for a diluent in patients who are being given combination therapy, and is more convenient.

8. Pulse, respiratory rate, and blood gases are the most important parameters to monitor over the first few hours. PEFR is the most important over the following days.

Frequent reassessment is essential in severe acute asthma, as rapid deterioration leading to death is a real possibility. Arterial blood gases must be checked initially and repeated to ensure that hypoxia has been controlled. The PaO_2 should be maintained at at least 8 kPa. Miss V's $PaCO_2$ was initially low/normal; a rising $PaCO_2$ should be viewed with alarm unless she is obviously improving. Although a young asthmatic such as Miss V will not have a depressed respiratory centre, severe airflow obstruction may lead to fatigue of the respiratory muscles after several hours; thus, a rising $PaCO_2$ may indicate exhaustion and is an indication of the need for artificial ventilation.

Pulse rate and respiratory rate should also be checked frequently. They should both fall if Miss V is improving. PEFR is less important in the severely ill patient, who may not be able to co-operate with the test. However, it becomes the most useful monitoring parameter during the recovery phase.

9. Inhaled beta$_2$-adrenoceptor stimulants, such as salbutamol, start to exert their effect almost immediately, reaching peak bronchodilation at 15 minutes. Ipratropium is slower, taking 30–45 minutes to reach peak effect. However, in a very severe case, such as Miss V, response to both drugs may be minimal. Corticosteroids, when given alone, take six hours to produce an improvement in PEFR, even when given intravenously. However, they can improve the response of the airways to bronchodilators at one hour after administration.

10. The choice lies between infusions of aminophylline or of a beta$_2$-adrenoceptor stimulant, such as salbutamol. There is not enough evidence to say which is the drug of choice for Miss V. Either intravenous aminophylline or intravenous salbutamol would be appropriate.

Aminophylline is the most widely used drug in these circumstances. Although its pharmacokinetics are now well understood, and allow for individualised dosage regimens, its effectiveness in severe acute asthma is not well proven. A meta-analysis of aminophylline trials in severe acute asthma was published in 1988. The conclusion was that aminophylline alone was inferior to beta$_2$-adrenoceptor stimulant therapy. Additionally, there was only a non-significant trend towards the combination of beta$_2$-adrenoceptor stimulant plus aminophylline therapy being superior to beta$_2$-adrenoceptor stimulant alone. All of the published trials compared obsolete regimens for beta$_2$-adrenoceptor stimulants.

The toxicity of aminophylline, however, is not in doubt. Numerous reports exist of vomiting, arrhythmias, convulsions, and deaths due to toxic levels of theophylline. These can only be avoided by care in individualisation of the dose.

Miss V has no history of theophylline ingestion. She can therefore be given a full loading dose of 6 mg/kg. She weighs around 50 kg, so the dose of aminophylline should be 300 mg, given as an infusion over 15 minutes. This loading dose should be followed by a continuous maintenance infusion of 0.6 mg/kg/hour. A maintenance dose of 30 mg/ hour would be appropriate for Miss V. This infusion rate may be a little conservative as, on average, adolescents have higher theophylline clearance than adults. Serum theophylline levels should ideally be checked half-an-hour after the loading dose, and again at around twelve hours into the infusion, to ensure that they are within the therapeutic range (10–20 mg/L). However, unless the results are available within a few hours, it is an academic exercise. There is no need to discontinue any of Miss V's other bronchodilator therapies when aminophylline is added.

Beta$_2$-adrenoceptor stimulant therapy has until recently been regarded as being no more effective when given intravenously than when given by nebuliser. However, this has been challenged by Cheong and co-workers. Their trial demonstrated increased effectiveness of intravenous salbutamol over nebulised salbutamol at the expense of some side-effects.

If this option is followed, Miss V should be started on an infusion of 8 micrograms/min. This dose can be adjusted up or down according to response. Some patients will respond to doses as low as 4 micrograms/min, whereas infusions of 12.5 micrograms/min (the dose used by Cheong) will be necessary in other patients. No loading dose is usually given, because of the short half-life of salbutamol. The main side-effect to monitor for is tachycardia, which may be severe and necessitate dosage reduction or even discontinuation of the infusion.

Potassium chloride (2 g) should routinely be added to the infusion fluids, as intravenous beta$_2$-adrenoceptor stimulants may cause a fall in serum potassium of up to 0.5 mmol/L by driving potassium into cells. Miss V should have her nebulised salbutamol discontinued during the infusion; however, the nebulised ipratropium should be continued.

Current evidence is insufficient to say categorically which of these options is better for Miss V. Either intravenous aminophylline or intravenous salbutamol is a reasonable alternative. The best advice in severe acute asthma is to reassess the patient frequently and, if the current therapy is not producing an adequate response, to try something different.

11. No. Inhaled bronchodilators will most likely be adequate during the recovery phase and long-term.

The most useful feature of oral sustained-release bronchodilators is their long duration of action. This enables a night-time dose to control nocturnal and early morning bronchospasm. Miss V appears to have this problem, judging by the morning dip in her PEFR; however, this is also a feature of the recovery phase from a severe acute attack, which is likely to improve after a few days or weeks anyway.

Sustained-release theophylline (the active component of aminophylline) has a proven track record of long-term effectiveness in preventing asthma attacks and in helping nocturnal symptoms, but it is inconvenient, requiring serum level monitoring to ensure optimum effect while avoiding toxicity. However, it is still the drug of choice if an oral bronchodilator is required. Miss V could be started on theophylline if her morning dipping persists.

Sustained-release beta$_2$-adrenoceptor stimulants have, until recently, been less effective than theophylline in preventing nocturnal symptoms. This was probably because of the inadequate duration of action of the available formulations. However, products have become available recently that use a laser-drilled osmotic release mechanism (e.g. Volmax®). Such products release salbutamol over nine hours, which is adequate to achieve good overnight levels. They also require less monitoring than theophylline therapy, but more research is required to establish their long-term effectiveness. There must be some concern as to whether tolerance will be a problem with these products.

12. No.

This type of request from a patient is not uncommon. Patients are often impressed by the "high-tech" look of the equipment and the instant relief it provides. They also tend to regard the nebuliser as the most important reason for their recovery in hospital. Much of the recent expansion in home nebuliser use has been demand-led by patients.

However, there are a number of problems with home nebulisers. Probably the most obvious are the expense of the equipment and its relative lack of portability. Other problems include an increase in side-effects, owing to the larger doses of drugs employed. Also, Miss V may be tempted to discontinue her preventative treatment in favour of irregular use of the nebuliser, thus worsening control of her asthma. A final reason for denying a home nebuliser is that patients may use repeated doses from their nebuliser in the face of worsening symptoms, and fail to summon medical attention in time.

There are very few asthmatics for whom the provision of a home nebuliser is justified. The largest group is of young children who cannot co-operate with other inhaler devices. These patients usually receive their preventative treatment through the nebuliser, in addition to bronchodilator therapy. In older children and adults with asthma, a nebuliser should only be recommended where all other inhaler devices have failed, and preventative treatment has been maximised. This is clearly not true in the case of Miss V. In addition, nebulisers should only be used along with regular monitoring of PEFR at home.

13. Miss V's airways are still very unstable and she is still on nebulised drugs.

During the recovery phase from severe acute asthma the PEFR is the most important monitoring parameter. In Miss V's case, although the PEFR is improving, it still shows wide fluctuations; this demonstrates that her airways are still very hyper-reactive. Even a mild irritant stimulus could pro-voke severe bronchoconstriction. In this state, discharge would be risky. There is an increased risk of death from asthma for three weeks after dis-charge from hospital for a previous severe attack. This may be due to this hyper-reactivity.

The second problem with immediate discharge is that she is still on regular nebuliser therapy. It is bad practice to re-start an asthmatic on their inhalers as they are discharged. The dose delivered from an inhaler is often less than 10% of that delivered by the nebuliser. A few patients are very dependent on the high dose administered by the nebuliser, and their PEFR will drop markedly when the nebulised bronchodilators are withdrawn. This is a problem if it occurs at home and can lead to readmission. Patients should be converted back to inhalers and their nebuliser therapy discontinued at least 24 h before discharge.

14. Salbutamol inhaler 100 micrograms, two puffs four times a day and when needed.

Beta$_2$-adrenoceptor stimulant bronchodilators are the most rapidly effective agents available for stable asthma. They cause few side-effects, the commonest being a fine tremor for a few minutes following the dose. In stable asthma they are effective for up to six hours. Extra doses can be taken prior to exercise, and to deal with any mild wheezing. There is little to choose between salbuta-mol, terbutaline and fenoterol. However, the avail-able fenoterol inhaler delivers a higher dose; this makes it appear longer-acting at the expense of an increased degree of tremor.

Ipratropium, though of great value during a severe attack, is of less use in chronic stable asthma. It is slower to act than beta$_2$-adrenoceptor stimu-lants and less able to prevent exercise-induced symptoms. Only a small fraction of patients benefit from it. Therefore it should be discontinued once Miss V's acute attack is over, unless reversibility testing indicates that benefit is still being achieved.

15. Yes.

Inhaled steroids should be the mainstay in the prevention of further asthma attacks in Miss V. They have the advantage of reducing airway inflam-mation, and hence reducing hyper-reactivity. Inhaled steroid therapy should replace the inhaled cromoglycate therapy she was receiving prior to admission, as the latter failed to prevent this attack, and in any case tends to become less effective with increasing age.

Inhaled steroids have little therapeutic effect in patients taking prednisolone in doses over 20 mg daily. However, starting the inhaled steroids prior to discharge allows inhaler technique to be checked, and any further counselling to take place. It also ensures that they are not forgotten as the oral steroid dose is reduced after discharge.

16. Miss V should be changed to beclometha-sone inhaler 100 micrograms, four puffs twice daily via a Volumatic®. She should be advised to rinse her mouth after each dose.

Side-effects of inhaled steroids are either systemic or local. Systemic effects are rare and are related to the total daily dose. For beclomethasone, the total daily dose should be kept below 1.5–2 mg if systemic effects are to be avoided.

Local side-effects, such as a hoarse voice and oral thrush, are more common. They are related to the amount of steroid deposited in the mouth and throat, and the frequency of exposure. This last point came to light in the steroid trials of the early 1980s, which compared traditional four-times-daily regimens with twice-daily regimens in stable asthma. Not only were the twice-daily regimens as effective, but the incidence of thrush was reduced, despite the total daily dose being the same. Thus, one sensible suggestion would be to change Miss V's dosage regimen to four puffs twice daily. This would reduce her chance of getting thrush, and might also help her compliance. An additional common-sense recommendation is for Miss V to take a drink of water after each dose in order to rinse her mouth out. However, there is no published evidence to show whether this tactic is successful or not.

Use of a large-volume spacer device also reduces steroid deposition in the oro-pharynx. Although these devices are bulky, patients may be persuaded to use them, provided the steroid regimen is only twice daily. This avoids the need to carry the device around. If the patient is using several puffs via the spacer it is more convenient to put the whole dose in and inhale, rather than inhale one puff at a time; however, a diminished fraction of each successive puff is available to the patient when the device is used this way. Thus, when advising Miss V about correct technique, it is necessary to balance convenience, and possibly compliance, against dose.

17. The prednisolone should be reduced slowly over three weeks from day 6.

It is important to note that the reason for tailing-off oral prednisolone therapy in asthmatics is not the fear of adrenal suppression; this does not become a problem until a patient has received at least three weeks of high dose therapy. The reason for not stopping suddenly is that a severe asthma attack may be provoked. Unfortunately, there is no one correct reducing dose regimen; it is rather a matter of judgement. Several factors need to be considered when designing such a regimen. Firstly, was the patient on maintenance prednisolone at home? This is important in helping determine the target dose to get down to. In Miss V's case she was not on regular oral steroids, so it is reasonable to reduce the prednisolone dose to zero.

The other factors that need to be taken into account are the overall severity of the attack, and the PEFRs during the recovery phase. These determine how quickly the steroids can be reduced and when to start reducing. It is advisable to maintain a high steroid dose until the PEFR has plateaued out at its usual value between attacks, and there is little dipping evident. In the case of a moderate attack which responds promptly to nebulised salbutamol, with the PEFR rising to normal over 24 hours with no dipping, the prednisolone may be reduced to zero over one week. In the case of a severe attack such as Miss V's, the prednisolone should be reduced over at least three weeks.

18. Very common.

Even with perfect inhaler technique only 10% of the dose from a pressurised aerosol is deposited in the conducting airways. This can be markedly reduced if technique is poor. Various figures for poor inhaler use are quoted in the literature. Patients who are given the inhaler with the instruc-

tion leaflet, but no verbal instruction, fail to use the inhaler optimally in 50–60% of cases. Demonstration of correct technique plus verbal instruction improves this figure. However, 10–15% of patients will still be unable to use the pressurised aerosol correctly. In practice, some errors in technique are easier to correct by counselling than others: activation of the inhaler at the end of inhalation is a particularly common error, and very difficult to correct. The best solution in these cases is for the pharmacist to recommend an alternative device.

19. The Rotahaler® or Diskhaler® would be suitable.

When considering alternative devices for a patient it is necessary to be aware of both the characteristics of the device and which drugs are available for use in it. These facts must be compared with an assessment of the patient's problems. It is often justifiable to change to another drug in the same class in order to be able to provide a more suitable inhalation device for a patient.

Miss V seems to have poor co-ordination between inhalation and activation of the inhaler. However, she seems to be reasonably dextrous and has no problem with grip strength. She is an active individual who needs to take her beta$_2$-adrenoceptor stimulant inhaler out and about with her. She will therefore need a device that is compact and convenient to use. Ideally, she should be able to use the same device for her inhaled steroid. However, if the steroid regimen is changed to twice daily, a more bulky device may be acceptable for that therapy (see answer 16).

The options for steroid devices are limited. The Spacer® (which takes budesonide) will not help grossly uncoordinated technique, and so should not be recommended for Miss V. The Nebuhaler® or the Volumatic® are large-volume tube spacers. These will help Miss V, but are too bulky to be carried around. One of them could be recommended only if the steroid regimen was changed to twice daily. In that case a different device would be needed for the bronchodilator.

In some respects a neater solution for Miss V would be to use a compact device through which both her steroid and bronchodilator could be delivered. Both the Rotahaler and the Diskhaler fall into this category. Both can be a little fiddly to load, but this is not usually a problem in younger patients. The Diskhaler has the advantage of being multi-dose. When designing a suitable regimen it should be noted that both of these dry powder inhalers deliver only about 5% of the drug to the conducting airways. This is about half that of a correctly used pressurised aerosol. Therefore, Miss V would need beclomethasone 400 micrograms four times a day, or 800 micrograms twice a day. Other devices that require little co-ordination are the Autohaler® and the Turbohaler®; these deliver salbutamol and terbutaline respectively. Both are compact and very simple to use, but no steroid is available for use in them. Their only value for Miss V would be as a replacement for the salbutamol pressurised aerosol.

After selecting the most suitable device it is necessary to confirm this choice by trying it out with the patient. Placebos of all these devices are available from the manufacturers on request.

20. The concepts of preventers, relievers, and crisis management need to be explained.

Miss V needs to be made aware of the differences in use between her two inhalers. Firstly, the salbutamol should be described as a "reliever". This is for quick relief of symptoms, but the effects do not last for more than a few hours. She should be encouraged to adjust the frequency of use according to how her chest feels. Some asthmatics are scared of using the inhaler too frequently; this fear is unfounded (but see below). It should be pointed out that whilst this reliever will help the majority of attacks it may not be able to deal with a very severe one.

Secondly, the steroid inhaler should be described as a "preventer", which will prevent many asthma attacks from occurring. It should be stressed that this inhaler is slow to work and will not provide quick relief in the case of an attack. Also, it should be used every day, even if the patient is feeling well. However, if the asthma is deteriorating day by day, then the patient should be encouraged to increase the dose for a couple of weeks, for instance by doubling up to four puffs four times per day. Counselling is particularly vital with steroid inhalers, as the most common problem with them is non-compliance. This occurs either because the patient feels no quick relief from a steroid inhaler, and therefore regards it as ineffective, or because they fail to recognise the need to continue usage between attacks.

Finally, crisis management needs to be discussed with Miss V, and, if possible, her parents. All should be aware that if the asthma gets so bad that the salbutamol fails to relieve it, or the relief only lasts for an hour or so, then they must summon medical assistance immediately, regardless of the time of day or night.

References and Further Reading

Anon., Acute asthma, *Lancet*, 1986, **1**, 131–133.

Cheong B. *et al.*, Intravenous beta agonist in severe acute asthma, *Br. med. J.*, 1988, **297**, 448–450.

Gross, N.J., Ipratropium bromide, *New Engl. J. Med.*, 1988, **319**, 486–494.

Horsley, M.G., Asthma, *Pharm. J.*, 1987, **239**, 552–554.

Horsley, M.G., Nebuliser therapy, *ibid.*, 1988, **240**, 22–24.

Horsley M.G. and Bailie G.R., Risk factors for inadequate use of pressurised aerosol inhalers, *J. clin. Pharm. Ther.* 1988, **13**, 139–143.

Littenberg B., Aminophylline treatment in severe acute asthma: a meta-analysis, *J. Am. med. Ass.*, 1988, **259**, 1678–1684.

Livingstone C. and Livingstone D., Inhalation therapy, *Pharm. J.*, 1988, **241**, 476–478.

O'Driscoll B.R. *et al.*, Nebulised salbutamol with and without ipratropium bromide in acute airflow obstruction, *Lancet*, 1989, **1**, 1418–1420.

Rogers A., Inhaler counselling, *Pharm. J.*, 1987, **239**, 652–653.

Sears M.R. *et al.*, Seventy-five deaths in asthmatics prescribed home nebulisers, *Br. med. J.*, 1987, **294**, 477–480.

Stead R.J. and Cooke N.J., Adverse effects of inhaled corticosteroids, *ibid.*, 1989, **298**, 405–406.

CHRONIC OBSTRUCTIVE AIRWAYS DISEASE

Peter D. Bramley

Principal Pharmacist (Clinical Services and Training), William Harvey Hospital, Ashford, Kent

Day 1 Sixty-five-year-old Mr L was admitted to a medical ward via casualty. He had suffered increasing dyspnoea and wheeze over the past five days. He had a cough productive of yellow sputum and swelling of the ankles. His wife said he had become too breathless to speak or eat, and today had been delirious. He could not walk further than from the chair to the toilet.

His current drug therapy was:

Frumil® (frusemide 40 mg, amiloride 5 mg), one tablet three times daily
Beclomethasone dipropionate inhaler (100 micrograms per inhalation), one puff four times a day
Salbutamol respirator solution, one 2.5 mg nebule up to four times a day when required
Simple linctus, 5 mL when required.

Mr L's wife admitted that her husband had not used his beclomethasone inhaler for some months because "it did not help". He was using bottled oxygen from two to four hours every day, whereas he used to use it only "in emergency".

Mr L had been a heavy smoker, but had stopped completely two years earlier. He lived with his wife in a bungalow and had retired from his job as a factory storekeeper at the age of sixty.

On examination he was centrally cyanosed. His chest was silent initially but, after one dose of salbutamol 2.5 mg by nebulisation, coarse crackles could be heard at the right base. He was diagnosed as having a right basal pneumonia with deterioration of his obstructive airways disease. An arterial blood sample was sent for analysis of blood gases, with the patient breathing 35% oxygen by face mask.

Mr L's blood gas results were:

Blood pH 7.163 (references range 7.32–7.42)
PaCO$_2$ 11.21 kPa (4.5–6.1)

PaO$_2$ 12.98 kPa (12–15)
Standard bicarbonate 29.2 mmol/ L (21–25)

In view of Mr L's serious condition he was transferred to the intensive therapy unit (ITU) for mechanical ventilatory support. He was sedated (midazolam 10 mg by intravenous bolus) and given a muscle relaxant (atracurium 40 mg by intravenous bolus) to enable tracheal intubation and commencement of intermittent positive pressure ventilation (IPPV). For maintenance sedation, propofol (120 mg intravenous bolus, then a variable dose continuous infusion of 20–50 mg/hour) was written up. Midazolam 2.5–5 mg intravenously when required was also written up, in case any further sedation was necessary. A central venous catheter was inserted via the right subclavian approach. He also underwent urinary catheterisation.

Mr L was thought to be fluid-depleted and was prescribed one unit of polygeline intravenous infusion to be given over 30 minutes, followed by two litres of dextrose/saline infusion, each litre to be given over eight hours.

The following drug therapy was written up:

Aminophylline 500 mg in 500 mL 5% dextrose infusion twice daily, each dose to be given by continuous intravenous infusion over twelve hours
Salbutamol (nebulised), 2.5 mg six times daily (every four hours)
Ipratropium bromide (nebulised), 250 micrograms six times daily (every four hours)
Hydrocortisone 100 mg intravenously six times daily (every four hours)
Cefotaxime 2 g intravenously three times daily (every eight hours)

Serum biochemistry and haematology results were:

Sodium 141 mmol/L (137–150)
Potassium 5.2 mmol/L (3.5–5.0)

Urea 5.4 mmol/L (2.5–6.6)
Haemoglobin 17.7 g/dL (14–18)
Haematocrit 0.57 (0.36–0.46)
White blood cells 18.1×10^9/L $(4–11 \times 10^9)$

1. What do Mr L's history, symptoms, and blood gases indicate about his respiratory disease?

2. What are the immediate priorities in Mr L's treatment?

3. Has the most appropriate sedative therapy been chosen for Mr L? How is the dose of propofol titrated?

4. Do you agree with the choice of agents to treat Mr L's respiratory condition? Comment on the doses prescribed.

5. What would you tell a nurse who had never administered salbutamol or ipratropium by nebuliser before?

6. What are the likely explanations for Mr L's abnormal serum biochemistry and haematology results?

Day 2 On examination of Mr L's respiratory system, very few rhonchi could be heard, and his blood gases were satisfactory. Urinary output was good (100–200 mL/hour) and a positive fluid balance had been achieved overnight. A repeat chest x-ray still showed some increased shadowing at the right base. The patient was noted to be shaking, and in response to this observation it was suggested on the ward round that the salbutamol dose should be reduced to 2.5 mg by nebuliser four times daily (every six hours), and that the aminophylline dose should be changed to 360 mg twice daily, as rectal suppositories.

7. Could Mr L's drug therapy be causing his tremor?

8. Are the suggested changes in treatment appropriate? If not, what recommendations would you make?

Mr L's salbutamol dosage was reduced as suggested. Aminophylline was continued by the intravenous route.

It was decided to raise Mr L's level of consciousness by gradually decreasing the rate of propofol infusion. The dose of hydrocortisone was reduced to 100 mg four times daily.

Day 3 Only scattered rhonchi could now be heard in both lungs. Bowel sounds were present, and so nasogastric feeding was commenced. Mr L was apyrexial, conscious, and alert.

Day 4 Mr L was improving rapidly and the IPPV rate was reduced to accelerate weaning. The propofol infusion was stopped at 9 a.m. and Mr L was extubated at 12 noon. The serum-theophylline concentration was reported to the ward as 15.8 mg/L (10–20).

9. How does reducing the mechanical ventilation rate help the weaning process?

10. Can drug therapy be helpful in the weaning process?

11. What action, if any, would you take after noting Mr L's theophylline level?

Day 5 Mr L's condition continued to improve, with no breathlessness or wheezing, minimal coughing and sputum production, and no cyanosis. Oxygen 28% was continuously administered through a face mask. Regular peak flow measurements were recorded, before and after bronchodilators, at 6 a.m., 2 p.m., and 6 p.m.

Day 6 Mr L was transferred to a general medical ward. It was noted that he still had some tremor, mild pitting oedema bilaterally, and some evidence of right ventricular strain on the electrocardiogram. He had a good urine output and was managing well without a catheter. His peak expiratory flow rate was 100 L/min before nebulised salbutamol and 120 L/min ten minutes after the 6 a.m. dose.

He was changed from intravenous hydrocortisone to oral prednisolone (30 mg once daily), and it was decided to reduce his aminophylline dose gradually.

Day 7 Mr L was changed from intravenous cefotaxime to oral cefaclor, 500 mg three times daily (every eight hours).

Day 8 Intravenous aminophylline was cancelled, and aminophylline 225 mg slow-release tablets, two tablets twice daily, written up; the theophylline level was to be measured in a few days.

Day 11 Since a degree of cor pulmonale was present, with ankle oedema and electrocardiogram abnormalities (large P waves and right axis deviation), Mr L was re-started on Frumil® at a dose of two tablets each morning.

12. Is this treatment appropriate for Mr L's cor pulmonale? Comment on alternative therapies that could be prescribed.

Day 12 A pre-dose serum theophylline level was reported as 19.6 mg/L (10–20). Mr L was noted still to have a significant tremor.

13. *Would you recommend any aminophylline dosage modification?*

Day 14 Mr L's respiratory condition was greatly improved and his ankle swelling had diminished significantly on Frumil. He was discharged on the following medication:

Frumil, two in the morning
Prednisolone 10 mg once daily, reducing to nil over one week
Aminophylline 350 mg slow-release twice daily
Salbutamol (nebulised), 2.5 mg four times daily

He was given a six-week out-patient appointment.

14. *Would there be any advantage in continuing Mr L's oral steroid therapy long-term? Would inhaled steroid therapy be more appropriate?*

15. *What changes might be made to his bronchodilator therapy?*

16. *What points would you discuss with Mr L when counselling him on his take-home medication?*

Day 56 Mr L attended the out-patient department. He was reasonably well, able to walk around the house, dress, and wash himself. He was still short of breath on exertion, with some ankle oedema and a few rhonchi at both bases. He was warned he might need antibiotics should he get another chest infection. He was written up for beclomethasone dipropionate inhaler (250 micrograms per inhalation), two puffs twice daily, and shown how to use a peak flow meter, to be used daily until the follow-up appointment in two weeks.

17. *Would you recommend that Mr L receive continuous prophylaxis against infection? If so, which agents would you recommend and at what dose?*

Day 70 Mr L's peak flow readings had improved since the last appointment, but he was now suffering from oral thrush. He was prescribed amphotericin, one lozenge five times daily for two weeks.

18. *What measures would you suggest to reduce the risk of Mr L suffering from oral thrush again?*

Answers

1. Mr L's rapidly increasing dyspnoea and general disability over the past few days suggest that his respiratory condition has deteriorated because of an acute event. His productive cough and discoloured sputum make a chest infection the most likely cause. His increasing use of oxygen, together with his symptoms of cyanosis, show that his lungs are failing to provide efficient gaseous exchange, and that he is in respiratory failure.

This can be confirmed by the blood gas results. The normal PaO_2 is misleading, since Mr L was given 35% oxygen on admission, before the first blood gases were measured. Usually a lower oxygen concentration (24%) is commenced, in order to avoid inhibiting the hypoxic ventilatory drive often present in chronic obstructive airways disease (COAD) patients. However, it was probably decided at an early stage that Mr L would need mechanical ventilation with a high oxygen concentration, so this risk was not significant.

The $PaCO_2$ is also markedly raised, which means that Mr L has Type 2 (ventilatory) failure, where alveolar ventilation is insufficient to prevent a rise in $PaCO_2$. This is in contrast to Type 1 (oxygenation) failure, where the PaO_2 falls below 8 kPa but a rise in $PaCO_2$ is counteracted by increased respiratory muscle drive. This relatively poor response to hypoxia puts Mr L in the "blue bloater" category of COAD patients. It should, however, be noted that he has emphysematous changes. The classical association of emphysema solely with the "pink puffer" category of COAD patient is now known to be incorrect.

Accumulation of carbon dioxide leads to respiratory acidosis with a low blood pH. The kidneys compensate for this by excreting more hydrogen ions into the urine (at the expense of potassium ions) and returning more bicarbonate ions to the circulation, thus causing a rise in plasma bicarbonate.

2. The immediate therapeutic aims are:
   (a) correction of acute respiratory failure, and
   (b) treatment of infection.

3. Mr L's sedative therapy is appropriate, but vecuronium is a more appropriate muscle relaxant for him.

The sedatives chosen for Mr L were the most appropriate of those available at the time of writing. A short-acting water-soluble benzodiazepine such as midazolam is a suitable sedative for intubation of Mr L, producing minimal effect on the cardiovascular system. The extent of respiratory depression caused by the sedative chosen to cover intubation is not an important consideration for Mr L, since the decision to ventilate him mechanically has already been made. Benzodiazepines also produce amnesia of the intubation procedure. As a single dose, it is doubtful whether midazolam has any advantage over diazepam; however, in this situation repeat doses can be required, and multiple doses of diazepam would be associated with a higher risk of drug accumulation and prolonged action.

When intubation has been accomplished the choice of sedative depends on the condition of the patient. If Mr L had been in pain, an opiate would have been required by continuous infusion, but prolonged use of opiate therapy can cause a significant degree of cardiovascular and respiratory depression, which may make weaning from the ventilator more difficult. As Mr L is not in pain, another agent is more appropriate. Although midazolam is a short-acting benzodiazepine, when it is given by continuous infusion accumulation will occur, and this can again prolong weaning, particularly in the elderly.

The main alternative to opiates and benzodiazepines currently available in ITUs for maintenance sedation is propofol, a short-acting anaesthetic agent which, at present, is not licensed for long-term infusion. Propofol also causes appreciable respiratory depression at sedative doses, but is associated with significantly less accumulation than the other agents available, and so rapid recovery occurs, which results in a shorter weaning time. The drug is highly lipophilic and is distributed rapidly from the blood into the tissues (half-life three minutes). There is then rapid metabolism to inactive metabolites and clearance from the body (half-life thirty minutes). A slow terminal elimination half-life (five hours) is thought to result from the slow return of propofol from poorly perfused tissue, but this third phase of elimination does not appear to affect recovery time.

The maintenance dose of propofol usually required for continuous sedation is 0.5–1.0 mg/kg/hour. The dose should be titrated according to Mr L's response. He should be calm but easily rousable (sedation scoring systems are available). The initial rate is set according to age and weight, and then adjusted by increments of 10–20 mg/hour, every four hours, until the patient is in the desired state. Bolus doses of midazolam or a short-acting opiate can be used to increase the level of sedation during periods of acute anxiety or stressful procedures, such as physiotherapy.

Finally, atracurium, a short-acting, non-depolarising muscle relaxant, is used during initiation of IPPV to relax the vocal chords and enable intubation to take place. Since it is associated with some histamine release it could exacerbate COAD; vecuronium would theoretically have been a better choice for Mr L.

4. (a) Antibiotic therapy. An antibiotic with a narrower spectrum of activity would have been more appropriate.

The cause of Mr L's acute respiratory failure is infection, so treatment with an appropriate antibiotic is very important. Sputum and blood samples should be sent off for culture and sensitivity, but the most likely causative organisms are *Haemophilus influenzae* or *Streptococcus pneumoniae*. Ampicillin, amoxycillin, erythromycin or trimethoprim would therefore usually be adequate; however, up to ten per cent of *H. influenzae* strains are now resistant to ampicillin and amoxycillin, and, bearing in mind the severity of Mr L's condition, the use of these agents is probably not appropriate without a sensitivity report. Augmentin® (1.2 g eight-hourly) would, however, have been a more suitable alternative for Mr L, as it is effective against penicillinase-producing bacteria that are resistant to amoxycillin.

Cefotaxime is effective against *H. influenzae* and *Strep. pneumoniae*, but the wide spectrum of a third-generation cephalosporin is unlikely to be necessary in this community-acquired infection, and may lead to supra-infection with another organism. Coliform pneumonias (Gram-negative, non-pseudomonal) are common in ventilated ITU patients, and cefotaxime should be reserved in case of this eventuality occurring at a later stage in Mr L's treatment.

The cefotaxime dose prescribed for Mr L (2 g eight-hourly) is, however, appropriate for a life-threatening infection.

(b) Bronchodilator therapy. It was appropriate to prescribe three bronchodilators for Mr L, but a loading dose of aminophylline should have been given.

Much of the airways obstruction of COAD is irreversible by bronchodilator therapy, since it is caused by mucus plugs and bronchiolar inflammation; however, some patients, like Mr L, have a reversible component and will obtain benefit from bronchodilators. Patients with COAD often have hypertrophy of bronchial smooth muscle and hyper-reactive airways. Although only small objective improvement can be measured (e.g. by peak flow measurement), this may be significant in someone with extremely poor respiratory function. The mode of action of beta$_2$-adrenoceptor stimulants is to increase smooth muscle cell cyclic AMP levels and stabilise mast cells. Salbutamol (or terbutaline) in nebulised form is acceptable. The maximum recommended dose for nebulised salbutamol is 5 mg four times daily, but since in severe airways obstruction the quantity of drug reaching the site of action may be limited, a smaller dose given more frequently can be more successful.

Ipratropium bromide is an anticholinergic agent, blocking the cholinergic reflex that causes bronchospasm. It is particularly useful in combination with beta$_2$-adrenoceptor stimulants in COAD patients, producing slightly greater bronchodilation than either agent alone. The onset of action of ipratropium is slower than for the beta$_2$-adrenoceptor stimulants and the duration of action longer (peak effect between one and two hours), and there is evidence that the combined therapy produces greater effect when the ipratropium is given at least two hours before the beta$_2$-adrenoceptor stimulant. The maximum recommended dose of nebulised ipratropium is 500 micrograms four times daily, but, as with salbutamol, a smaller dose given more frequently can be more successful.

In addition to causing relaxation of bronchial smooth muscle, there is some evidence that theophylline may have other beneficial actions in COAD. It is thought to act as a respiratory stimulant, reduce respiratory muscle fatigue, improve right ventricular performance, and increase mucociliary clearance. Another advantage is that, unlike the other two bronchodilators in the regimen, intravenous aminophylline does not depend on penetration of the obstructed bronchioles to exert its effect. Although clinical evidence for these properties is inconclusive, intravenous aminophylline should be added to the bronchodilator therapy of a COAD patient like Mr L who has severe acute respiratory failure.

The aminophylline dosage regimen prescribed for Mr L was not optimal. He was given an arbitrary maintenance dose (MD) of 42 mg/hour. Since he was not taking oral theophylline or aminophylline before admission, he should have received a loading dose (LD) to achieve a therapeutic concentration rapidly. The normal half-life of theophylline in adults is eight hours, and so steady state can only be achieved after approximately thirty-two hours. With a suitable LD of 5 mg/kg (or worked out by pharmacokinetic calculation) administered over twenty to thirty minutes, a therapeutic concentration would have been achieved far more rapidly. After loading is completed, the MD should be started. Ideally the MD should be determined using pharmacokinetic calculation, which takes into account those factors that affect theophylline clearance, such as smoking history.

The plasma concentration of theophylline should then be monitored to maintain therapeutic levels (between 10 and 20 mg/L). As no LD was given, the earliest time usefully to measure Mr L's plasma concentration would be twelve to twenty hours after starting the infusion, which represents twice the normal half-life. Even at this time, the concentration can only be a guide as to whether the dose is too high or too low, since steady state will not have been reached. If an LD had been given, it would have been worthwhile to check the level after six to eight hours, and to adjust the dose up or down if necessary.

(c) Corticosteroid therapy.

The value of intravenous corticosteroids in Mr L's condition is not in doubt in the short term, when inflammation plays a significant part in the airways obstruction, but after the first few days the role of steroids becomes more controversial. The dose of hydrocortisone prescribed for Mr L is commonly used, and should be reduced as his condition improves, with a change to oral prednisolone as soon as practicable.

5. (a) Volume of nebulised solution.

Nebulisers have a dead volume, usually of just under 1 mL, which will not be available to the patient; so the larger the fill volume, the greater the fraction of drug released. However, increasing the volume increases the time for nebulisation. In hospital a volume of 4–5 mL is an acceptable compromise, producing an administration time of fifteen to thirty minutes. As Mr L is written up for 2.5 mg of salbutamol (one 2.5 mL nebule) and 250 micrograms of ipratropium (1 mL from a 2 mL nebule) every four hours, it is convenient to mix the two in the nebuliser, making a total volume of 3.5 mL. This is common practice on wards, although the stability of the two solutions combined has not been fully evaluated. Unpublished work carried out on the stability of the mixture using the preserved formulations suggested that they would be compatible when mixed in this way, but both formulations are now preservative-free, which could theoretically affect the results. Where the volume of fluid is insufficient and dilution is required, normal saline (e.g. Normasol® sachets) should be used, since hypotonic solutions may provoke bronchospasm.

(b) Driving gas.

The driving gas may be air or oxygen at a rate of 6–8 L/min. In patients with COAD who may have low oxygen tolerability the driving gas should be air; however, as Mr L is ventilated and on 35% oxygen already, the choice is not so critical and oxygen is acceptable as a driving gas.

(c) Administration in ventilated patients.

The ventilator itself affects the delivery of nebulised drug. With some ventilators, connecting the nebuliser to the inspiratory arm of the tubing leads to a proportion of the drug being drawn back into the ventilator during the expiratory phase, since the nebulised drug is continually fed into the tubing by the driving gas. Some ventilators have a synchronised nebuliser cycle, which electronically opens a valve to allow the nebulised drug to pass into the inspiratory arm only during the inspiratory phase. When the ventilator does not have this facility, the patient should be disconnected from the machine and "bagged" while the drug is administered, to prevent loss of drug into the machine.

Administration of nebulised drug via the ventilator tubing takes longer than in a non-ventilated patient, since the ventilator delivers less breaths per minute than a patient breathing spontaneously.

6. Mr L's raised serum potassium concentration is likely to be a result of his respiratory acidosis, which is caused by accumulation of carbon dioxide. Sodium conservation by the kidney and the sodium pump at the cell wall both involve the exchange of sodium for potassium or hydrogen, the latter two ions being in free competition. In acidotic states there is an excess of hydrogen ions in the blood, and so they are cleared in preference to potassium at these two sites. The clearance of potassium is consequently reduced, and hyperkalaemia results.

Mr L also has a raised haematocrit and white blood cell count. Secondary polycythaemia occurs as a response to chronic hypoxia, causing a raised haemoglobin and also a raised haematocrit (an indicator of red cell volume). The raised white blood cell count indicates that Mr L has an infection.

7. Yes.

Salbutamol is known to cause a fine tremor of skeletal muscle, along with other manifestations of sympathetic stimulation such as an increase in heart rate, and peripheral vasodilation. These effects occur particularly when large doses are inhaled. Aminophylline can also cause tremor, but in most cases only at plasma concentrations above the therapeutic range.

8. No. If the doses of both drugs are changed simultaneously, it will be impossible to determine which is causing the problem. It is more appropriate to reduce Mr L's salbutamol dose as suggested, and to measure his serum theophylline level.

If a serum theophylline concentration were available it would give a clearer indication of what is causing Mr L's tremor. In the absence of a level, pharmacokinetic calculation indicates that it is unlikely that Mr L's theophylline concentration is above the therapeutic range, so a reduction in salbutamol dose would be a reasonable response to his symptom of tremor. However, if Mr L's serum theophylline level is found to be in the toxic range, an appropriate adjustment in intravenous infusion rate can be determined by pharmacokinetic calculation.

Furthermore, changing from intravenous to rectal aminophylline therapy would not be a logical step. Since aminophylline is absorbed slowly and highly unreliably by the rectal route, this change would be likely to result in wide fluctuations in plasma concentration throughout the dosage interval.

9. Reducing the ventilation rate reduces the clearance of carbon dioxide, causing the $PaCO_2$ to rise. This helps to stimulate respiratory drive by transferring control of breathing from the ventilator back to the patient.

10. Yes. Although respiratory stimulants have fallen from general use in recent years, they have a limited place in the treatment of respiratory failure.

It is very important that a patient's clinical situation is carefully assessed before the decision to use this type of drug is made. If, during weaning, Mr L (a "blue bloater") failed to respond to a rising pCO_2 by increasing his spontaneous respiratory rate, then a trial of respiratory stimulant would be indicated. However, in a patient who is already fighting for breath (a "pink puffer"), further respiratory stimulation could actually lead to a dangerous situation where more carbon dioxide is produced metabolically than the compromised lungs can eliminate.

The only useful respiratory stimulant available at present in the UK is doxapram. Other alternatives, such as nikethamide, are now considered too toxic. Doxapram is thought to act principally on the peripheral chemoreceptors to produce an increase in tidal volume, and, to a lesser extent, an increase in respiratory rate. The dose is between 1.5 and 4.0 mg/min by continuous intravenous infusion, depending on the condition and response of the patient. An interaction, presenting as agitation and increased skeletal muscle activity, has been reported between doxapram and aminophylline.

11. Since the plasma concentration is in the middle of the therapeutic range no adjustment in infusion rate is necessary.

The infusion has been running for over forty-eight hours at a constant rate so steady state will have been achieved, and as it is a continuous intravenous infusion, the sampling time is not critical. As always when interpreting drug level data, the result should also be judged in the light of the patient's clinical response: if the current dose is ineffective or toxicity has occurred, a change of dose should be considered, even if the reported level is in the therapeutic range.

If Mr L had been changed to rectal aminophylline therapy, it would have had to be ensured that at least twenty-four hours had elapsed between changing the route of administration and taking the sample, to ensure that steady state was approached. As absorption from the rectal route is so variable, a pre-dose (trough) concentration would have been the most reliable for interpretation.

12. Yes, provided Mr L's serum potassium level is first checked. Treatment of the respiratory failure, supplementation with oxygen, and diuretic therapy are the mainstays of the treatment of cor pulmonale. Other drugs, for example vasodilators, may be helpful as second-line agents.

Cor pulmonale is fluid retention and heart failure associated with diseases of the lung. It is initiated by pulmonary artery hypertension, which produces a high afterload and consequently right ventricular hypertrophy. There is no intrinsic abnormality of the heart, and initially there may be sufficient functional reserve to maintain cardiac output at normal values; however, eventually the right ventricle fails to compensate for the hypertension and venous pressure becomes elevated.

It is now believed that pulmonary hypoxic vasoconstriction, rather than anatomical damage to the capillary bed, causes the rise in pulmonary artery pressure. Erythrocytosis (occurring as a response to hypoxia, and causing a rise in haematocrit, increased resistance to flow, and an increase in red cell clumping) can also play a part. As hypoxia is the causative factor, treatment of Mr L's respiratory failure is vital. Episodes of frank heart failure frequently appear during infective episodes. Supplementation with oxygen reduces hypoxia and there is now good evidence that long-term oxygen therapy reduces mortality, morbidity, and frequency of hospital admission in such patients. The oxygen must, however, be given for at least fifteen hours per day.

Diuretic therapy will reduce oedema, improve peripheral circulation and may improve gaseous exchange in the lungs if pulmonary congestion is present. It should be remembered that, as Mr L recovers from the acute exacerbation of his pulmonary disease, the cor pulmonale is also likely to improve and his diuretic requirement may thus decrease.

The potency of a loop diuretic will be valuable in the acute treatment of Mr L's cor pulmonale. Also, since he has a raised serum potassium, the greater capacity of loop diuretics for lowering potassium levels acutely may be advantageous. During long-term use, however, thiazides have a greater potential for causing hypokalaemia, and as patients with COAD tend to have low total body potassium, a loop diuretic would also appear to be more appropriate as long-term therapy. Furthermore, a potassium-sparing diuretic can be added to the treatment to avoid exacerbation of this problem, for which there is no current satisfactory explanation. Spironolactone has traditionally been used (as raised aldosterone levels are frequently present, owing to hepatic congestion), but fears of carcinogenicity have limited the use of this drug. Amiloride is a suitable alternative, but before it is prescribed for Mr L it is important to check that his serum potassium has returned to normal. Whichever diuretics are chosen, it is important that their effect on Mr L's electrolyte balance is monitored.

Digoxin is thought to be of little value in cor pulmonale unless atrial fibrillation needs to be controlled. Pulmonary vasodilators are theoretically useful additions to therapy, but are not yet of proven value; hydralazine, calcium-channel blockers, and angiotension-converting enzyme (ACE) inhibitors are examples. ACE inhibitors offer particular hope as they block the renin-angiotensin system, which leads to vasodilation and decreased aldosterone formation.

13. Yes. Mr L's dose of slow-release aminophylline should be reduced to 350 mg twice daily (every twelve hours).

The sample was taken on the third day after changing to slow-release tablets, so steady state has been reached. Since the level is from a pre-dose sample, it is likely that the peak theophylline concentration (four to six hours post-dose) is above 20 mg/L. This observation, combined with Mr L's continued tremor, which is a side-effect associated with high serum theophylline levels, leads to the recommendation of dosage reduction.

14. No. Continuation of Mr L's systemic corticosteroid therapy indefinitely would not be appropriate at this point. A formal trial of oral or inhaled steroids is, however, warranted.

It is not possible to predict which COAD patients will benefit from long-term systemic steroid therapy. A formal trial should thus be carried out when Mr L has recovered from the acute exacerbation of his condition. The following regimen is appropriate for an oral steroid therapy trial: high-dose oral prednisolone (e.g. 40 mg daily) should be given for two to three weeks, combined with regular objective monitoring (such as peak expiratory flow rates) and subjective assessment of respiratory function. If worthwhile improvement is achieved, lower-dose maintenance treatment may be started, for example prednisolone 10 mg daily.

Prior to admission Mr L had been prescribed a beclomethasone inhaler, but he had not used it for several months because he felt it did not help. This is a common observation by patients with COAD (and asthma) but is very misleading. On further questioning it can frequently be established that the patient did not realise that regular, continuous therapy was required for benefit, and that he or she had stopped using it because no immediate relief was obtained on a "when required" basis. A formal trial of inhaled steroids may thus be warranted for Mr L before long-term oral steroid therapy is evaluated. It should be noted that negative results from this trial would not rule out the possibility of Mr L gaining benefit from oral steroids.

15. Mr L could have been changed to a salbutamol inhaler before discharge, to simplify his treatment at home.

The change from nebulised to inhaled therapy should be made at least a few days before discharge, so that the effect on respiratory function can be determined. However, since Mr L already has a nebuliser at home, it is likely that inhaler therapy is no longer considered adequate for him.

Nebulised ipratropium could also be prescribed for home use, but it is expensive; before instituting its long-term use in a COAD patient the effects of such therapy should also be assessed by formal trial as an out-patient.

Since Mr L's aminophylline dose has been

adjusted immediately before discharge, his plasma theophylline concentration should be checked at his first out-patient appointment, or preferably earlier by his general practitioner.

16. (a) Salbutamol.

The nebulised therapy is the most complex part of his treatment and must be explained to Mr L in detail, with emphasis on the importance of using the correct fill volume and flow-rate of gas. If possible, Mr L should be observed using his own equipment. He must also know who to contact if the machine breaks down.

(b) Prednisolone.

The tailing-off of the prednisolone dose should be explained, ensuring that Mr L understands that he is to stop taking this drug after one week. In addition, in view of Mr L's previous belief that steroids were of no benefit, he must be counselled before starting any formal trial of inhaled or oral steroids. This counselling should cover the importance of taking or using steroids regularly, and the delay in obtaining useful effect with this type of medication.

(c) Frumil®.

The dose should be taken regularly in the morning, and Mr L should continue taking these tablets until told otherwise.

(d) Aminophylline.

The tablets should be swallowed whole, at regular intervals, and preferably after food, with a cold drink. The concept of sustained release should be explained. Mr L should realise that this therapy will continue indefinitely, and that he will need occasional blood tests to check that the dose is right for him.

(e) General.

If, in the future, Mr L is given a course of antibiotics to take when required, he must understand when to start treatment (e.g. when his sputum is discoloured) and at what point to get medical help.

17. No. This hospital admission was Mr L's first serious acute exacerbation due to infection; however, if he has further severe infective episodes, this option should be seriously considered.

There is no general agreement as to the ideal drug for prophylactic antibiotic therapy, but wide-spectrum antibiotics such as amoxycillin and cefaclor, which have activity against *Strep. pneumoniae* and *H. influenzae*, are commonly chosen and prescribed

at the normal therapeutic dose for mild to moderate infections (e.g. amoxycillin 250 mg three times daily). Rotating two drugs at monthly intervals throughout the winter may reduce the risk of emergence of resistant organisms, and antibiotics that are not currently in use as first-line treatment of infection in hospitals are most suitable (for example, tetracyclines).

If a patient has bronchiectasis, prophylactic ciprofloxacin may be prescribed by a chest physician, as this condition is commonly associated with pseudomonal infections. However, since this drug is not very active against *Strep. pneumoniae* it is advisable to rotate its use with one of the other drugs mentioned. It should also be remembered that ciprofloxacin may cause a significant increase in plasma theophylline levels, which must therefore be monitored carefully, and theophylline or aminophylline dosage reduction may be required.

Finally, Mr L is in the group of patients highly vulnerable to influenza, and vaccination should be considered.

18. Mr L should use a spacer device with his inhaler, and rinse out his mouth after each dose.

This problem is caused by deposition of the steroid in the mouth and throat. Two measures may reduce the risk of it recurring. Firstly, Mr L can rinse out his mouth with water after each administration although the benefits of this measure are not proven. Secondly, most of the drug that stays in the mouth is deposited when the inhaler is fired; if a spacer device is used, this deposition occurs in the device itself. Using a spacer device should also help to overcome Mr L's poor inhaler technique, which has probably contributed to this problem in the first place. Beclomethasone dipropionate is also available as a suspension for nebulisation, but it is relatively inefficient because of the product's poor solubility. When counselling on these points, Mr L should also be instructed to use the steroid inhaler ten minutes after a dose of salbutamol, to improve steroid penetration.

References and Further Reading

Horsley M., Nebuliser therapy, *Pharm. J.*, 1988, **240**, 22–24.

Hyde J. and Wilson A., *Clinical Pharmacy Handbook*, 2nd edn, Welwyn Garden City, Smith Kline & French, 1989.

Kay E.A., Chronic obstructive airways disease, *Br. J. Pharm. Pract.*, 1989, **11**, 228–234.

Kucers A. and Bennett N.McK., *The Use of Antibiotics*, 4th ed, London, William Heinemann, 1987.

Mann K.V., Leon A.L. and Tietze J., Use of ipratropium bromide in obstructive lung disease, *Clin. Pharm.* 1988, **7**, 670–680.

Weatherall D.J., Ledingham J.G.G. and Warrell D.A. (eds), *Oxford Textbook of Medicine*, 2nd edn, Oxford, Oxford University Press, 1987.

Winter M.E., *Basic Clinical Pharmacokinetics*, 2nd edn, Vancouver, WA, Applied Therapeutics, 1983.

Young, L.Y. and Koda-Kimble M.A. (eds), *Applied Therapeutics—the Clinical Use of Drugs*, 4th edn, Vancouver, WA, Applied Therapeutics, 1988.

EPILEPSY

Michael G. Spencer

Principal Pharmacist, Patient Services, St James's University Hospital, Leeds

Day 1 Mr U was a 73-year-old man who had lived alone since the death of his wife three years earlier. He was an ex-accountant who led a relatively independent life. He received support from neighbours and nearby relatives.

He had been referred to hospital by his general practitioner because of a three-year history of "small strokes". Mr U described these attacks (as observed by others) as being occasions where he developed a vacant, staring look followed by a period of lip-smacking and chewing movements. A period of confusion followed. Initially the attacks had been infrequent, but they had now increased in frequency to three or four times weekly.

Mr U was admitted to a medicine for the elderly ward. On examination, he was noted to be a well-dressed and well-spoken man who weighed 60 kg and was well nourished. He was alert and responsive but clearly troubled by his condition. He had a ten-year history of angina which was reasonably well controlled by glyceryl trinitrate patches and occasional sublingual glyceryl trinitrate. His blood pressure was satisfactory for his age and his past medical history and examination was unremarkable.

A referral was made to the neurology department and a diagnosis of complex partial seizures made.

1. What is epilepsy and what are the main types of seizures?

2. What is the importance of seizure classification?

3. What are the therapeutic aims of drug therapy?

4. Why is monotherapy generally preferred for the treatment of epilepsy?

5. Which anticonvulsant drug(s) would you recommend for Mr U? Explain how you arrive at this decision.

Day 3 It was decided to start Mr U on phenytoin therapy.

6. What are the relevant pharmacokinetic characteristics of phenytoin that influence its clinical use?

7. Are there any specific phenytoin dosage recommendations for elderly patients?

8. What dose of phenytoin would you recommend for Mr U? Is a loading dose required?

9. How should Mr U be monitored?

10. What are the main potential adverse effects of phenytoin therapy?

Day 9 After seven days of phenytoin therapy a blood sample was taken for phenytoin assay. The laboratory reported a plasma level of 9 mg/L. Clinically Mr U was a little improved, although he continued to have seizures three or four times a week. He was still distressed by them.

His other serum biochemistry results of relevance were:

Albumin 51 g/L (reference range 33–50)
Creatinine 83 micromol/L (44–150)

There was no evidence of renal impairment in excess of the likely age-related reduction in glomerular filtration rate. His liver function tests were all within the reference ranges for his age.

11. What is the target range for phenytoin plasma levels?

12. When should blood samples be taken for phenytoin assay?

13. What information is necessary before plasma levels of phenytoin can be interpreted fully?

14. What recommendations would you make regarding Mr U's drug therapy?

Day 16 After a further seven days on phenytoin

therapy a blood sample was taken for phenytoin assay. The reported level was 15 mg/L. The sample had been taken before the evening dose, and was regarded as a "trough" level. Mr U had had one seizure during the week following the dose increase.

15. What recommendations would you make on the basis of this level?

Day 18 Mr U was discharged from hospital on phenytoin 250 mg at night. He was asked to return to the out-patient clinic after seven days for a further level to be measured.

16. What advice should be given to Mr U on discharge?

Day 25 Mr U returned to the out-patient clinic. A blood sample was taken for phenytoin assay, 16 hours after the previous dose. Clinically he was much improved and had had no seizures the preceding week. The plasma phenytoin level was reported as 17 mg/L. The dose of phenytoin was left at 250 mg daily.

Week 12 Mr U was seen in out-patients. A plasma level taken 17 hours post-dose was 15 mg/L, and seizure control was satisfactory. Phenytoin 250 mg daily was continued.

Week 24 Mr U was admitted via the accident and emergency department after having a grand mal seizure while out shopping. On admission he was drowsy and confused, ataxic, and grossly uncoordinated. Nystagmus was also present. A phenytoin plasma level was reported as 28 mg/L. Phenytoin toxicity was diagnosed.

17. Can elevated phenytoin levels cause grand mal seizures?

18. What might account for Mr U's very high plasma phenytoin concentration?

Mr U's neighbours brought in his current medication, and it was noted that he had no phenytoin 50 mg tablets. After discussion with Mr U, it was thought likely that he had run out of 50 mg tablets and had taken three 100 mg tablets daily for several days before admission.

19. How would you recommend Mr U's phenytoin therapy be managed?

On the ward round two days later it was decided that, because of the potential dangers of phenytoin toxicity if a similar event occurred again, Mr U should be transferred to carbamazepine therapy.

20. Is carbamazepine the best alternative for Mr U?

21. What are the main pharmacokinetic features of carbamazepine?

22. How should carbamazepine therapy be initiated in Mr U?

23. Can carbamazepine be given once daily?

24. Should Mr U's phenytoin therapy be discontinued at the same time as carbamazepine therapy is initiated?

25. How should Mr U's carbamazepine therapy be monitored?

Week 28 Mr U was now on carbamazepine 400 mg twice daily, and phenytoin therapy had been withdrawn. His plasma carbamazepine level was 7.5 mg/L and he was having infrequent seizures.

Week 36 Mr U was seen in the out-patient department complaining of an increase in seizure frequency. A carbamazepine plasma concentration was reported as 4 mg/L. The sample had been taken six hours after the last dose.

26. How should Mr U be managed now?

Week 38 Mr U was now taking carbamazepine 600 mg twice daily. He complained of an unacceptable level of adverse effects on this regimen. A dose of 400 mg three times daily was considered, but it was felt that this might compromise compliance.

27. What alternative formulations are available that might enable twice-daily dosing of high-dose carbamazepine?

Answers

1. Epilepsy can be defined as a continuing tendency towards epileptic seizures – a seizure being a sudden, brief, abnormal discharge of cerebral neurones, which is accompanied by motor, sensory, autonomic or behavioural symptoms.

Many different terms have been used to describe the various types of epilepsy; however, most neurologists now use the classification produced by the International League Against Epilepsy. In this classification, seizures are divided into two types: generalised and partial (or focal). An abbreviated version of the classification is as follows.

(a) *Generalised seizures:*

(i) Absence seizures (petit mal): brief episodes of unconsciousness with little or no motor accompaniment.

(ii) Myoclonic seizures: single or multiple sudden or uncontrollable jerks.

(iii) Tonic/clonic seizures (grand mal): unconsciousness and generalised tonic/clonic convulsions.

(b) *Partial (focal) seizures:*

(i) Simple partial seizures: without impairment of consciousness. Symptoms may be motor, sensory, aphasic, cognitive, and so on, depending on the anatomical site of seizure discharge.

(ii) Complex partial: may have simple partial onset, followed by impaired consciousness, or impairment of consciousness at onset.

2. To facilitate choice of the most appropriate drug therapy.

While there are some "all-purpose" anticonvulsant drugs, the majority of currently used agents are particularly effective against specific types of seizure; drug choice is thus usually governed by a knowledge of the type of seizure involved.

3. To suppress seizures with the minimum of side-effects.

A diagnosis of epilepsy is usually considered when an individual has had two or more seizures in a short interval, although initiation of anticonvulsant treatment after a single seizure may be considered (depending on individual circumstances such as age, type of seizure, or implications of further fits on social and/or employment prospects).

When anticonvulsants are used the overall aim is to completely suppress seizures without producing troublesome side-effects, in a regimen that is as simple as possible. This then allows the patient to live as normal a life as possible.

4. To minimise side-effects, maximise compliance, and facilitate therapy monitoring.

As with most drug therapy, the administration of more than one drug to a patient increases the likelihood of adverse reactions and produces a potential for drug interactions. In addition, patient compliance may be reduced with the prescribing of increasing numbers of drugs.

In the treatment of epilepsy there is no evidence that the use of several drugs in low dosage will produce additive therapeutic effects without additive toxicity. In addition, the interpretation of plasma levels of drugs becomes more difficult when two drugs are given concurrently, since most therapeutic ranges have been determined using monotherapy. Two drugs may, however, be useful in patients with mixed seizure types, such as myoclonic jerks and tonic/clonic fits appearing together.

In general, therapy should be initiated with one drug, and the dose adjusted until seizures are controlled and/or levels within the therapeutic range are achieved. If seizures are not controlled despite adequate plasma levels, the dose of drug should be gradually reduced and an alternative agent introduced.

5. Phenytoin.

Drug choice is generally determined on the basis of seizure type. Often the efficacy of two or more drugs may be similar, and relative toxicities and pharmacokinetic properties may then be important. Patient factors such as age, sex (e.g. likelihood of pregnancy), and liver and renal function may also be important in decision-making, as may concurrent drug therapy and the possibility of drug interactions.

For complex partial seizures the first-choice drugs are usually considered to be phenytoin or carbamazepine, with sodium valproate as a second-line drug. Phenytoin and carbamazepine are thought to be equally effective in the treatment of complex partial seizures. Phenytoin displays a wider range of adverse effects than carbamazepine; however, its efficacy and toxicity appear to correlate better with measured plasma levels than do carbamazepine's. Mr U lives alone and will have to manage his own drug therapy. Phenytoin is therefore most appropriate for him, both for the greater ease of monitoring therapy and because it can be given as a single daily dose, which will probably aid his compliance.

6. (a) Absorption.

Absorption of phenytoin is slow after oral administration, with a bioavailability of over 85%. Oral forms may contain phenytoin sodium or phenytoin acid: the conversion factor from sodium salt to acid is 0.92 (108 mg to 100 mg). Peak levels are achieved three to twelve hours after a dose.

(b) Distribution.

Phenytoin is approximately 90% bound to albumin in plasma under normal conditions. Protein binding can be significantly reduced, and hence the proportion of unbound "free" phenytoin significantly increased, when there is a decreased serum albumin concentration (such as in cirrhosis, or nephrotic syndrome), or when there is an apparent decrease in the affinity of serum albumin for phenytoin (such as in renal failure, or severe jaundice).

(c) Metabolism.

Phenytoin is transformed primarily by metabolism in the liver to several inactive hydroxylated metabolites, some of which are subsequently conjugated before elimination in urine. The capacity of the hepatic mono-oxygenase system to convert phenytoin is limited, and at therapeutic concentrations can become saturated. Phenytoin demonstrates zero-order kinetics at therapeutic concentrations and shows a non-linear relationship between dose and plasma concentration. In particular, there is a disproportionate increase in the plasma phenytoin concentration as the daily dose is increased.

The maximum rate of metabolism (Vm) and the concentration at which the rate is half of the maximum (Km) vary widely from patient to patient. Vm can range from 100 to 1000 mg/day and Km from 1 to 15 mg/L. Problem patients tend to have low values of Km.

Because of the saturable metabolism, the half-life of phenytoin varies as the steady-state plasma concentration changes. At low plasma concentrations it may be around 13 hours, rising to over 46 hours at the top end of the therapeutic range.

7. No.

No specific information is available on the use of phenytoin in elderly patients, although it has been estimated that the rate of phenytoin metabolism is reduced with increasing age, and that the elderly require maintenance doses 20% less than younger patients to maintain levels in the target range.

8. Phenytoin 200 mg daily. A loading dose is unnecessary.

The generally accepted "target" concentration for phenytoin plasma levels is about 15 mg/L. Allowing for the variability in half-life, but assum-

ing that at that concentration it may be around 24 hours, it would take about five days to reach steady-state levels. Whether this is acceptable depends on the clinical situation. If a patient is suffering frequent tonic/clonic seizures, or is in status epilepticus, then a loading dose may be needed. This should be administered by a slow intravenous injection, as large oral doses of phenytoin can cause gastro-intestinal problems and absorption may be very slow.

If, like Mr U, the patient suffers infrequent fits or the seizures are not severe, then the gradual increase in levels achieved by daily administration of a maintenance dose will probably be acceptable. The maintenance dose of phenytoin necessary for adult patients ranges from 150 to 600 mg daily. In most patients, including the elderly, it is advisable to commence therapy at 200 mg daily and to adjust the dose as necessary after clinical and plasma level monitoring.

9. By clinical and plasma level monitoring.

The main aims of antiepileptic therapy are to reduce or abolish seizures, and to avoid toxicity. Clinical observations of changes in seizure frequency and careful monitoring for adverse effects are of utmost importance.

Plasma level monitoring is a particularly useful adjunct to clinical monitoring because:

(a) The saturable metabolism of phenytoin makes it difficult to predict the dose or dose increment needed to achieve a chosen target plasma level, and to avoid excessively high levels.

(b) Phenytoin toxicity may be difficult to diagnose clinically if it presents in an unusual or unexpected way, such as with neuropsychiatric symptoms, encephalopathy or an increase in seizure frequency.

(c) In some instances, patient compliance may be poor.

(d) Levels may change when drugs with the potential to interact with phenytoin are started or stopped.

(e) In pregnancy, phenytoin clearance may increase, causing a fall in plasma levels.

10. (a) Acute idiosyncratic reactions.

These include rashes, Stevens-Johnson syndrome, blood dyscrasias (such as agranulocytosis or aplastic anaemia, and immunological reactions (such as systemic lupus erythematosus and hypersensitivity reactions).

(b) Concentration-dependent adverse effects.

These are mainly symptoms of neurotoxicity,

such as nausea, vomiting, drowsiness, ataxia, and tremor. Nystagmus is often the earliest sign. High plasma phenytoin concentrations can increase the frequency of fits by producing paradoxical, irreversible peripheral nerve or cerebellar damage. Intellectual blunting, depression, psychomotor slowing and behavioural changes may be associated with chronic neurotoxicity.

(c) Chronic adverse effects.

These include gum hypertrophy, folate-dependent megaloblastic anaemia, acne, gingival hyperplasia, hirsuitism, and coarsening of the facies and osteomalacia.

11. 10–20 mg/L.

Early studies in small numbers of patients with severe epilepsy demonstrated that control was improved with levels over 10 mg/L, and dose-related toxicity was more common at levels greater than 20 mg/L. Thus a target range of 10–20 mg/L was proposed and almost universally accepted. However, some patients require levels greater than 20 mg/L, whilst other patients are well controlled at levels less than 10 mg/L; for this reason, some neurologists do not like the concept of a lower level, since it may lead to the decision to increase a patient's dose, in the absence of clinical necessity.

12. (a) With regard to achievement of steady state.

As indicated earlier, it may take between five and 14 days to reach steady state, depending on the final plasma concentration. Samples taken early (e.g. after five to seven days) can be of value, even if steady state has not been achieved, since if they are high they may indicate that unexpected, excessive accumulation is occurring. Subsequent samples at around 10–12 and 12–14 days will confirm whether steady state has been reached, and will indicate the steady-state level.

(b) With regard to time of dose.

Fluctuation in phenytoin plasma levels at steady state should be minimal. Even on once-daily dosing, the slow absorption and long half-life of phenytoin suggest that at therapeutic plasma levels fluctuation will only be ±10%, being lower at higher concentrations, and higher at lower concentrations. Timing of samples is therefore not critical, although it is useful to standardise it as far as practical for an individual patient, for example while they are in hospital.

13. A number of factors must be considered.

(a) The patient's dose regimen (of phenytoin and other drugs).

(b) The patient's serum creatinine and serum albumin levels (to assess any effect on protein binding).

(c) Some indication of the patient's liver function, or of other disorders that may affect phenytoin kinetics.

(d) All concurrent drug therapy (for the presence of any interacting drugs).

(e) Time of sample (i.e. number of days on therapy, time of last dose).

In addition, the patient's clinical condition must be considered. It is important that the patient is treated, not the plasma level.

14. Increase his daily dose to 250 mg and re-sample after 7–14 days.

Mr U's plasma level is below the lower end of the generally accepted therapeutic range. Although, as discussed in answer 11, some neurologists are unhappy about the concept of a lower end to the therapeutic range, Mr U's seizures are still not controlled satisfactorily and a dosage increase is therefore warranted. Dosage increments of phenytoin should be small, because of the drug's non-linear pharmacokinetics. In addition, there is significant inter-patient variability in Km and Vm (see answer 6) and it can be difficult to estimate an appropriate increment for an individual.

Several methods are available for estimating appropriate phenytoin doses. Using the Richens nomogram, which requires one steady-state level achieved on a known dose, Mr U requires a dose of 240 mg daily to achieve a plasma level of 15 mg/L. This can be rounded up to 250 mg daily. The nomogram assumes a Km of 6 mg/L and therefore will only give adequate results if Mr U's Km is close to this figure.

15. Keep the dose at 250 mg daily and re-sample in seven days.

Mr U's plasma level is now within the therapeutic range and he is clinically improved; however, it is not yet clear whether this level represents a steady-state concentration. The dose-dependent pharmacokinetics of phenytoin mean that the usual method of estimating whether a patient is at steady state (i.e. four to five times the half-life of the drug) is of limited use, as the half-life of phenytoin increases with increasing dose and plasma concentration. The time to steady state is therefore difficult to predict. A nomogram or a pharmacokinetic equation can be used, either to estimate the time to steady state, or to confirm whether a measured value represents a steady-state concentration, but in practice it is advisable to confirm by measurement at five- to seven-day intervals whether accumulation is taking place.

It is possible that Mr U's level does not yet represent steady state and that the drug will continue to accumulate, therefore his plasma level should be measured again in seven days. As Mr U is keen to return home, his therapy can be monitored in the out-patient clinic.

16. The importance of the drug therapy in preventing seizure recurrence should be stressed, and Mr U should be warned of the danger of running out of tablets. He should be advised to take his daily dose at around the same time each night. If he forgets to take a dose he should take it as soon as possible within the next 24 hours, but should not double-up a dose.

Mr U could also be told about how the British Epilepsy Association was formed to help people who suffer from epilepsy, and their families and friends. It provides professional advice and counselling services and back-up support for self-help groups around the country. It also publishes a variety of information leaflets and booklets about epilepsy.

17. There have been reports of high plasma levels of phenytoin causing seizures, or an increase in fit frequency, both in epileptic patients and in those with no previous history of seizures.

In the absence of a high plasma phenytoin level the possibility that disease progression had occurred would have had to be considered.

18. Several possibilities might account for Mr U's high plasma phenytoin level, such as changes in his compliance or in the dosage form of phenytoin he is taking, a drug interaction, or the fact that phenytoin accumulation had occurred since his discharge.

The pharmacokinetic profile of phenytoin can result in very large increases in plasma level after relatively small changes in dose, or in phenytoin availability or metabolism. The following possibilities should thus be considered.

(a) Drug interactions. Several drugs can cause an elevation of plasma phenytoin levels, either through enzyme inhibition or by another mechanism. Drugs that may increase phenytoin levels include amiodarone, azapropazone, cimetidine, and co-trimoxazole. Mr U's recent and current drug history must therefore be reviewed.

(b) Steady state. The possibility that Mr U was not at steady state on discharge should be considered. Previous compliance, sample timing, and sample interpretation should be reviewed.

(c) Patient compliance. The possibility of over- or under-compliance by Mr U, at the present time and earlier, should be investigated.

(d) Brand of phenytoin. The bioavailability of phenytoin may vary from brand to brand. The brands taken by Mr U should be ascertained, if possible, and any instances of brands being changed noted.

19. Omit the next day's dose and measure his plasma-phenytoin level 48 hours after admission. When the plasma level is back in the therapeutic range, re-institute phenytoin at a dose of 250 mg daily.

Allowing a drug-free interval will permit the phenytoin level to fall. Again, because of the non-linear pharmacokinetics of the drug, predicting when the level will be back within the therapeutic range is difficult. There has been no evidence that a dose of 250 mg daily is too high for Mr U; therefore it should be continued.

20. Yes. Carbamazepine is at least as effective as phenytoin in the treatment of complex partial seizures.

While carbamazepine has a number of adverse effects, it is less pharmacokinetically complex than phenytoin, and has taken over as drug of first choice for many indications.

21. (a) Absorption.

Absorption of carbamazepine from the gastro-intestinal tract is slow, with peak plasma concentrations occurring four to eight hours after a dose. Absorption may also be dose-dependent, with a smaller fraction being absorbed after larger doses. Bioavailability is generally good, and is thought to be about 90%.

(b) Metabolism.

The metabolism of carbamazepine takes place in the liver, the major metabolite being carbamazepine-10,11-epoxide, which also has anticonvulsant activity. Carbamazepine also induces enzymes within the liver, and increases its own metabolism and that of some other drugs. Carbamazepine half-life after a single dose is around 24–36 hours, but this falls to 10–20 hours on chronic dosing. Thus, dose requirements are likely to increase with time as carbamazepine clearance increases. The full effect of this enzyme induction may not be seen for up to one month after the start of therapy.

22. He should be started on 200 mg twice daily, to be increased by 200 mg weekly until optimal clinical effects are obtained.

Carbamazepine is likely to cause neurotoxic adverse effects (such as nausea, headache, drowsiness, sedation, ataxia, and diplopia) if therapy is started with full maintenance doses. The drug is therefore usually introduced at a low dose (e.g. 200 mg twice daily) and increased in increments of 200 mg weekly until optimal clinical effects are obtained. The usual maintenance dose for monotherapy is in the range 10–20 mg/kg/day.

23. No.

The reduction in carbamazepine's half-life on chronic dosing means that once-daily dosing results in sub-therapeutic levels for a large portion of the day. In addition, central nervous system toxicity is often unacceptably severe after large doses (even when the total daily dose is given in two aliquots). Conventional preparations need to be given a minimum of two times a day; often, when high daily doses are necessary, adverse effects necessitate administration three or even four times a day.

24. No.

As Mr U is obtaining clinical benefit from phenytoin, it would be advisable to decrease his phenytoin dose slowly (by 50 mg each week) while carbamazepine therapy is being introduced and slowly increased.

25. By clinical and plasma level monitoring.

(a) Clinical efficacy. Mr U was clinically reasonably well controlled on phenytoin therapy; therefore an increase in seizure frequency on carbamazepine therapy would be unacceptable. Close clinical monitoring of seizure control and of possible additive neurotoxicity should be carried out, especially while carbamazepine therapy is being introduced and phenytoin therapy withdrawn.

(b) Toxicity. At the initiation of therapy neurotoxicity can occur, but this can be minimised if the dose is increased gradually. Rashes may occur in up to 5% of patients at the start of therapy.

Leucopenia may occur but is usually mild, and is often reversible despite continued drug administration. Routine white blood cell counts are considered to be unnecessary. Blood dyscrasias such as aplastic anaemia and agranulocytosis have been reported but are rare. Hepatotoxicity has been reported rarely.

Carbamazepine can stimulate the release of antidiuretic hormone from the pituitary, and, as a result, can cause mild, symptomless hyponatraemia. The effect is thought to be dose- and concentration-dependent, and occasionally confusion, fluid retention and serum sodium levels below 120 mmol/L may occur. Routine laboratory monitoring is generally not considered necessary in patients on carbamazepine, but all patients treated with the drug should be advised to report unusual symptoms to their doctor.

(c) Plasma concentrations. The commonly quoted therapeutic range for carbamazepine is 4–12 mg/L. Interpretation of carbamazepine plasma concentrations is made more difficult by the presence of the 10,11-epoxide metabolite, which can contribute to both therapeutic effects and toxicity. In addition, the much-reduced half-life of carbamazepine on chronic therapy leads to inter-dose fluctuation in plasma concentration of up to 100%. Many patients require plasma concentrations significantly higher than 12 mg/L for optimal therapeutic effect.

Samples for carbamazepine plasma concentration should be taken after the absorption phase, and trough concentrations are often used.

26. His carbamazepine dose should be increased to 600 mg twice daily.

It is possible that, if Mr U's compliance with therapy is good, and in the absence of any drug therapy that could cause a reduction in carbamazepine levels, the enzyme-inducing effect of carbamazepine has resulted in a lowering of carbamazepine plasma levels, and break-through seizures. A dose increase is therefore indicated. The relationship between dose and plasma concentration is thought to be linear for carbamazepine, and a dosage increase of about 50% should bring about seizure control.

Unfortunately, increasing Mr U's dose to a level sufficient to regain seizure control may cause dose-related adverse effects (such as diplopia, headache, nausea, dizziness, and tiredness).

27. A controlled-release carbamazepine preparation (Tegretol® Retard) is now available.

The preparation is based on a crystalline matrix and is said to reduce intra-dose fluctuations of carbamazepine plasma levels. Bioavailability has been shown to be similar to that of plain Tegretol® tablets. It is possible that this preparation would be suitable for Mr U, and enable him to take his daily dosage in two aliquots.

References and Further Reading

Anon., Carbamazepine update, *Lancet*, 1989, **2**, 595–597.

Brodie M.J. and Hallworth M.J., Therapeutic monitoring of carbamazepine., *Hosp. Update*, 1987, **13**, 57–63.

Culshaw M., Epilepsy and its treatment, *Pharm. J.*, 1989, **242,** 138–140.

Hallworth M.J. and Brodie M.J., Therapeutic monitoring of phenytoin, *Hosp. Update*, 1987, **13,** 830–840.

Hopkins A. (ed.), *Epilepsy*, London, Chapman and Hall, 1987.

Hopkins A., Epilepsy, in Weatherall D.J., Ledingham J.G.G. and Warrell D.A. (eds), *Oxford Textbook of Medicine*, 2nd edn, Oxford, Oxford University Press, 1987, 21.53–21.67.

Laidlaw J. *et al.* (eds), *A Textbook of Epilepsy*, 3rd edn, Edinburgh, Churchill Livingstone, 1988.

Marshall P. and Marshall K., Epilepsy: counselling the patient, *Pharm. J.*, 1989, **242,** 168.

Richens, A., Clinical pharmacokinetics of phenytoin, *Clin. Pharmacokinet.*, 1979, **4,** 153–169.

Winter M.E. and Tozer T.N., Phenytoin, in *Applied Pharmacokinetics: Principles of Therapeutic Drug Monitoring*, 2nd edn, Evans W.E., Schentag J.J. and Jusko W.J. (eds), Spokane, Applied Therapeutics, 1986, 493–540.

PARKINSON'S DISEASE

Michael G. Spencer

Principal Pharmacist, Patient Services, St James's University Hospital, Leeds

Day 1 Mr E, a 62-year-old retired accountant, was admitted to the neurology ward. His presenting complaints included an increasing frequency of dystonic limb movements, severe inertia of movement, and difficulty in manipulating small objects.

Two years earlier friends had commented that he had begun to limp, while he had noticed that he had difficulty in relaxing his grip after using a knife and fork, especially with his left hand. These symptoms had gradually worsened over the next eighteen months and he had also developed a resting tremor in his left hand and left leg.

His general practitioner had diagnosed Parkinson's disease.

1. What are the main symptoms of Parkinson's disease?

2. What biochemical defects are thought to be present in a patient like Mr E?

3. Which drugs are generally used as first-line agents for patients with Parkinson's disease, and what are their modes of action?

4. What treatment would you recommend for Mr E, and why?

Day 2 Mr E was started on benzhexol 1 mg three times daily. Over the next few days the dose was gradually increased to 4 mg three times daily. Benzhexol therapy improved his tremor but had little effect on his other symptoms, so Sinemet-Plus®, one tablet three times daily, was added. This produced some improvement in his remaining symptoms.

5. How should Mr E's levodopa therapy be adjusted to optimise response?

6. What are the most frequent side-effects of anticholinergic and levodopa therapy? How can the incidence of such side-effects be minimised?

Day 14 Mr E was discharged on Sinemet-275® three times daily, plus benzhexol 4 mg three times daily.

Month 85 Mr E was admitted for reassessment.

Day 1 of readmission Mr E's therapy and symptoms had remained unchanged until recently, when he had begun to notice a "tremor" or "shaking" occurring about one hour after each dose of Sinemet. The "tremor" lasted for about 45 minutes and then abated. In addition, one year prior to this readmission Mr E had begun to develop a painful flexion of the right hip early in the morning, to prevent which he had tried taking an extra late-night Sinemet, a strategy that was sometimes successful. He also stated that his mobility was significantly impaired for two or three hours before he was due to take his doses during the day.

Examination revealed facial impassivity and a resting tremor of both hands and legs. "Cog-wheel" rigidity was found in all four limbs. Plantar reflexes were flexor. When asked to write, Mr E demonstrated micrographia. He appeared to have difficulty in initiating speech and complained of a dry mouth. It was noted that he had difficulty in rising from a chair, and had a "Parkinson's shuffle" when he walked.

Mr E complained that he had occasional falls, that he was unable to leave the house, and that his wife had to do everything for him. He was very depressed about his condition.

There was no other medical history of note. Laboratory values of routine tests were all within normal limits. His drug therapy was Sinemet-275 and benzhexol 4 mg at 7.00 a.m., 1.00 p.m., and 5.00 p.m. and, occasionally, Sinemet-275 at 10.30 p.m.

7. Which of the long-term complications of levodopa therapy does Mr E appear to be suffering from?

8. What alterations to his therapy would you recommend in order to try to minimise these effects?

9. *How could you monitor and assess his response to these therapy changes?*

10. *Can you suggest any non-drug management that might benefit Mr E?*

Day 2 Mr E's therapy was changed from Sinemet-275 three times daily to one-and-a-half Sinemet-110 tablets at 6 a.m., 10 a.m., 2 p.m., 6 p.m. and 10 p.m. His benzhexol therapy was not altered. The nursing staff were asked to complete an hourly mobility chart. The mobility chart records for Day 1 and Day 5 were:

	Day 1 (275, 3 × daily)	Day 5 (110, 5 × daily)
6 a.m.	+2	+1 (dose)
7 a.m.	+2 (dose)	−1
8 a.m.	−1	0
9 a.m.	−1	0
10 a.m.	−2	+1 (dose)
11 a.m.	+1	−1
12 noon	+1	0
1 p.m.	−1 (dose)	0
2 p.m.	−1	0 (dose)

Although Mr E's mobility and dyskinesia were improved, he remained depressed about his condition.

11. *Might bromocriptine or selegiline therapy benefit Mr E?*

12. *Which antidepressant would you recommend for Mr E?*

Day 7 It was decided to start Mr E on bromocriptine. He was prescribed 1 mg at night for one week, and discharged on bromocriptine 2.5 mg at night, with instructions to his general practitioner to increase the dose by 2.5 mg daily every five to seven days, according to response.

Day 65 Mr E was admitted as an emergency by his general practitioner, after having had two spells of hallucinations. Two weeks earlier he had complained, for five days, that he was continuously hearing voices discussing him, and that he was being controlled by radio-waves from a neighbour's burglar alarm. Immediately prior to admission his disease symptoms had deteriorated, and he had also complained that he could hear a motor-cycle revving continuously. On admission he was taking one Sinemet-110 five times daily, benzhexol 4 mg three times daily, and bromocriptine 15 mg daily.

13. *Which drugs might have contributed to Mr E's symptoms.*

14. *What adjustments would you recommend be made to his therapy?*

Day 66 The recommendations were carried out. Mr E's hallucinations resolved and did not recur. His mobility did not deteriorate significantly and he was discharged.

15. *What is the long-term outlook for Mr E?*

Answers

1. The four main symptoms found in patients with Parkinson's disease are tremor, rigidity, bradykinesia, and postural abnormalities.

Onset of Parkinson's disease is usually insidious, and progression slow. Many patients notice a resting tremor first. This usually affects the hands initially, and may be unilateral. The tremor disappears on movement and during sleep and may worsen under stress.

Rigidity manifests as an increased resistance to passive movement and is classically termed "cogwheel" rigidity, a ratchet-like phenomenon felt at the wrist on passive movement of the hand.

Bradykinesia is reflected in immobile features and a fixed, staring appearance, and, together with the rigidity, is responsible for the typical abnormalities of gait: difficulty in starting and finishing steps, which results in shuffling; a stooped head; flexed neck, upper extremities and knees; and a lack of normal arm swing.

Loss of postural reflexes leads to postural imbalance and sometimes to frequent falls. Other common symptoms include micrographia, drooling of saliva, constipation, difficulty in swallowing, and speech alteration. Symptoms increase in number and severity as the disease progresses.

2. Several biochemical defects are thought to be present in patients with Parkinson's disease.

A combination of cholinergic (excitatory) and dopaminergic (inhibitory) mechanisms, acting in the striatal tracts of the basal ganglia of the brain, are thought to be responsible for the smooth control of voluntary movements. Imbalances in the neurotransmitters lead to movement disorders. In patients with Parkinson's disease, dopamine concentrations in the three major parts of the basal ganglia are reduced to a fraction of normal. Compensatory mechanisms operate, and symptoms are not noted until a severe loss of dopaminergic neurones has occurred. The severity of some symptoms, such as bradykinesia, has been found to correlate with striatal dopamine levels; however, abnormalities of other neurotransmitters, including noradrenaline, 5-hydroxytryptamine, and gamma-aminobutyric acid, have also been reported. The full relevance of these changes is as yet unclear.

3. First-line therapy for Parkinson's disease is usually either an anticholinergic drug, or levodopa, or a combination of both.

Anticholinergic drugs (e.g. benzhexol, benztropine and orphenadrine) are thought to act by correcting the relative central cholinergic excess brought about by dopamine deficiency. Anticholinergics are considered to have more effect on tremor and rigidity than on bradykinesia, and are sometimes useful as sole therapy when function is only mildly impaired. They act synergistically with levodopa preparations.

Dopamine deficiency cannot be rectified by the administration of dopamine, since dopamine does not cross the blood–brain barrier; however, levodopa does cross the blood–brain barrier and is converted to dopamine in the basal ganglia. Levodopa is thus thought to act primarily by increasing brain dopamine concentrations.

If levodopa is administered alone, over 95% of a dose is decarboxylated peripherally, which results in reduced amounts being available to cross the blood–brain barrier, and an increase in peripheral side-effects (such as nausea, vomiting, anorexia, and postural hypotension). Levodopa is therefore usually administered with a decarboxylase inhibitor, either carbidopa or benserazide. The decarboxylase inhibitor does not cross the blood–brain barrier, and enables smaller daily doses of levodopa to be administered (thereby reducing the incidence of peripheral side-effects). Levodopa therapy is particularly helpful in controlling symptoms of bradykinesia or akinesia.

4. Mr E should first be prescribed a low dose of an anticholinergic, such as benzhexol 1 mg three times daily. The dose should be gradually increased until an optimal balance of therapeutic and side-effects is achieved.

A trial of anticholinergic therapy alone is warranted in Mr E, but his overall symptom picture indicates that he is also likely to require levodopa therapy. If anticholinergic therapy alone does not produce sufficient symptom control, levodopa plus a decarboxylase inhibitor should be introduced, again starting with a low dose (e.g. Sinemet-Plus® three times daily), and increasing gradually according to response.

There has been considerable controversy over whether levodopa therapy should be started early or withheld until disability is reasonably severe. Fears that effectiveness decreases, and side-effects increase, after a few years of levodopa therapy led to suggestions that it should be withheld for as long as possible. Although there are still proponents of both early and late initiation of levodopa therapy, many clinicians believe that levodopa can help patients at all stages of the disease, and that it does not lose effectiveness over time, nor halt progression of the disease. This latter observation generally results in attempts to increase dosage as the disease progresses, and consequently to an increase in levodopa side-effects.

5. Mr E should be started on a low dose of levodopa/decarboxylase inhibitor therapy (e.g. Sinemet-Plus – 100 mg levodopa plus 25 mg carbidopa), which should be increased gradually until optimal effects are achieved.

At the commencement of levodopa therapy, the effects of a dose usually last for four to eight hours, so the tablets may be prescribed three times daily. The dose should be increased by one tablet every two to three days until optimum effects are seen or adverse effects occur. If daily doses of less than 70 mg carbidopa are used the peripheral decarboxylase will not be saturated, and Mr E will be more likely to suffer from nausea and vomiting. Most patients are initially controlled on 400–800 mg levodopa daily.

6. (a) Anticholinergic side-effects.

The adverse effects of all the anticholinergics used for the treatment of Parkinson's disease are similar, and are due mainly to peripheral cholinergic receptor blockade. Such effects are well known and easily recognisable, and include blurred vision, dry mouth, constipation, and urinary retention, the latter being especially common in men with prostatic hypertrophy. Although often classed as "minor", these effects can be particularly troublesome to elderly patients and can significantly reduce their quality of life.

Central adverse effects of anticholinergics include delerium, disorientation, anxiety, agitation, and hallucinations. Such effects are particularly likely at high doses and/or in elderly patients.

Side-effects of anticholinergics can be minimised by introducing the drug gradually, and increasing the dose slowly. If side-effects are troublesome, a gradual reduction of dose may help, but anticholinergic therapy should not be stopped suddenly in patients with Parkinson's disease, as this may result in a sudden increase in disability.

(b) Levodopa side-effects.

The peripheral side-effects of levodopa are significantly reduced by combining levodopa with a decarboxylase inhibitor (see answer 3); however, peripheral side-effects may still occur. Levodopa therapy is thus best started at a low dose and the daily dosage increased gradually. In addition, the incidence of nausea and vomiting can be reduced still further by ensuring that the drug is taken with food.

Unfortunately, combining levodopa with a decarboxylase inhibitor does not reduce, and indeed usually increases, the incidence of levodopa's adverse effects on the central nervous system (such as depression, delerium, agitation and aggression). Auditory and visual hallucinations may occur. These effects are more common in patients over 60, patients with underlying dementia, and those with severe Parkinson's disease. If central nervous system side-effects do occur, reduction of levodopa dosage may be necessary but, as with anticholinergic therapy, levodopa therapy should not be stopped suddenly.

7. Mr E appears to be suffering from end-of-dose akinesia and dyskinesias.

Most patients will demonstrate a slow improvement in response during the first 12–18 months on levodopa therapy. Symptoms are then adequately controlled for a period of about three to five years. After this time, around 50% of patients develop fluctuations in motor performance or drug-induced dyskinesias. If appropriate action is not taken, these effects may become as disabling as the disease itself.

End-of-dose akinesia is the term used when the therapeutic effects of a dose of levodopa are lost. This commonly occurs first thing in the morning (after the longest dosage interval) or just before or after a dose during the day. Patients may become immobilised and unable to do anything except wait for the next dose. After prolonged treatment, gradual deterioration in symptoms may occur between one and three hours after a dose.

Dyskinesias can occur in 60–90% of patients and are usually dose-related. They are generally worst when the response to a dose of levodopa is maximal, and have been correlated with high levodopa plasma levels; they are therefore commonly seen after a dose has been taken. Symptoms include grimacing, gnawing, and involuntary rhythmic jerking movements.

A third effect of long-term levodopa therapy is the "on-off" phenomenon. The patient develops a sudden loss of effectiveness ("off") when "freezing" occurs, which may last for only one minute or for up to several hours before normal function returns ("on"). Dyskinesias are frequently seen in the "on" period of patients who develop this phenomenon.

8. Increase the frequency of levodopa administration to four-hourly and reduce the amount of levodopa given with each dose.

End-of-dose bradykinesia or akinesia is thought to be caused by a progression of the underlying disease or an unexplained occurrence of symptoms of dopamine deficiency after an initial response to each dose. Although there is no change in the plasma half-life of levodopa, it appears that the pharmacological half-life is reduced. End-of-dose akinesia has been shown to be corrected by levodopa infusions; however, these are not a genuine therapeutic option, as levodopa must be infused in large volumes, owing to its acidity, and it also commonly causes thrombophlebitis. The initial approach taken to minimise the end-of-dose effect is to try to decrease the levodopa dosage interval. It has also been proposed that a levodopa/benserazide controlled-release preparation (Madopar CR®, levodopa 100 mg and benserazide 25 mg), which has recently become available, may reduce end-of-dose akinesia. The manufacturers claim that the preparation produces a more sustained and prolonged levodopa plasma concentration. The time to peak, and peak plasma levodopa concentrations, are reduced and the bioavailability, compared with the standard Madopar 125® preparation, is 60%.

Dyskinesias are of central origin and reflect the success of carbidopa in allowing adequate amounts of levodopa to reach the central nervous system. As dyskinesia is usually dose-related, a reduction in levodopa dose may be beneficial.

A reasonable initial strategy for Mr E would be merely to give his present total daily dose of 750 mg levodopa in five, rather than three, aliquots.

9. By charting Mr E's mobility regularly.

Most neurology wards have some type of mobility chart on which an indication of a patient's mobility is recorded at suitable intervals. Such charts can be a valuable aid to the manipulation of drug administration in order to optimise therapy. One version of a scoring system is described below. In addition to a score, a brief description of the patient's condition is usually added.

Score	Description
−2	Severe dyskinesia
−1	Occasional involuntary movements
0	No rigidity, mobilising well
+1	Mild rigidity, with or without tremor. Needs help to mobilise
+2	Severe rigidity, with or without tremor. Unable to mobilise

10. Mr E may benefit from some remedial therapy, such as speech therapy, physiotherapy or occupational therapy. In addition, specialist disability equipment may help.

Mr E and his relatives should also be made aware of the existence of the Parkinson's Disease Society,

which can provide education and general advice, and the Disabled Living Foundation, which can provide information about aids.

If Mr E has difficulty in handling his tablets or opening bottles, consideration should be given to obtaining a tablet dispenser from Merck Sharp & Dohme. This is available free of charge.

11. Either agent could benefit Mr E.

Bromocriptine acts in Parkinson's disease by stimulating dopamine receptors. Although it can be effective when used alone, the doses necessary often cannot be tolerated, and it is therefore usually used as an adjunct to levodopa therapy. It can benefit patients who have demonstrated a deteriorating response to levodopa and may reduce Mr E's end-of-dose akinesia.

Selegiline is a monoamine-oxidase-B inhibitor; this drug can also be used in combination with levodopa to reduce end-of-dose akinesia. It is also useful in patients with on-off phenomena.

The addition of selegiline to Mr E's regimen may improve his symptoms by prolonging the action of levodopa, but the effects are usually short-lived; consideration would then need to be given to prescribing a direct-acting dopamine agonist such as bromocriptine. It is therefore probably more appropriate to start Mr E on bromocriptine.

Bromocriptine should be started in a low dose (e.g. 2.5 mg at night) and gradually increased by 2.5 mg increments until an optimal response is achieved. The dose of levodopa will need to be reduced because of the possibility of additive side-effects.

12. Lofepramine, trazodone or doxepin.

Depression is relatively common in patients suffering from Parkinson's disease. Choice of an antidepressant, when this is clinically indicated, is essentially the same as in any other situation, although older agents with pronounced anticholinergic effects should probably be avoided in patients already taking anticholinergics.

13. All three drugs prescribed for Mr E can cause the psychiatric complications described.

Anticholinergics and levodopa cause a variety of psychiatric symptoms, including hallucinations, while central nervous system effects such as hallucinations and confusion can also occur with bromocriptine. The psychiatric complications of all three drugs are especially common in the elderly, and concomitant administration of the drugs can result in additive effects on the central nervous system.

14. Reduce his doses of bromocriptine and benzhexol.

The psychiatric complications of most anti-Parkinson drugs are dose-related, and often respond to a reduction in dosage. As Mr E's problems have occurred since the introduction of bromocriptine, dosage reduction of this agent (e.g. to 10 mg daily initially) is appropriate. Dosage reduction of benzhexol is also appropriate (e.g. to 2 mg three times daily). If the therapeutic effects of the regimen are also reduced, then very cautious dosage increments of, in the first place, bromocriptine are warranted, until the optimal balance of therapeutic effects versus adverse effects is achieved.

15. It is likely that Mr E's condition will again start deteriorating after two to two-and-a-half years, as the duration of efficacy of bromocriptine when added to levodopa therapy is usually around this time.

End-of-dose akinesia and bradykinesia may continue to be a problem for Mr E, and further dose manipulation may be necessary. If "on-off" fluctuations prove to be a problem, some new therapeutic strategies have recently become available.

The controlled-release preparation Madopar CR, discussed in answer 8, may be of value. In patients with "on-off" fluctuations, substitution of an appropriate dose of Madopar CR for a conventional release form can reduce fluctuation and cause an increase in "on" time. Dose frequency is unlikely to be significantly reduced.

Subcutaneous injection or infusion of apomorphine has recently been shown to be of value in patients with "on-off" fluctuation in response. Apomorphine is a potent dopaminergic agent. Its oral use is limited because of its short-lived effect, and side-effects such as nausea, vomiting, postural hypotension, and sedation. Domperidone (a peripheral dopamine antagonist) can control the adverse effects, and the effect of apomorphine can be prolonged by continuous subcutaneous infusion. Intermittent subcutaneous doses have been used successfully in patients with only a small number of "off" periods per day, and are usually effective within 10–15 minutes.

Although levodopa therapy does not halt the pathological changes in patients with Parkinson's disease, it does appear to increase life-expectancy, when compared with the life-expectancy of untreated patients. Unfortunately, the effectiveness of levodopa and other currently available drugs appears to decrease with time, and management of symptoms becomes increasingly difficult as the disease progresses. Death is usually due to respiratory complications, especially infection.

References and Further Reading

Eadie M.J., Neurological diseases, in *Avery's Drug Treatment: Principles and Practice of Clinical Pharmacology and Therapeutics*, 3rd edn, Speight T.M. (ed.), Edinburgh, Churchill Livingstone, 1989, 1106–1112.

Erwin W.G. and Turco T.F., Current concepts in clinical therapeutics: Parkinson's disease, *Clin. Pharm.*, 1986, **5**, 742–753.

Gibberd F.B., Clinical algorithms: management of Parkinson's disease, *Br. med. J.*, 1987, **294**, 1393–1396.

Marsden C.D., Movement disorders, in *Oxford Textbook of Medicine*, 2nd edn, Weatherall D.J., Ledingham J.G.G. and Warrell D.A. (eds), Oxford, Oxford University Press, 1987, 21.218–21.225.

McEvoy G.K. (ed.), *AHFS Drug Information 90*, Bethesda, American Society of Hospital Pharmacists, 1990, 2181–2186.

Quinn N.P. and Husain F.A., Clinical algorithm: Parkinson's disease, *Br. med. J.*, 1986, **293**, 379–382.

Robertson D.R.C. and George C.F., Drug therapy for Parkinson's disease in the elderly, *Br. med. Bull.*, 1990, **46**, 124–146.

TUBERCULOUS MENINGITIS

Robert Horne

Principal Pharmacist/Lecturer, Clinical Pharmacy Unit, Brighton Health Authority/School of Pharmacy

Day 1 Mr Q was admitted via the emergency and accident department. He was a 65-year-old Bengali gentleman, who had been resident in the UK for 18 months. He was a widower and lived with his 28-year-old daughter, her husband, and their two children (aged two and three years). Mr Q's understanding of English was limited and his medical history was taken with the help of his daughter, who had accompanied him to the hospital.

Mr Q presented with a four-week history of lethargy, intermittent headaches, fever, and night sweats. His symptoms had gradually increased in severity during this time, and in the three days prior to admission he had become progressively drowsy and slightly confused. He did not drink alcohol or smoke tobacco. His past medical history was unremarkable.

On examination he was found to be thin, feverish and pale. His temperature was 38.5°C. He appeared to be drowsy and slightly disorientated, with a short concentration span. He complained of headache and exhibited slight neck stiffness. Examination and reflex tests revealed a mild right hemiparesis. Apart from paracetamol (1 g every six hours when required for headache), he was taking no medication.

His serum urea and electrolyte levels, haemoglobin level, and liver function tests (LFTs) were all within normal limits. A computerised tomography (CT) scan was normal, with no evidence of raised intracranial pressure, oedema or hydrocephalus. A lumbar puncture was therefore performed, and a sample of cerebrospinal fluid (CSF) sent for analysis. Mr Q's chest x-ray showed evidence of apical fibrosis consistent with previous pulmonary tuberculosis (TB). CSF, sputum, blood, and urine samples were sent for microbiological examinations.

His lumbar puncture results were:

	Mr Q's CSF	Normal CSF
Appearance	Colourless and clear	Colourless and clear
Polymorphic neutrophils	$50/\mu L$	Absent
Lymphocytes	$180/\mu L$	0–5
Protein	0.8 g/L	0.1–0.4
Glucose	1.2 mmol/L	2.5–4.2
Acid-fast bacillus	Absent	Absent

Mr Q's fasting blood glucose at the time of his lumbar puncture was 5.8 mmol/L (reference range less than 6). (CSF glucose is usually approximately half the value of blood glucose. Simultaneous blood and CSF glucose estimations should thus be performed.) His blood, urine, and sputum samples were negative for acid-fast bacillus.

Because of Mr Q's x-ray result and his non-specific presentation, a Mantoux test 1 in 10,000 (1 unit of tuberculin PPD in 0.1 mL) was ordered. A diagnosis of tuberculous meningitis (TBM) was made, based on his previous medical history, chest x-ray, lumbar puncture results and clinical presentation.

Mr Q (who weighed 62 kg) was prescribed:

Isoniazid 600 mg orally daily
Rifampicin 600 mg orally daily
Pyrazinamide 2 g orally daily
Streptomycin 750 mg intramuscularly daily

1. Was the presentation of Mr Q's TB typical for his age and ethnicity?

2. Was the correct Mantoux test chosen? How would you recommend the test be carried out?

3. Was it appropriate to start treatment before the results of microbiological culture were known?

4. Why were four antituberculants prescribed for Mr Q?

5. Would you have recommended the agents chosen for Mr Q?

6. Were the prescribed doses appropriate? How should the drugs be administered?

7. Would you recommend additional therapy at this stage?

8. How should Mr Q's treatment be monitored biochemically?

Day 2 Mr Q still had a low-grade fever (temperature 38.2°C). He complained of headache and neck pain. Apart from slight right hemiparesis, neurological signs were still absent. A CT scan revealed no evidence of cerebral oedema or hydrocephalus. He was not eating but was taking fluids and managing to swallow his medication.

9. Should Mr Q be prescribed corticosteroid therapy?

10. Would it be appropriate to add intrathecal streptomycin to his regimen?

11. What changes would you recommend to his treatment regimen if he should become unable to tolerate oral medication?

Day 3 Mr Q's condition was stable. He continued to appear vague and occasionally a little confused. A low-grade fever remained, but his fluid balance and serum electrolytes were within normal limits. A palpable induration of 12 mm diameter, at the site of his earlier Mantoux test, indicated a positive response to tuberculin PPD 1 in 10,000.

12. What is the significance of the positive Mantoux test?

13. What other skin tests are used in the diagnosis of TB? What are their advantages and disadvantages?

14. Should Mr Q's grandchildren and their mother be allowed to visit him at this stage?

15. Is prophylactic treatment indicated for Mr Q's grandchildren? If so, which agent(s) and dosage regimen would you recommend?

16. Mr Q's daughter is two months pregnant. Which, if any, prophylactic agents should she receive?

Day 5 Mr Q's headache was abating. He felt better and his temperature was settling (37.6°C). Although still drowsy, he had become progressively less confused. His serum urea and electrolyte levels and blood counts remained within normal limits, but the results of his LFTs were:

Alanine aminotransferase (ALT) 78 units/L (reference range 7–35)
Aspartate aminotransferase (AST) 80 units/L (7–40)
Alkaline phosphatase 47 units/L (25–90)
Bilirubin (total) 12 micromol/L (less than 17)
Bilirubin (direct) 2 micromol/L (less than 6)

Mr Q was not jaundiced, and clinical signs of hepatic disease were absent.

17. What might have caused Mr Q's abnormal LFTs? What action would you recommend?

Day 12 Mr Q had improved steadily. His LFTs had returned to normal. His right-sided hemiparesis was still present, but he was able to sit up in bed and converse normally with his daughter. It was decided to discharge him in three days' time if progress was maintained.

18. For how long is treatment likely to be necessary?

19. What are the major points you would want to convey to Mr Q during discharge counselling?

20. What general measures could you adopt to encourage his compliance?

21. If it was suspected at a later date that Mr Q was not complying with his treatment regimen, what alternative strategies would you recommend? What additional monitoring may be necessary?

Answers

1. Mr Q's presentation is atypical with respect to the British population as a whole, but is typical when the sub-group of Asian or African immigrants is considered.

It is first important to distinguish between TB infection and disease. Primary infection usually occurs when droplets of infected sputum are inhaled into the lungs. When first exposed, the host lacks acquired immunity and the bacteria may spread rapidly from the lungs to the lymph, and possibly other tissues, such as the kidney and joints.

Widespread symptomatic infection is usually prevented by the development of acquired resistance to the mycobacterium. Macrophages engulf the bacteria and later coalesce to form clumps or tubercules, which may become calcified. Primary infection, therefore, rarely produces any symptoms except perhaps a fever or mild illness, and may even go unnoticed. An exception is in infancy, when infection may be fatal if it becomes disseminated or uncontrolled.

Primary infection may be followed by post-primary disease if the subject becomes re-infected or the primary disease is reactivated. The likelihood of this depends on the patient's age, general health, nutritional and immune status, and on the virulence of the organism.

In adults post-primary disease most commonly surfaces in the lungs, but may focus on other organs (such as the kidneys, lymph nodes, or joints), or may be disseminated (miliary TB). TBM is more common in children between the ages of three months and three years. However, in Britain, adult Asian and African immigrants often present atypically, and TBM is more common in this group than in the endogenous adult population.

2. The correct Mantoux test was chosen, as it was strongly suspected that Mr Q was tuberculin sensitive.

The Mantoux test involves the intradermal injection of a small quantity of tuberculin purified protein derivative (PPD). Previous or current infection with *Mycobacterium tuberculosis* produces an allergic type IV response, which results in a zone of induration (localised skin thickening due to oedema), the size of which depends on the degree of hypersensitivity. In the UK, a zone of induration greater than 5 mm diameter, measured 72 hours after injection of 10 units tuberculin PPD, is usually recognised as a positive result.

Tuberculin PPD is available in three strengths.

For the Mantoux test, the amount injected is always 0.1 mL. The usual testing dose is 10 units, or 0.1 mL of a 1 in 1000 dilution (100 units/mL). If there is any doubt about the zone size, a higher dose of 100 units (0.1 mL of a 1 in 100 dilution) may be given after two days. In order to avoid severe local reaction and tissue damage, a person who is suspected to be tuberculin-sensitive should be given a low dose of 1 unit (0.1 mL of a 1 in 10,000 dilution).

The test should be applied as follows. After cleaning the skin of the volar surface of the arm with alcohol, 0.1 mL of the tuberculin PPD test solution should be injected intradermally, using a needle number 25 or 26. The results should be read 72 hours later. Only areas of induration should be measured. Erythema should be ignored. Young children should usually be given half the adult dose.

3. Yes. The infecting organism can be difficult to identify and culture, and a delay in treatment can increase the morbidity and mortality associated with the disease.

The onset of TBM is often insidious and the disease may be well advanced before symptoms arise, which even then may be non-specific. In Western countries, a diagnosis of TBM is associated with a 15–30% mortality rate. The mortality rate in untreated patients approaches 100%. If treatment is not started early, severe neurological complications may occur: these can include blindness, deafness (cranial nerve damage), hemiplegia or paraplegia (spinal cord damage), hydrocephalus, and intellectual impairment. Prompt treatment is imperative to save life or avoid debilitating sequelae.

Mycobacterium tuberculosis is notoriously difficult to identify in the CSF, or to culture in the laboratory (culture may take weeks). In addition, failure to cultivate acid-fast bacillus from the CSF does not guarantee absence of the organism. Treatment must often begin before the results of a Mantoux test or microbiological culture are available. Mr Q's presentation, ethnicity, and the results of his chest x-ray, which indicated possible previous TB infection, justify early treatment.

4. It is necessary to combine treatments in order to:

(a) minimise the risk of treatment failure due to existing or emergent bacterial resistance, and

(b) widen the scope of attack to maximise bacterial kill.

Isoniazid is the most potent bactericidal agent and is active against large numbers of growing bacteria. Along with rifampicin it also prevents the emergence of drug resistance by suppressing resistant mutants within the bacterial population. Rifampicin and pyrazinamide are most effective at killing "bacterial persisters". These are slowly metabolising organisms that exist in a semi-dormant state. Failure to eradicate these could result in re-emergence of the disease. Streptomycin is a bactericidal drug which is most effective in the alkaline environment outside cells. This is in contrast to pyrazinamide which is effective against organisms in the acidic intracellular environment.

5. Yes. The serious nature of TBM, and the likely degree of central nervous system (CNS) penetration of the agents chosen, justifies the use of this regimen.

Most specialists within the UK now recommend initial treatment with isoniazid, rifampicin, and pyrazinamide, with the possible inclusion of ethambutol or streptomycin. The suitability of this combination has been demonstrated by several large studies in patients with pulmonary TB. To date, no such studies exist for other forms of TB, but this proven efficacy seems to be extrapolated in clinical practice, and similar regimens are generally prescribed on this basis. However, although a starting regimen of isoniazid, rifampicin, and pyrazinamide are usually considered to be sufficient for pulmonary TB, four drugs are often used for the initial treatment of TBM.

The ability of agents to cross the blood–brain barrier is an important consideration in the choice of treatment for TBM. Drug penetration into the CNS is usually enhanced by inflammation of the meninges. Isoniazid is widely distributed to all body tissues, including the CNS. Rifampicin crosses the blood–brain barrier when the meninges are inflamed, and gains access to the CSF for the first one or two months of treatment. Pyrazinamide readily crosses into the CNS and this, coupled with its effect against persisters, makes it an essential addition to the regimen. Streptomycin does not normally cross the blood–brain barrier, but some penetration may occur when the meninges are inflamed. Intramuscular injections of streptomycin may thus be a worthwhile addition during the early stages of treatment; however, they may be stopped when drug treatment begins to reduce the effects of infection, which may be within ten days of starting treatment. Ethambutol crosses the inflamed meninges but is bacteriostatic, so is unlikely to increase the efficacy of the regimen.

6. The prescribed doses are appropriate.

Similar doses and regimens are used to treat most other forms of TB. For patients like Mr Q, with normal renal and hepatic function, the higher dose of isoniazid (10–12 mg/kg/day) used to treat TBM is needed to increase the likelihood of optimal penetration of the drug into the CNS. The doses of rifampicin, streptomycin and pyrazinamide are appropriate for Mr Q's age and weight.

Initially, all the drugs prescribed for Mr Q should be given as a single daily dose. In this way the maximal plasma concentrations obtained will favour penetration of the drugs into the CNS.

Rifampicin is best absorbed on an empty stomach and, together with isoniazid, should be given half to one hour before breakfast, with a full glass of water. When advising on administration of the drug it should be remembered that rifampicin may stain body fluids pink. It is therefore important to inform Mr Q and all those caring for him of this harmless, but potentially distressing, effect.

Pyrazinamide tablets (500 mg) are large, and Mr Q may find them difficult to swallow. The drug may irritate the gastric mucosa and, for this reason, it is often prescribed in three or four divided doses, with or immediately after food. Although Mr Q is eating little, his pyrazinamide therapy should initially be given in a single daily dose (to enhance CNS penetration) at the same time as rifampicin and isoniazid. If he complains of gastric irritation, the pyrazinamide dose could be changed to 500 mg four times a day, taken with milk, at least one hour after the dose of rifampicin.

Care should be taken during the preparation and administration of intramuscular streptomycin. The drug has a significant displacement value (1 g in solution displaces 0.82 mL). The addition of 1.2 mL of water for injection to a vial containing 1 g streptomycin powder produces a 500 mg/mL solution. Mr Q should receive 1.5 mL of this solution, as a slow intramuscular injection, into the right upper quadrant of the gluteal muscle.

7. Mr Q should receive pyridoxine 50 mg daily.

Isoniazid may cause a reversible peripheral neuritis, which is attributed to an effect of isoniazid on vitamin B_6 (pyridoxine) metabolism (isoniazid interferes with enzymic reactions in which pyridoxal phosphate acts as a co-enzyme).

Isoniazid is eliminated mainly by hepatic acetylation. The population is split into fast and slow acetylators, slow acetylators being more prone to isoniazid-induced peripheral neuritis. Acetylator status is genetically determined and there are clear ethnic differences: Orientals and Innuits are predominantly fast acetylators and may therefore require larger doses of isoniazid, while Caucasians and Asians tend to have equal proportions of fast and slow acetylators. Although the acetylator status of an individual can be demonstrated by a laboratory test, widespread testing is not justified when prophylaxis can be so easily and safely administered to all individuals.

For the majority of patients, prophylaxis with low doses of pyridoxine (e.g. 10 mg daily) is enough to reduce the incidence of isoniazid-induced neuritis from 20% to less than 1%. However, some sources, particularly in the USA, recommend higher doses, of 50–100 mg pyridoxine daily. As Mr Q is receiving a high dose of isoniazid, it would be prudent to administer a larger dose of pyridoxine. Pyridoxine 50 mg daily is likely to be a safe and effective prophylactic measure.

8. By routine monitoring of his hepatic and renal function, and by regular monitoring of his serum streptomycin levels.

(a) Routine LFTs. Rifampicin, isoniazid and pyrazinamide may all produce hepatotoxicity, which can range in severity from mild sub-clinical alterations in LFTs, to more serious reactions producing clinical jaundice or, rarely, fatal hepatitis. Experts are divided as to when LFTs should be monitored. Routine LFTs should be performed before starting treatment, and during the initial few weeks of treatment; thereafter, regular monitoring of LFTs is usually only necessary if the patient is over 50, regularly consumes large quantities of alcohol, has existing liver disease, or is receiving other hepatotoxic drugs. Since Mr Q is over 50 and is taking isoniazid, his LFTs should be monitored weekly for the first four weeks and monthly for three months afterwards.

(b) Routine renal function tests. The elimination of all four drugs used to treat Mr Q is to some extent dependent upon renal function. This is especially true of streptomycin, which is eliminated almost entirely by the kidneys. Renal function should be monitored before starting treatment and at intervals during treatment. As Mr Q's renal function on starting treatment was normal, standard doses of his prescribed drugs were justified. The dose of isoniazid should, however, be reduced in severe renal impairment. Reduced renal elimination of rifampicin may be compensated for by increased biliary excretion.

(c) Streptomycin monitoring. In common with other aminoglycosides, streptomycin may produce ototoxicity and renal damage. Streptomycin has a specific action on the eighth cranial nerve, and vestibular damage resulting in defects of balance is more common than auditory impairment. Vestibular damage is dose-related and permanent, but if the drug is stopped early enough the damage may be small enough to allow the patient to develop compensatory ocular or proprioceptive mechanisms. A simple test of asking the patient to walk along a straight line, first with eyes open, and then closed, can be used to detect vestibular damage. However, streptomycin serum levels should be monitored in order to optimise dosage and minimise toxicity. This is particularly true for Mr Q, who is bed-bound and over 50 years of age. Owing to the short half-life of streptomycin (two to three hours in patients with normal renal function), steady-state serum concentrations can be obtained soon after starting treatment, and a loading dose is not required. Trough concentrations should not exceed 2 mg/L. As with other aminoglycosides, the drug may accumulate during chronic treatment. Mr Q should receive streptomycin serum monitoring at three and ten days after starting treatment.

It should also be remembered that the appearance of vomiting, headache, flushing or hypotension soon after the injection of streptomycin may indicate allergy to the drug, and sensitisation tests should be performed if this occurs.

9. Corticosteroid treatment is not justified at present.

The use of corticosteroids in the treatment of TB is controversial. These drugs may suppress cell-mediated immunity and so worsen the disease; however, if they are given with appropriate antituberculous therapy their anti-inflammatory effect may reduce local tissue damage, and they may also improve patient well-being as a result of their "mood-elevating" effects. In TBM, steroids can reduce life-threatening cerebral oedema and hydrocephalus, and are generally used if there is clinical evidence of these. However, it is possible that by returning the blood–brain barrier to normal status, steroids limit the passage into the CNS of poorly lipid-soluble drugs, such as rifampicin, streptomycin and ethambutol.

In view of Mr Q's CT scan results, and in the absence of clinical evidence of cerebral oedema or hydrocephalus, corticosteroids may be omitted at this stage of his disease, but if his condition were to deteriorate, or if signs of cerebral oedema become apparent, he should be given prednisolone in a dose of 40–60 mg daily. Large doses are necessary to offset the effects of rifampicin on corticosteroid elimination. Rifampicin is arguably the most potent drug inducer of liver enzymes. Concurrent treatment with rifampicin reduces the serum levels of many hepatically metabolised drugs, such as corticosteroids, oral hypoglycaemic agents, anticonvulsants, and the contraceptive pill. This effect is usually seen within a few days and may persist for up to two to three weeks after rifampicin treatment is stopped.

10. Not unless Mr Q's condition deteriorates further.

The use of intrathecal streptomycin is controversial. The dangers of injecting a drug directly into the intrathecal space are obvious, and are likely to outweigh the benefits of this route of administration if the meninges are inflamed, as in this situation sufficient concentrations of streptomycin and other antituberculants are likely to be present in the CSF after systemic administration of the drugs.

Mr Q's treatment has fortunately begun at an early stage. His symptoms are relatively mild and there is no evidence of severe neurological impairment. Intrathecal streptomycin is therefore not indicated at present; however, if his clinical or neurological status should deteriorate, or if corticosteroid therapy is initiated, then the addition of intrathecal streptomycin in a dose of 1 mg/kg/day would become justifiable.

11. Rifampicin and isoniazid may be given by intravenous and intramuscular injection respectively. Pyrazinamide is only available as tablets; however, in the short term it may be possible to replace pyrazinamide by morphazinamide, an antituberculous agent which is chemically related to pyrazinamide and which is available as an intravenous injection.

12. A positive response to the Mantoux test demonstrates hypersensitivity to tuberculoproteins, which usually indicates that the subject has been previously infected with *Mycobacterium tuberculosis* or has received a BCG vaccination (it is impossible to differentiate between these two).

It is likely that the degree of tuberculin sensitivity after infection is related to the size of the infecting dose, the virulence of the organism, and the subject's immune status. A negative response usually indicates the absence of infection, and that the subject is suitable for BCG vaccination.

In some cases, a negative response to tuberculin testing may occur in someone who is strongly suspected of being infected by *M. tuberculosis*. Possible explanations for this are:

(a) One to three per cent of patients infected with *M. tuberculosis* are negative tuberculin reactors.

(b) If the test is performed within six weeks of infection, hypersensitivity may not have had time to develop.

(c) The test has been incorrectly performed or read.

(d) A higher concentration of tuberculin may be necessary.

(e) The person may be taking immunosuppressant drugs, such as corticosteroids, which may suppress the subject's sensitivity to tuberculin.

(f) The person is suffering from a disease that may suppress tuberculin sensitivity. Such diseases include some cancers, such as Hodgkin's lymphoma, leukaemia, and bronchial carcinoma (sensitivity may be unaffected if the cancer is not far advanced), and sarcoidosis.

(g) The infection may be with an atypical mycobacterium. In this case, the patient may show a weak positive response to tuberculin PPD testing. This is particularly important in immunocompromised patients or those with HIV disease, in whom atypical infections are more commonplace.

(h) Tuberculin sensitivity seems to diminish with time, and elderly people previously infected with *M. tuberculosis* may be tuberculin-negative unless they have active lesions.

13. The Heaf test, Imotest® and Tine test.

The Mantoux test is the most commonly used tuberculin PPD test in the UK. Variants include:

(a) The Heaf Test. An apparatus is used which consists of six pre-set needles (2 mm for adults and older children, 1 mm for children under three years old). A drop of tuberculin is placed on the patient's arm. The apparatus (Heaf gun) is placed over the thin film of tuberculin formed, and the needles are released while holding the patient's arm taut. The test can be read after three days, but the results are usually still visible after a week. This is convenient when groups of people are being tested. The size of the zone of palpable induration indicates the grade of positivity. It is recommended that the Heaf test apparatus is sterilised after each use by dipping the end in methylated spirits and flaming. This test has become less popular because of the theoretical risk of transmission of HIV or viral hepatitis.

(b) The Imotest®-Tuberculin (Servier). This is similar to the Heaf test but has the advantage of being a disposable plastic unit.

(c) The Tine test. This is a disposable plastic unit with four prongs. The test must be carefully applied and read in order to avoid false results. Some physicians argue that the Tine test produces inconsistent results, but others maintain that if it is carefully applied it provides a simple and reliable screening test.

14. Yes.

The usual source of TB infection is the sputum of patients with active pulmonary TB. In such cases bacilli are usually detectable in sputum smears. Mr Q is sputum-negative, and he has no clinical evidence of pulmonary TB. His TBM is unlikely to be an infection risk and visits can be allowed.

As a precautionary measure, Mr Q's household contacts may be given a Mantoux test and chest x-ray in order to ascertain whether they are infected by *M. tuberculosis*. This is particularly important in the case of young children, because in this group primary disease is more likely to lead to miliary TB or TBM. Prompt treatment is essential in order to avoid the high degree of mortality and morbidity associated with these conditions.

15. Preventative treatment is warranted if the tuberculin-sensitivity of the child indicates that he or she is at risk of developing active disease, for example, if the results of tuberculin testing are clearly positive with a normal chest x-ray and the absence of clinical symptoms.

Contacts of patients with non-pulmonary disease are at low risk of developing TB. However, owing to the incidence of the disease in Asian families in the UK, and the severe nature of TB in children, Mr Q's grandchildren should undergo tuberculin testing. The Imotest® should be used. The reaction produced is graded on a scale of 1–4, according to the tuberculin sensitivity of the individual. Subsequent management depends on the results. If the reaction is graded 0–1, BCG vaccination should be offered. If the child has been vaccinated in the past, a follow-up chest x-ray should be taken in three months' time. If the reaction is graded 2–4, a chest x-ray should be taken and prophylaxis with isoniazid 5–10 mg/kg/day for 6–12 months should be prescribed. In this case, the child should be followed up with chest x-rays for two years.

16. The decision must rest on the results of tuberculin testing and on the interpretation of her clinical picture.

The decision to administer any drug during the first trimester of pregnancy is complicated by the fact that safety can never be guaranteed, and that there is a lack of correlation between drug effects in humans and those observed in animal studies. It is rarely possible to give a "black or white" verdict of "safe or not safe" during pregnancy. In deciding to use an anti-infective agent during pregnancy, the potential teratogenic effects of the drug must be balanced against the risks to mother and foetus of withholding treatment.

Most authorities now consider that the use of isoniazid, pyrazinamide and ethambutol during the first trimester can be justified, if there are good clinical indications. The use of rifampicin is more controversial: large doses of the drug are teratogenic in rats and the drug manufacturers consider it to be contra-indicated during the first trimester; however, the World Health Organization states that "There is no evidence that the doses of rifampicin used in clinical practice have a teratogenic effect". Streptomycin is best avoided because of the risk of ototoxicity to the foetus.

The decision of whether to treat should therefore depend on the results of tuberculin testing and the clinical picture. A negative tuberculin test and the low infective potential of Mr Q would probably be enough to rule out prophylaxis. A positive test and normal chest x-ray would indicate the need for preventative treatment with isoniazid, 300 mg as a single daily dose for six to twelve months. Clinical evidence of active disease would warrant treatment with normal adult doses of isoniazid, rifampicin and pyrazinamide. Extra pyridoxine (e.g. a dose of 50–100 mg daily) should be given with the isoniazid, as pregnant women have an increased requirement for this vitamin.

17. It seems likely that Mr Q's drug therapy has caused his abnormal LFTs, but no action is required at present.

Isoniazid, rifampicin and pyrazinamide are potentially hepatotoxic. However, it is often difficult to attribute a hepatitis directly to drug treatment, or to decide which antituberculant is responsible, as the drugs are nearly always used in combination.

Isoniazid may produce a hepato-cellular damage that resembles hepatitis (elevated serum levels of ALT and AST, but little change in alkaline phosphatase and bilirubin). This is usually mild and subclinical, and disappears even if therapy is continued. However, a proportion of people (0.1–1%) develop acute hepatic injury, which in about 10% of these patients progresses to a chronic active hepatitis. The exact mechanism is unknown, but is thought to have an auto-immune basis and to be linked to the production of a toxic metabolite. Pre-existing liver disease, alcoholism, and age over 50 are predisposing factors. The reaction usually occurs between two and 12 months after starting treatment.

Rifampicin may produce two types of liver damage:

(a) A dose-related cholestasis resulting from interference with the uptake and excretion of bilirubin.

(b) An idiosyncratic hepato-cellular damage. This reaction usually occurs three to five weeks after starting treatment. It is rare, but may pose a risk in alcoholics, the elderly, or patients with pre-existing liver disease.

The hepatitis produced by pyrazinamide is dose-related and is limited if doses are kept below 40 mg/kg/day.

In the absence of a clinical explanation, Mr Q's abnormal LFTs may be attributed to his drug treatment. Mild, transient elevations in LFTs are common during the first two months of antituberculous therapy. Treatment should be stopped if there is clinical evidence of liver damage (e.g. jaundice, hepatic enlargement, anorexia, and malaise), but if clinical signs are absent, it will, in most cases, be safe to continue treatment. Exceptions to this rule of thumb include those who consume large quantities of alcohol, the elderly, the very young, or those with pre-existing liver disease. Large (e.g. more than three or four times normal) or persistent elevations in ALT or AST serum levels may necessitate a break in therapy. Mr Q's LFTs are only slightly raised. His treatment should thus be continued with careful monitoring of his LFTs. If they continue to increase, or if he develops clinical signs of liver damage, *all* his antituberculants should be stopped, as it is not possible to identify the agent responsible for Mr Q's abnormal results (however, the normal serum bilirubin result indicates that rifampicin therapy is a less likely cause). The antituberculants should then be re-introduced one at a time, each drug being given for about a week before another is added. This should be accompanied by regular monitoring of LFTs and close clinical supervision, so that the drug responsible may be identified by a recurrence in symptoms. The offending drug could then be omitted from the regimen, or replaced by ethambutol.

18. The treatment of TB is usually split into two phases: an initial intensive phase, and a "consolidation" phase. Because there have been no large specific trials, the treatment of TBM is based on treatment regimens for pulmonary TB.

The British Thoracic Society currently recommends treatment for pulmonary TB with three or four drugs (isoniazid, rifampicin, and pyrazinamide, plus, in some cases, streptomycin or ethambutol) for the initial two months, followed by four months' treatment with two drugs (usually rifampicin and isoniazid). Treatment of TBM is similar, except that ethambutol is not recommended and the second phase is often extended to twelve or twenty-four months in order to prevent recurrence.

Because of Mr Q's rapid recovery, streptomycin is no longer indicated. He should receive isoniazid, rifampicin and pyrazinamide for a further six weeks. The duration of the next phase of treatment is debatable: preliminary data from a recent trial seem to support the efficacy of short-course treatment (i.e. a second phase of seven months); however, until further evidence is available, Mr Q is likely to receive isoniazid and rifampicin for a further twelve months. For the second phase, the dose of rifampicin and isoniazid can be reduced to 450 mg and 300 mg daily, respectively.

19. (a) The importance of compliance.

It is better for a patient to stop taking the whole drug regimen than to regularly omit one or two drugs, as the latter strategy might lead to the development of resistance to the remaining agent(s). This would preclude future use of these drugs, and necessitate the inclusion of more toxic second-line agents such as cycloserine, capreomycin, prothionamide and kanamycin.

(b) The need to continue therapy until told otherwise.

In order to "keep the disease at bay", he must continue treatment even though he may feel well.

(c) When and how to take his medicines.

All three drugs may be taken together, with a full glass of water, about an hour before breakfast. To lessen the risk of gastric irritation, the pyrazinamide dose can be split to 500 mg every six hours, but if this is likely to lessen compliance, it should be taken as a single dose of 2 g in the morning.

(d) To always give his doctor or pharmacist a list of drugs he is taking.

This is to prevent interactions which may occur between rifampicin and many other drugs, such as corticosteroids and oral hypoglycaemic agents.

20. (a) Use combination preparations wherever possible.

In Mr Q's case, his high-dose isoniazid therapy prevents the use of combination preparations during the initial phase of treatment.

(b) Encourage a drug-taking routine by fitting medication into activities of daily living.

(c) As Mr Q's English is limited, he should be counselled with his daughter present as translator.

She and her husband may then be willing to

supervise and help with the administration of Mr Q's treatment regimen, particularly if compliance seems likely to be a problem.

(d) After the dosage regimen is explained, Mr Q should be asked to relate the information back, as a check that he has understood the instructions.

(e) Tablet bottles should be labelled clearly in simple English, and Mr Q provided with a Bengali translation as a written reminder, if one can be obtained from a member of the hospital staff. Merrell Dow has produced information leaflets in Arabic, Hindi, Gujarati, Urdu, Punjabi and Bengali.

21. An intermittent, supervised drug regimen may be used, with the drugs being given twice or three times a week under full out-patient supervision.

The rifampicin dose should not exceed 600 mg twice weekly, as high-dose intermittent use is associated with an increased incidence of a flu-like syndrome (in about 1% of patients) and of thrombocytopenia. Platelet counts should be monitored and therapy changed to 300 mg daily if thrombocytopenia occurs. The isoniazid dose should be adjusted to 15 mg/kg twice a week, pyrazinamide to 3 g twice a week, and pyridoxine to 50 mg twice a week.

Acknowledgments

I would like to thank Jane Hough, Principal Pharmacist (Clinical Services) at the London Hospital, for her help with organising this chapter, Dr Albert Ferro, Medical Registrar, the London Hospital, for advice on clinical aspects, and Pat Knight and Susan Myer for typing the manuscript.

References and Further Reading

Anon., Chemotherapy of pulmonary tuberculosis in Britain, *Drug Ther. Bull.*, 1988, **26**, 1–3.

Anon., Management of contacts of tuberculosis, *ibid.*, 1990, **28**, 21–22.

Dodds L., Interactions with antitubercular drugs, *Pharm. J.*, 1988, **240**, 182.

Farrar K., Tuberculosis and its treatment, *ibid.*, 149–151.

Grosset J.H., Present status of chemotherapy of tuberculosis, *Rev. infect. Dis.*, 1989, **II**, S347–S352.

Jacob R.F. and Abernathy R.S., Management of tuberculosis in pregnancy and the newborn: infectious complications of pregnancy, *Clinics Perinatol.*, 1988, **15**, 305–319.

Joint Tuberculosis Committee of the British Thoracic Society, Control and prevention of tuberculosis: a code of practice, *Br. med. J.*, 1983, **281**, 1118–1121.

Marshall P., Patient compliance with TB treatment, *Pharm. J.*, 1988, **240**, 183.

Ormerod L.P., Chemotherapy and management of tuberculosis in the United Kingdom: recommendations of the Joint Tuberculosis Committee of the British Thoracic Society, *Thorax*, 1990, **45**, 403–408.

Ross J.D. and Horne N.W., *Modern Drug Treatment of Tuberculosis*, 6th edn, London, Chest, Heart and Stroke Association, 1983.

Subcommittee of the Joint Tuberculosis Committee of the British Thoracic Society, Control and prevention of tuberculosis in Britain: an updated code of practice, *Br. med. J.*, 1990, **300**, 995–999.

Traub M. *et al.*, Tuberculosis of the central nervous system, *Quart. J. Med.*, 1983, **209**, 81–100.

CHEMOTHERAPY-INDUCED NAUSEA AND VOMITING

Pamela S. Warrington and Margaret Nicolson

Clinical Pharmacists, Western General Hospital, Edinburgh

Day 1 Thirty-five-year-old Mr G was admitted to the medical oncology unit for treatment of his advanced malignant teratoma. He had a six-month history of epigastric discomfort and post-prandial fullness, and was complaining of increasing shortness of breath. He was not taking any regular medication and had no significant past medical history, other than a possible history of orchidopexy on the left side and a recent episode of painless haematuria. He worked on a farm, was married, and had three children. He did not smoke and only drank socially.

On examination Mr G was found to have a mass in his left testicle. Ultrasound investigations confirmed the presence of a testicular mass, and also showed a renal mass and hepatic metastases. Aspiration cytology from the renal mass showed malignant cells suggestive of metastatic testicular teratoma. A chest x-ray revealed bilateral pulmonary metastases.

Mr G's full blood count and biochemical investigations were normal, except for the following:

Lactate dehydrogenase (LDH) 620 u/L (reference range 72–395)
Human chorionic gonadotrophin (HCG) 3250 iu/L (<5)
Alpha-fetoprotein (AFP) 1457 iu/mL (2–6).

Human chorionic gonadotrophin and alpha-fetoprotein are not normally produced by males but may be secreted by germ cell tumours, making them useful indicators of tumour presence. Mr G's creatinine clearance, determined by a 24-hour urine collection, was 160 mL/min (80–120).

A diagnosis of stage 4 bulky disease teratoma was confirmed. In view of his extensive disease it was decided to treat Mr G initially with combination chemotherapy. The following regimen was prescribed:

Vincristine 2 mg intravenous bolus on day 1
Methotrexate 200 mg intravenous bolus on day 1
Methotrexate 400 mg intravenous infusion over 12 hours on day 1
Bleomycin 15 mg intravenous infusion over 24 hours on days 2 and 3
Cisplatin 240 mg intravenous infusion over one hour on day 4

In order to avoid hyperuricaemia and possible urate nephropathy, which can follow lysis of malignant cells, Mr G was also started on allopurinol 300 mg daily. Folinic acid therapy, commencing 24 hours after the start of the methotrexate therapy, was given to avoid toxicity due to methotrexate.

1. What patient and drug factors should be taken into consideration when selecting anti-emetics for patients receiving cancer chemotherapy?

2. How do these factors influence your choice of anti-emetic(s) for Mr G?

Day 4 Mr G was tolerating his chemotherapy well, although he did admit to feeling very anxious. At 3 p.m. he received cisplatin with appropriate pre- and post-cisplatin hydration. Metoclopramide and dexamethasone were prescribed as anti-emetic therapy.

Mr G slept throughout most of the day. He ate very little but experienced no vomiting and only slight nausea. He had two episodes of diarrhoea for which he was given loperamide.

3. Why was more than one anti-emetic prescribed?

4. Do you agree with the choice of metoclopramide and dexamethasone for Mr G?

5. What doses of dexamethasone and metoclopramide would you recommend, and how should they be given?

6. *Would you have recommended any additional anti-emetic therapy for Mr G?*

Day 5 Mr G slept well overnight but was unable to eat any breakfast. He was discharged from the ward later in the morning, and given an appointment to return in two weeks' time.

Day 17 Mr G was admitted for his second cycle of chemotherapy. He reported feeling tired for about a week after the first course. He also admitted that he had vomited on a couple of occasions on the day he was discharged from hospital, and had felt nauseated for a further three days. Since then he had felt well and was complaining of no new symptoms.

7. *Could the nausea and vomiting he reported after discharge be attributed to the chemotherapy?*

8. *What discharge medication would you recommend after future courses of cisplatin?*

Day 18 Mr G's HCG level had fallen to 25 iu/L and his AFP to 195 iu/mL, indicating that he was responding to chemotherapy. The results of routine biochemistry and haematology tests were normal. His creatinine clearance of 100 mL/min was satisfactory, and the previous cycle of chemotherapy was repeated with dexamethasone and metoclopramide given as before.

Day 21 Mr G did not tolerate this cycle of chemotherapy as well as the first course. He felt very nauseated and started to vomit about three hours after receiving cisplatin. As before, he slept through most of his treatment and again experienced quite profound diarrhoea. He also complained of being very restless towards the end of his treatment, and of having a feeling of tightness in his jaw which he found very distressing.

9. *Could any of Mr G's symptoms be related to his anti-emetic therapy?*

10. *How should these symptoms be managed?*

11. *What alternative anti-emetic therapy could be prescribed with future courses of cisplatin?*

12. *What objective criteria can be used to evaluate the efficacy of an anti-emetic regimen?*

13. *What metabolic and electrolyte abnormalities can occur in patients who have experienced severe vomiting?*

14. *What measures should be taken to correct them?*

Day 33 Mr G was due his third cycle of chemotherapy, which was to be given on an out-patient basis:

> Etoposide 200 mg intravenous infusion over 30 minutes on day 1
> Etoposide 400 mg orally on days 2–5
> Actinomycin D 500 micrograms intravenous bolus on days 3–5
> Cyclophosphamide 1 g intravenous infusion over 30 minutes on day 5

On arrival at the clinic Mr G was feeling very nauseated, and began to retch while awaiting the results of his blood counts.

15. *What measures can be taken to avoid anticipatory nausea and/or vomiting occurring on future occasions?*

16. *What additional factors need to be taken into consideration when designing an anti-emetic regimen suitable for out-patient use?*

17. *What anti-emetic therapy would you recommend this time and why?*

18. *What points would you cover when counselling Mr G on his anti-emetic therapy?*

Mr G tolerated his chemotherapy well as an out-patient. It was planned to reassess his disease before making any decisions on his future management.

Answers

1. In selecting anti-emetic therapy for patients receiving chemotherapy, it is necessary to consider the emetic potential of the cytotoxic agents prescribed, their putative mechanism(s) of inducing emesis, and the time to onset and duration of symptoms. It is also vital to take into consideration certain patient characteristics.

(a) The emetic potential of the cytotoxic drug. The likelihood of vomiting occurring after administration of cytotoxic agents varies according to the agent prescribed, and may be dose- or schedule-dependent. Not all cytotoxic drugs cause nausea and/or vomiting, and those that do are generally classified as mildly, moderately or severely emetogenic.

(b) The mechanism of cytotoxic drug-induced nausea and vomiting. This is not clearly defined and probably differs between drugs. Centrally, the chemoreceptor trigger zone and the emetic centre are important, but receptors in the peripheral nervous system are also implicated. The identification of receptors within the brain has resulted in investigation of anticholinergics, antihistamines, antidopaminergics, encephalins and 5-hydroxytryptamine-modulating drugs as anti-emetics. In the future it may be possible to tailor an anti-emetic regimen to target the underlying mechanism of emesis of a specific cytotoxic agent.

(c) The time to onset and duration of symptoms. This also varies considerably between different cytotoxic drugs. Patients may experience nausea and/or vomiting within an hour of receiving cisplatin therapy, whereas with cyclophosphamide the onset of symptoms can be delayed for up to 12 hours.

(d) Patient characteristics. Specific anti-emetic agents may be contra-indicated because of a patient's age, underlying medical conditions, or concomitant medication. Previous exposure to chemotherapy will adversely affect a patient's response to anti-emetic therapy, and, in general, males respond better than females.

2. Consideration of the factors outlined in the previous answer leads to the recommendation that anti-emetics need only be prescribed on day 4 of Mr G's chemotherapy regimen.

The cytotoxic drugs that Mr G will receive on days 1–3 are only mildly emetogenic, and he need not be given anti-emetics prophylactically on these days with his first course of treatment. In contrast, cisplatin is one of the most emetic drugs, and without the use of anti-emetics vomiting would occur in virtually every patient. There is an acute phase with cisplatin, which begins within one to six hours of starting treatment and lasts for approximately 24 hours. From his medical history it would appear that there are no specific contra-indications to any anti-emetic agent, so Mr G should be given prophylactic anti-emetics on day 4 of treatment.

3. To increase the efficacy of the regimen.

When given as single agents, the currently available anti-emetics do not provide reliable control of symptoms caused by severly emetogenic drugs (such as cisplatin). The use of drugs in combination to achieve an additive or synergistic effect has thus been developed, and, in general, such combinations have proved to be superior to single agents. Ideally, anti-emetics used in combination should have different sites of action and toxicity profiles.

4. Yes.

Given in high doses, metoclopramide has been shown to be superior, or at least equivalent, to other anti-emetic regimens used to prevent cisplatin-induced nausea and vomiting. Conventional doses (such as 10 mg three times daily) are ineffective at controlling symptoms, but the introduction of "high-dose" intravenous metoclopramide (at doses of 1–10 mg/kg) was a major breakthrough in the control of cisplatin-induced nausea and vomiting.

Metoclopramide is thought to act by inhibiting dopamine receptors in the chemoreceptor trigger zone, and, at high doses, by blocking 5-hydroxytryptamine type 3 receptors. Although it is difficult to compare the results of different anti-emetic studies, the combination of high-dose metoclopramide with dexamethasone is recognised as being one of the most effective therapies currently available for patients receiving cisplatin, and would thus be an appropriate choice for Mr G. The mechanism of action of the glucocorticoids as anti-emetics is at present uncertain. Although in theory there is the potential for an interaction between glucocorticoid therapy and chemotherapy, this has not been shown to be a problem clinically.

5. (a) A single dose of dexamethasone sodium phosphate 20 mg in 50 mL 0.9% sodium chloride, as a 15-minute infusion, starting 30 minutes before the cisplatin.

(b) A loading dose of 3 mg/kg metoclopramide in 50 mL 0·9% sodium chloride over 15 minutes, given before cisplatin, and followed immediately by a continuous infusion of 4 mg/kg in 500 mL 0.9% sodium chloride over eight hours, to give a total dose of 7 mg/kg metoclopramide.

When prescribed as an anti -emetic, the optimal dose and schedule of administration of dexamethasone remains controversial: doses ranging from 4 to 60 mg have been advocated. Administration as a short infusion avoids the side-effect of perineal discomfort experienced with an intravenous bolus of dexamethasone.

Initially, intermittent infusions of metoclopramide were used, but the suggestion that the effectiveness of this agent is related to the plasma level has resulted in the use of a loading dose to achieve a therapeutic level, then a maintenance infusion to sustain this concentration. This has proved to be at least as effective, and is more convenient than, intermittent infusions of the drug.

The optimal dose and schedule of administration of metoclopramide still needs further investigation, for example, to determine whether control could be further improved by giving the drug for a longer period of time. A number of alternative routes of administration are also being investigated, such as high-dose oral and rectal preparations.

6. No.

Additional anti-emetic therapy is not necessary at this stage of Mr G's treatment. Although highly effective anti-emetic regimens containing up to five drugs have been reported in the literature, the addition of further agents to Mr G's regimen at this stage would increase the risk of side-effects and the potential for interactions, and would have to be balanced against any modest increase in anti-emetic effectiveness.

7. Yes.

Although the risk of cisplatin-induced emesis is greatest in the first 24 hours, late nausea and vomiting has been reported in 20–68% of patients receiving the drug. This may last from one to 14 days after treatment, although delayed emesis is not usually as severe as that suffered in the acute phase.

8. Oral dexamethasone 8 mg twice daily for two days, then 4 mg twice daily for two days, plus oral metoclopramide 0.5 mg/kg four times daily for four days.

The effective treatment of cisplatin-induced delayed emesis still requires further investigation, but the combination of oral dexamethasone and metoclopramide has been found to be more effective than dexamethasone alone in reducing the incidence of delayed emesis.

9. Yes.

The drowsiness and diarrhoea experienced by Mr G are probably due to the metoclopramide, although cisplatin therapy can itself cause diarrhoea. Mild sedation is the most common side-effect suffered with high-dose metoclopramide therapy, being reported in up to 76% of patients.

The tightness in the jaw that Mr G experienced probably represents an extrapyramidal reaction to metoclopramide. Acute dystonic reactions, such as muscle spasm and oculogyric crisis, are most common in patients under the age of thirty and in women. These effects are unrelated to plasma concentrations of metoclopramide. Tardive dyskinesia is more likely to develop in elderly patients, especially those receiving long-term therapy, and is potentially irreversible.

Restlessness or akathesia has also been reported after high-dose oral metoclopramide therapy.

10. Prophylaxis should be prescribed to prevent acute dystonic reactions occurring during future courses of high-dose metoclopramide therapy, but Mr G's diarrhoea should be controlled symptomatically.

Mr G is being treated as an in-patient, and the fact that he is drowsy while receiving treatment should not be a problem, as the nursing staff will check that he remains rousable to avoid the risk of inhalation of vomit.

Acute dystonic reactions can be reversed by the administration of a benzodiazepine, such as diazepam (5–10 mg), or the anticholinergic agents benztropine (1–2 mg) or procyclidine (5 mg). These agents are usually given parenterally. The anticholinergics can also be given prophylactically before starting anti-emetic therapy in patients thought to be at risk. A suitable regimen would be intravenous benztropine 1 mg prior to metoclopramide, followed by 1 mg at the end of the infusion. Such therapy does not result in any loss of anti-emetic activity.

Antidiarrhoeal agents can be given for the symptomatic relief of diarrhoea.

11. Combination therapy with nabilone and prochlorperazine.

Although other anti-emetic agents, such as the phenothiazines, nabilone, and the butyrophenones, are usually inferior to high-dose metoclopramide in cisplatin-induced emesis, they may be useful in cases where metoclopramide is contra-indicated. The selection is largely a matter of prescriber preference. Should Mr G require further treatment with cisplatin, the combination of nabilone and prochlorperazine could be tried.

The synthetic cannabinoid nabilone has proved useful against a range of cytotoxics, including low-dose cisplatin. The usual dose is 1–2 mg orally the night before treatment, then 1–2 mg orally 12-hourly on the day of chemotherapy. The addition of prochlorperazine (in normal therapeutic doses) helps to reduce some of the side-effects (such as euphoria, dysphoria, and hallucinations) that limit nabilone's use, particularly in older patients. Dexamethasone plus lorazepam could also be considered as an alternative therapy for Mr G.

At higher-than-usual doses, prochlorperazine is showing evidence of improved efficacy against chemotherapy-induced nausea and vomiting. Single intravenous doses of up to 1.2 mg/kg, or 120 mg in three divided doses, have been given in preliminary trials and have generally been well tolerated. Doses have been given over 20–30 minutes, with the patient recumbent, in order to avoid hypotension. The main side-effects observed have been sedation and a dry mouth.

The most promising new development in the field of anti-emetics has been the discovery of a new group of agents, such as granisetron and ondansetron, that are specific antagonists of 5-hydroxytryptamine type 3 receptors. These agents appear to have activity superior to high-dose metoclopramide therapy, but are free from extrapyramidal side-effects. The side-effects that have been seen so far include transient increases in liver enzymes, headache, sedation, and diarrhoea.

12. The time to onset and duration of symptoms, the number of emetic episodes, and the volume of emesis produced.

The outcome of anti-emetic therapy is dependent on so many variables that it is difficult to compare individual studies of anti-emetics. The problem is compounded by the fact that there is no standardised approach to the assessment of anti-emetic therapy.

The aspects of vomiting and retching that can be quantified are: the time to onset and duration of symptoms; the number of episodes; and the volume of emesis. Ideally these assessments should be carried out by the same trained observer. The patient's own assessment of subjective responses such as nausea can be measured using visual analogue scales or ordinal scales (e.g. none, mild, moderate, severe). Whatever the scale selected it should be simple for the patient to use and the results must be reproducible. Particular care is required when agents with sedative or amnesic properties are used, as the patient may not recall symptoms clearly. The patient's own evaluation of the anti-emetic therapy is particularly important. A constant feeling of nausea may bother a patient much more than acute vomiting.

13. Severe or prolonged vomiting can lead to dehydration, malnutrition, and a number of metabolic and electrolyte imbalances.

Dehydration can occur as a result of gastric losses and/or reduced fluid intake. Although vomitus contains relatively little potassium (5–10 mmol/L), hypokalaemia can occur under these circumstances. Further potassium may be lost through the renal tubules, where it is exchanged for sodium in an effort to conserve sodium. Loss of hydrochloric acid in vomit contributes to the development of metabolic alkalosis.

14. The initial goal is to correct fluid deficits. In most cases three litres of sodium chloride 0.9%, given over 24 hours, should be sufficient. In cases of severe deficit greater volumes may be required.

The fluid therapy required should initially be given at a rate of one litre over four hours. Potassium chloride can be added to the infusion fluid if required. Caution is required in cases of hepatic, renal, or congestive heart failure, where infusion of large volumes of fluid could result in fluid overload.

15. Lorazepam therapy could be added to Mr G's future anti-emetic regimens (recommended dose: 1 mg on the morning of treatment, repeated four- to six-hourly as required). In addition, it is vital to try to ensure effective anti-emetic regimens are prescribed in the future.

Anticipatory nausea and vomiting, where symptoms start before the administration of chemotherapy, is a significant problem. The sight of the hospital, or staff, or particular smells, can be enough to trigger vomiting, especially in patients with previous poor emetic control. For this reason it is important to take an aggressive approach to anti-emetic therapy from the outset of chemotherapy.

The benzodiazepine lorazepam, with its sedative and anxiolytic properties, helps make treatment more tolerable for patients. Its amnesic properties mean that even when the patient does experience vomiting, this fact may not be recalled. As an anti-emetic, lorazepam has only limited activity.

Relaxation techniques or hypnosis can also be useful to help patients overcome anticipatory nausea and vomiting.

16. In addition to the factors discussed in answer 1, particular attention must be given to the route of administration of the anti-emetics, and to their side-effects.

Continuous parenteral infusions or intermittent injections are not practical for out-patient therapy, and this generally prevents severely emetogenic drugs from being given in the out-patient setting. Bolus doses of parenteral anti-emetics, such as low- or moderate-dose metoclopramide, prochlorperazine or dexamethasone, may, however, be given just prior to chemotherapy, and oral therapy continued for the next 24–48 hours as appropriate. When oral therapy is not suitable, for example in patients with established vomiting, then sublingual or rectal administration should be considered. However, if patients are thrombocytopenic the rectal route should be avoided because of the risk of bleeding.

In the out-patient setting it is also important that the anti-emetic agents themselves cause the minimum of side-effects. In particular, drowsiness can be a problem for patients having to travel after receiving their chemotherapy.

17. Lorazepam 1 mg orally in the morning before coming to clinic, and oral dexamethasone 2 mg four times each day for the duration of the course.

Although etoposide is generally only mildly emetic, Mr G has already experienced chemotherapy-induced nausea and vomiting, and this factor increases the chances of it occurring again. Both actinomycin D and cyclophosphamide have moderate emetic potential, causing emesis in 60–90% of patients. A number of anti-emetic drug combinations have been used successfully with cytotoxics that are moderately emetogenic, including lorazepam plus dexamethasone, nabilone plus prochlorperazine, and dexamethasone plus Motival® (fluphenazine hydrochloride 500 micrograms, nortriptyline 10 mg).

The dopamine antagonist domperidone is also useful against moderately emetogenic drugs at a dose of 10–20 mg orally or 60 mg rectally, repeated four- to eight-hourly. As it does not produce acute extrapyramidal side-effects, domperidone can be given to younger patients, or patients who have reacted adversely to metoclopramide. However,

since the withdrawal of the intravenous formulation in 1984 because of ventricular arrhythmias following high intravenous dosing, a parenteral preparation is no longer available.

In view of the anticipatory nausea and vomiting displayed by Mr G, the combination of lorazepam and dexamethasone is most appropriate. If vomiting does occur, then anti-emetics will have to be given parenterally or rectally.

18. The counselling points that should be covered are:

(a) Anti-emetics should be taken regularly, as they are more effective in preventing emesis than in treating established symptoms.

(b) Anti-emetics should be taken 30 minutes before the oral etoposide therapy.

(c) The hospital should be informed if vomiting occurs within one hour of taking an oral dose of etoposide.

(d) Lorazepam therapy will cause drowsiness, and you should not drive after taking the medication. Also, the stated dose should not be exceeded.

(e) Dexamethasone is being given as an anti-emetic and is only to be used for a short course of treatment. A further supply should not be obtained from your general practitioner.

References and Further Reading

Allan S.G., Mechanisms and management of chemotherapy-induced nausea and vomiting, *Blood Rev.*, 1987, **1**, 50–57.

Finley R.S., Nausea and vomiting, in *Applied Therapeutics – the Clinical Use of Drugs*, 4th edn, Young L.Y. and Koda-Kimble M.A. (eds), Vancouver, WA, Applied Therapeutics, 1988, 85–99.

Martin J.K. and Norwood M.B., Pharmacist management of antiemetic therapy under protocol in an oncology clinic, *Am. J. Hosp. Pharm.*, 1988, **45**, 1322–1328.

Merrifield K.R. and Chaffee B.J., Recent advances in the management of nausea and vomiting caused by antineoplastic agents, *Clin. Pharm.*, 1989, **8**, 187–199.

Olver I.N., Simon R.M. and Aisner J., Antiemetic studies: a methodological discussion, *Cancer Treat. Rep.*, 1986, **70**, 555–563.

Kris M.G. *et al.*, Controlling delayed vomiting: double-blind, randomized trial comparing placebo, dexamethasone alone, and metoclopramide plus dexamethasone in patients receiving cisplatinum, *J. clin. Oncol.*, 1989, **7**, 108–114.

TREATMENT OF INFECTION IN THE IMMUNOSUPPRESSED PATIENT

Maxwell Summerhayes

Oncology Pharmacist, ICRF Clinical Oncology Unit, Guy's Hospital, London

Day 1 Sixty-five-year-old Mr R was admitted from his local hospital, where he had been receiving supportive care during CAPOMET chemotherapy for Stage IVB non-Hodgkin's lymphoma.

CAPOMET is a treatment protocol which, like the majority of current chemotherapy regimens, incorporates a number of antineoplastic agents from different therapeutic classes (the alkylating agent, cyclophosphamide; the cytotoxic antibiotic, doxorubicin; the antimitotic agents, vincristine and etoposide; the antimetabolite, methotrexate; and the steroid, prednisolone). Combination treatments are designed to maximise the chances of including drugs to which the patient's disease is sensitive, to prevent the emergence of drug-resistant tumour-cell populations, and to enable lower, less toxic doses of individual agents to be used than would be the case during monotherapy.

In CAPOMET, the drugs are administered intermittently over a four-week period, with the intention of repeating the cycle twice. This gives a total treatment duration of 12 weeks. The limiting toxicity of the regimen is usually bone-marrow suppression due to cyclophosphamide, doxorubicin, etoposide, and, to a lesser extent, methotrexate. The objective of Mr R's treatment with CAPOMET was to induce a prolonged remission in his disease.

Ten days earlier, Mr R had been seen in the lymphoma clinic with a view to administering the day 15 portion of his third and final course of CAPOMET (methotrexate 500 mg and etoposide 200 mg, administered intravenously via Mr R's permanently implanted Hickman catheter). This was deferred because of his low blood neutrophil count of 1.9×10^9/L (reference range $2.2-7.0 \times 10^9$) and clinical evidence of a chest infection and pleural effusion. He was referred to his local hospital for drainage of the effusion and antibiotic treatment. Here he remained pyrexial after three days on ceftazidime 2 g three times daily, but his temperature settled when antitubercular therapy was added: Rifinah 300® (rifampicin 300 mg, isoniazid 150 mg) two each morning, ethambutol 600 mg each morning. However, he had continued to feel weak and unwell, had little appetite for food (his weight had declined by 10 kg to 68 kg in 11 weeks), and was anxious to return to this hospital for further treatment.

On arrival Mr R was afebrile but felt short of breath at rest and had a cough productive of white sputum. Examination revealed abnormal breath sounds suggestive of a left-sided chest infection. The hepatomegaly noted at previous out-patient appointments could not be felt.

In addition to ceftazidime and antitubercular treatment, Mr R was taking the following therapy:

Nystatin mouthwash, 2 mL orally four times daily
Amphotericin lozenges, two four times daily
Bendrofluazide 5 mg orally each morning
Propranolol 20 mg orally twice daily
Naproxen 500 mg orally when required for an arthritic big toe.

Mr R stated that he had given up smoking 39 years ago, and rarely consumed alcohol.

His serum biochemistry and haematology results were:

White blood cells 9.1×10^9/L (reference range $4-11 \times 10^9$)
Neutrophils 7.55×10^9/L ($2.2-7.0 \times 10^9$)
Sodium 134 mmol/L (134–148)
Potassium 3.9 mmol/L (3.4–5.0)
Urea 6.4 mmol/L (2.5–7.5)
Creatinine 104 micromol/L (50–130)
Calcium 2.29 mmol/L (2.1–2.6)
Phosphate 1.23 mmol/L (0.8–1·5)
Liver function tests: Within normal limits

His antibiotic and antitubercular therapies were stopped, and a bronchoscopy arranged for the next day, with washings and biopsy samples to be sent for cytology and bacteriology.

1. What is the aim behind prescribing two oral antifungals for Mr R? What instructions would you give to the patient on the use of his antifungal preparations?

2. Would you have recommended the antifungals prescribed? What alternative oral antifungal preparations are available?

Day 2 Mr R remained apyrexial. Bronchial washings were found to contain fungal hyphae but did not stain for acid-fast bacilli. Samples were to be cultured overnight and, in view of Mr R's poor condition, systemic amphotericin treatment was to be started in the interim.

3. What starting dose of amphotericin would you recommend?

4. Is amphotericin suitable for monotherapy in this patient?

5. Do you anticipate any interactions between amphotericin and Mr R's other medications?

6. How should amphotericin be administered?

7. What parameters would you want to monitor during Mr R's amphotericin treatment?

Day 3 Overnight cultures confirmed that the bronchial washings contained viable *Candida albicans*, sensitive to amphotericin and resistant to flucytosine. Mr R was due to receive his second daily dose of 50 mg amphotericin; the dose was increased to 100 mg the following day.

Day 7 Mr R was still very poorly and being fed via a nasogastric tube. He was on the fifth day of amphotericin therapy (100 mg once a day, infused over six hours).

Serum biochemistry results were:

Sodium 136 mmol/L (134–148)
Potassium 3.0 mmol/L (3.4–5.0)
Urea 21.7 mmol/L (2.5–7.5)
Creatinine 315 micromol/L (50–130)
Calcium 1.92 mmol/L (2.1–2.6)
Phosphate 1.93 mmol/L (0.8–1.5)

8. What do these laboratory results indicate?

9. Is any modification to Mr R's treatment appropriate?

Day 8 Mr R's amphotericin therapy was discontinued, and replaced by fluconazole 150 mg orally every 48 hours for four doses. Sando-K® (effervescent potassium chloride 600 mg, potassium bicarbonate 400 mg, providing potassium 12 mmol and chloride 8 mmol), two tablets four times daily, was added to Mr R's treatment.

Day 17 Mr R was discharged. He was feeling much better, eating normally, breathing easily and with an almost normal and still improving chest x-ray. His renal function had improved, but was still impaired, with a creatinine clearance of 30 mL/min, calculated from his serum creatinine level.

Day 60 Mr R was readmitted after his lymphoma had relapsed. He had been started on HOPE chemotherapy two weeks earlier. HOPE is a regimen of doxorubicin, vincristine, prednisolone and etoposide. It lacks the cyclophosphamide and methotrexate components found in CAPOMET. It had been anticipated that, while HOPE still includes several of the drugs to which Mr R's tumour had originally responded, the less intensive nature of the regimen would allow treatment to proceed without the delays, ascribable to low white cell counts, that had interfered with Mr R's CAPOMET. Such delays are extremely prejudicial to the successful treatment of high-grade lymphomas.

On attending the lymphoma clinic for his day 8 chemotherapy, Mr R had a very low white cell count of 2.0×10^9/L ($4–11 \times 10^9$), with neutrophils 0.6×10^9/L ($2.2–7.0 \times 10^9$), although he felt well. He was prescribed ciprofloxacin 250 mg twice daily prophylactically, and asked to return in one week. When he did return he was febrile, anorexic, dehydrated, and generally unwell. Consequently, he was admitted to hospital for antibiotic treatment. Blood samples were taken for culture, and it was decided to start Mr R on piperacillin 4 g four times daily, and gentamicin, pending culture results, as well as giving 3 L of normal saline to rehydrate him.

Serum biochemistry and haematology results were:

WBC 2.0×10^9/L ($4–11 \times 10^9$)
Neutrophils 0.6×10^9/L ($2.2–7.0 \times 10^9$)
Sodium 145 mmol/L (134–148)
Potassium 4.3 mmol/L (3.4–5.0)
Urea 9.0 mmol/L (2.5–7.5)
Creatinine 170 micromol/L (50–130)
Liver function tests: Within normal limits

10. Was the prophylactic antibiotic regimen of ciprofloxacin 250 mg twice daily appropriate? If so, why did Mr R become infected?

11. Is the in-patient antibiotic regimen an appropriate one for Mr R?

12. Suggest an appropriate loading dose, and maintenance dosing regimen, for Mr R's gentamicin therapy.

13. *Why might the gentamicin doses you suggest prove inappropriate?*

14. *How would you monitor Mr R's therapy?*

Day 63 Mr R's blood cultures were all reported to be negative. He was feeling a little better, but still had a fever with a temperature spiking to 39.2°C. While talking to the pharmacist, Mr R complained of a "prickly-heat rash" around his waist, and wanted to know if he could have some calamine lotion for it.
  Serum biochemistry results were:

  Gentamicin peak (30 minutes post-dose) Off scale (5– 10 mg/L)
  Gentamicin trough 15 mg/L (less than 2 mg/L)
  Sodium 139 mmol/L (134–148)
  Potassium 4.0 mmol/L (3.4–5.0)
  Urea 8.5 mmol/L (2.5–7.5)
  Creatinine 155 micromol/L (50–130)

15. *Should antibiotic treatment be continued in view of the negative blood cultures and failure of the patient to respond to antibiotics?*

16. *Why are the gentamicin levels so high, and what should you do about them?*

17. *Are any of Mr R's other blood parameters a cause for concern?*

18. *Is it appropriate to ask the House Officer looking after Mr R to prescribe calamine lotion?*

Day 64 In view of the possibility that Mr R had a *Staphylococcus epidermidis* infection, further blood samples were sent to the microbiology department for culture, and his gentamicin treatment was replaced by vancomycin at a dose of 250 mg intravenously four times daily. There were no further instructions on the drug chart relating to this drug. Mr R was also started on acyclovir 800 mg five times daily by mouth.

19. *Is the vancomycin dose appropriate?*

20. *Are the dosage instructions for vancomycin adequate?*

21. *How should Mr R's vancomycin therapy be monitored?*

22. *Should his acyclovir therapy be given intravenously?*

23. *Is there a place for topical idoxuridine therapy in Mr R's regimen?*

Day 65 Mr R's fever was subsiding and he was feeling much better. His shingles rash was starting to turn crusty but was not getting any bigger.
  Serum biochemistry results were:

  Vancomycin peak (one hour post-dose) 30 mg/L (25– 30)
  Vancomycin trough 7 mg/L (5–10)
  Urea 8.7 mmol/L (2.5–7.5)
  Creatinine 170 micromol/L (50–130)

24. *Would you recommend any modification to Mr R's vancomycin therapy?*

Day 68 Mr R continued to improve. His laboratory results were substantially unchanged.

Day 70 After five days of vancomycin and acyclovir therapy Mr R felt much better, and both drugs were discontinued. His renal function had not deteriorated further. He still had a low neutrophil count of 1.22×10^9/L. A bone marrow biopsy confirmed that this was probably due to marrow infiltration by lymphoma cells. He was discharged with a view to recommencing "gentle" chemotherapy as an outpatient.

25. *What discharge medication and counselling should Mr R receive?*

Answers

1. The aim of combination local antifungal therapy is to maximise the time during which the mucous membranes of the oropharyngeal area are exposed to effective concentrations of antifungals.

Mr R is at risk of developing oral thrush for two reasons: firstly, he is immunosuppressed as a consequence of his chemotherapy; secondly, he has been treated with broad-spectrum antibiotics, which disrupt the normal bacterial flora of the oropharynx, and make overgrowth by *Candida* more likely.

The potential consequences of a candidal infection for Mr R are serious. He is immunocompromised, and there is a risk that his local infection may develop into a systemic one, especially since his chemotherapy regimen includes methotrexate, a drug that is particularly prone to producing oral ulceration, and thus breaching the barrier between the mouth and the circulation. It is therefore important to treat Mr R's candidiasis aggressively, and to ensure that he knows how to use his antifungal medicines correctly.

Mr R should be told to keep the nystatin mouthwash in his mouth for as long as is comfortable (at least three minutes), and to "swish it around" to ensure the whole mucosal surface is treated before swallowing the liquid. He should then refrain from eating or drinking for half-an-hour. The amphotericin lozenges should be allowed to dissolve slowly in his mouth. The doses of both medications should be spread out and taken alternately throughout the day. This may require liaison with Mr R's doctor to ensure that the charted times of administration of the medications are appropriate, or that Mr R keeps them at his bedside for self-administration.

Finally, if Mr R wears dentures, he should soak them overnight in 1% sodium hypochlorite solution.

2. Yes.

The regimen Mr R is receiving combines two different antifungals, both of which are relatively inexpensive, in a way that gives regular peaks of antifungal activity with nystatin, plus prolonged exposure to amphotericin. Miconazole is also available in topical formulations (gel and tablets for dissolution), but it does not offer any obvious advantage to Mr R, and is more expensive than topical preparations of nystatin or amphotericin. However, the gel may be useful for a patient who is too moribund to co-operate in his treatment, or whose mouth is too sore to suck lozenges.

If Mr R's treatment fails to control his candidiasis he may require systemic antifungal therapy, especially if the infection spreads to the oesophagus, where topical treatment is difficult. Until recently, ketoconazole was the only systemic antifungal available for oral administration. As well as having a tendency to cause nausea and vomiting (in 3–10% of patients) and gynaecomastia, this drug can, rarely, cause serious hepatotoxicity. This may be especially significant for Mr R, who, until recently, exhibited hepatomegaly as a result of his lymphoma. The recent introduction of fluconazole offers an effective oral treatment (greater than 95% cure) which seems to be devoid of serious hepatotoxicity and effects on steroidogenesis, and is generally well tolerated. This would thus be the treatment of choice for Mr R if local therapy fails.

3. He should receive a test dose of 1 mg amphotericin infused over two hours, and then, in the absence of serious problems, he should be started on 250 micrograms/kg (20 mg approximately) on day 1, escalated over five days to a maximum of 100 mg daily, depending upon his response.

Amphotericin is a toxic drug, and patients receiving it will undoubtedly experience adverse reactions. The commonest problems are headache, fevers, chills, nausea, anaemia, epigastric pain, thrombophlebitis at the injection site, and nephrotoxicity. Nephrotoxicity is the most serious problem with amphotericin treatment, and is seen in 80% of patients. It is probably dose-related, and is a less serious problem if the initial dose is kept low and increased stepwise over five days to an absolute maximum of 1.5 mg/kg once daily. However, in life-threatening infections, the maximum dose can be given on the first day of treatment.

Amphotericin is also capable of producing hypotensive reactions, so a test dose should be administered prior to the commencement of treatment.

Considering these factors, and Mr R's condition, it is reasonable to recommend the regimen described.

Since adverse effects can be expected during amphotericin therapy, thought should be given to the co-administration of agents to ameliorate its toxicity.

(a) Febrile reactions. Many drugs have been suggested for the control of such reactions, including pethidine, antihistamines, non-steroidal anti-inflammatory drugs (NSAIDs), and steroids. Few of these agents have been systematically evaluated and all of them are probably beneficial to some patients. If Mr R experiences febrile reactions to his amphotericin it would be reasonable to prescribe a combination of regular paracetamol (1 g four times daily), infused hydrocortisone (50 mg at the same time as his amphotericin infusion), and a 10 mg intramuscular injection of chlorpheniramine immediately prior to the antifungal, this regimen being modified according to subsequent response.

(b) Renal toxicity. Attempts have been made to minimise amphotericin-induced renal damage by the administration of mannitol, and by "sodium-loading" patients with sodium chloride. Mannitol is used as an osmotic diuretic to flush amphotericin rapidly through the renal tubules, while "sodium-loading" appears to be based on the premise that patients who are not sodium-depleted are less vulnerable to the toxic effects of amphotericin. Neither approach can be recommended on the evidence currently available. Amphotericin-induced renal damage often manifests itself as a systemic acidosis. This must be corrected by administration of sodium bicarbonate. Uncorrected renal tubular acidosis will result in further renal damage, and, possibly, the deposition of calcium phosphate within the kidney tubules. The amount of bicarbonate to be administered depends upon measurements of blood bicarbonate. If the supplementation needed is moderate, oral therapy may be adequate, otherwise parenteral treatment must be instituted.

(c) Thrombophlebitis. It has been suggested that the addition of 500–1000 units of heparin to amphotericin infusions minimises the incidence of thrombophlebitis. Controlled studies of this use of heparin are lacking, but it may be worth trying if phlebitis proves to be a problem.

4. Yes, at least initially.

Amphotericin is often used in conjunction with flucytosine, with which it has a synergistic action, for the following reasons:
(a) to produce greater antifungal activity;
(b) to reduce drug toxicity by allowing lower doses of both agents to be used; and
(c) to achieve better penetration of areas like the cerebrospinal fluid (CSF), which are poorly penetrated by amphotericin (levels of amphotericin in the CSF are 3% of the serum concentrations).

Although Mr R was very unwell at the start of his systemic antifungal treatment, the (possibly unnecessary) addition of a drug to which resistance is common seems unwise, especially since flucytosine has significant bone marrow toxicity. Mr R's marrow is only just recovering from cytotoxic therapy and would be expected to be especially vulnerable to this adverse effect.

5. Possibly, but they are probably only theoretical.

(a) Bendrofluazide. Bendrofluazide may produce hypokalaemia, which may worsen the hypokalaemia that characterises amphotericin-induced renal damage.

(b) Naproxen. Like all NSAIDs, naproxen has the potential to cause renal damage. This is believed to be due to renal vasonconstriction, a mechanism thought to be at least partly responsible for amphotericin-induced renal toxicity. In practice, NSAIDs are frequently given with amphotericin to ameliorate the influenza-like symptoms it induces (see answer 3). No change in Mr R's treatment need be recommended.

6. Mr R's amphotericin should be infused in 5% dextrose through his Hickman catheter. The solution should have a pH greater than 4.2, and an amphotericin concentration less than 0.1 mg/mL. It should pass through a filter with a mean pore diameter greater than 1 μm, and be protected from light.

Amphotericin is administered as a colloidal dispersion, which has very specific physico-chemical requirements if aggregation is to be prevented. Amphotericin is incompatible with sodium chloride, and many drugs, and should only be infused in 5% dextrose. Addition of other drugs to the infusion should be avoided, with the exception of heparin and hydrocortisone, which may be co-infused (see answer 3). Amphotericin is pH-sensitive and should only be administered in dextrose that has a pH greater than 4.2. In the absence of pH-tested dextrose, phosphate buffer can be added to untested dextrose.

Even under ideal conditions, aggregates of amphotericin may form. Therefore, the drug should be administered via an in-line filter with a mean pore diameter greater than 1 μm. This will retain aggregates but allow colloid infusion.

Adequate dilution of the infused drug reduces both aggregation and thrombophlebitis. Local vascular damage can also be minimised by using a central venous line, such as Mr R's Hickman catheter, for drug administration. This ensures rapid removal of drug from the injection site and dilution in the blood. If peripheral injection sites are used, they should be changed frequently. Toxicity is further lessened by slow infusion. Six hours is an appropriate administration period.

The drug's manufacturer recommends that amphotericin should be protected from light. Although it is doubtful that significant photodegradation occurs during a six-hour infusion, this instruction should be complied with.

7. Blood chemistry and blood cell count.

(a) Blood chemistry. Urea, creatinine, and electrolyte levels should be monitored at least each alternate day for signs of drug-induced nephrotoxicity; modification of amphotericin dosage should be considered if significant toxicity is seen. Amphotericin-induced hypokalaemia and hypomagnesaemia should be watched for, and electrolyte supplementation recommended if required. Bilirubin and alkaline phosphatase levels should also be observed for signs of liver damage, which is a rare complication of amphotericin therapy that may require drug discontinuation.

(b) Blood cell count. A full blood count is required each week. Various haematological abnormalities are associated with amphotericin treatment. Normochromic, normocytic anaemia occurs in up to 90% of patients treated. This is usually reversible and can be managed supportively while therapy continues.

8. Mr R is suffering from very significant amphotericin-induced renal damage. This is indicated by his falling potassium and calcium levels, and his rising urea, creatinine and phosphate concentrations. Using the Cockroft and Gault equation, where:

Creatinine clearance (CrCl) =
(in males)

$$\frac{1.2\,(140-age)\times wt}{\text{Serum creatinine concentration}}$$

it can be calculated that Mr R's creatinine clearance has fallen to around 20 mL/min from 87 mL/min when he was admitted to hospital (reference range 50–130).

It should be noted that the Cockroft and Gault equation is only reliable when applied to patients whose renal function is in steady state. It should not be used for patients whose serum creatinine levels are fluctuating by more than about 40 micromol/L/day. Mr R's renal function is deteriorating steadily and fairly rapidly, and a creatinine clearance based on his serum creatinine concentration should thus be viewed with caution.

9. Yes. Fluconazole therapy should be substituted for amphotericin, and an oral potassium supplement (100–150 mmol daily) should be added to Mr R's treatment until his serum potassium has returned to normal.

Mr R is only on his fifth day of treatment and his renal function is already markedly impaired. Amphotericin doses have probably been elevated too high, too fast. At this point there are two options for treating Mr R's fungal infection.

(a) Modify his amphotericin treatment. It would be reasonable to omit one dose of the drug and then resume treatment at a lower dose (say 500 micrograms/kg/day), giving the reduced dose on alternate days. Alternate-day dosing has been associated with lower toxicity. For Mr R, this would mean giving 70 mg on alternate days, though it might be prudent to lower this even further, perhaps to 50 mg on alternate days, and gradually increase the dose if the infection is not resolving and if renal function allows. Although this dose seems very low, especially when coupled with a long dose interval, it should still produce therapeutic blood levels of the drug. Amphotericin is only slowly excreted via the kidneys, especially in patients like Mr R who have renal impairment. This results in drug accumulation, so that reduced doses are sufficient to produce adequate blood levels.

(b) Change antifungal. It is now known that Mr R's chest infection is due to *C. albicans* that is resistant to flucytosine. This leaves only one other injectable antifungal: miconazole. This agent is relatively non-toxic (compared with amphotericin), but can cause anaphylactoid reactions, various blood abnormalities, nausea, pruritus, and disturbances of blood electrolytes and lipids. Furthermore, its penetration of sputum is poor. By contrast, the newer agent fluconazole*, though not available in an injectable form, shows excellent sputum penetration (same concentrations as in plasma) and is generally very well tolerated. It is also well absorbed orally (greater than 90%) and has good anticandidal activity. Fluconazole, therefore, seems the best therapeutic option for Mr R. In view of the drug's long half-life (28 hours) and its renal excretion, together with Mr R's poor renal function, a course of four doses of 150 mg orally, given at intervals of 48 hours, is appropriate, based on information provided by the manufacturers.

10. It was probably appropriate, and the reason for its failure is unclear.

Several studies have shown that ciprofloxacin 500

---

* At the time of treating Mr R, fluconazole injection was not available, and the oral formulation was licensed only for the treatment of oropharyngeal and vaginal candidiasis. The recent introduction of injectable fluconazole and the extension of its licensed indications to cover systemic candidiasis will almost certainly influence the treatment given to patients like Mr R in the future.

mg twice daily is effective in reducing the incidence of infection in leukaemic patients, or those undergoing autologous bone marrow transplantation. These groups of patients both receive very intensive chemotherapy and experience profound and prolonged neutropenic episodes. Good information on chemoprophylaxis in less severely neutropenic patients is sparse, but it seems reasonable that ciprofloxacin should also afford such patients protection. The reason for the failure of prophylaxis in Mr R's case is unclear: the ciprofloxacin dose (250 mg twice daily) may have been inadequate; a ciprofloxacin-resistant organism may have infected Mr R; or his compliance with treatment may have been poor.

11. Yes.

Blind treatment of presumed infection in neutropenic patients requires a broad-spectrum regimen that will be active against the most likely sources of infection, such as faecal coliforms and skin commensals. Most oncology units have a preferred regimen for this purpose, which takes into account local resistance problems. At this hospital, Mr R would normally have received ceftazidime 2 g twice or three times daily. This has the advantage of low toxicity, and simplicity. However, monotherapy does carry the theoretical risk of selecting out resistant strains of bacteria. Since Mr R has been treated with ceftazidime recently, he may be carrying a ceftazidime-resistant organism. It is therefore appropriate to give him second-line treatment with piperacillin and gentamicin. This is a good antimicrobial treatment, but carries the risk of aminoglycoside toxicity. Substituting the possibly less nephrotoxic netilmicin for gentamicin might avoid aggravating Mr R's renal impairment, though the evidence that netilmicin is substantially less nephrotoxic in clinical use is scant.

12. A loading dose of 140 mg followed by a maintenance dose of 80 mg twelve hourly.

The loading dose of a drug needs no adjustment in renal failure. It is the amount of drug that, when distributed evenly through the volume of distribution of that drug, produces the required drug concentration. It is independent of drug clearance. For gentamicin the volume of distribution is 0.25 L/kg body weight (but see answer 13). The weight used in this calculation is the "ideal body weight". Since Mr R is not obese, and currently has no collections of effusion fluid, this is the same as his actual body weight (67 kg). Any dose of gentamicin given to him will thus be diluted in $67 \times 0.25 = 16.75$ L (say 17 L). To obtain a suitable peak concentration of 8 mg/L,

a loading dose of $8 \times 17 = 136$ mg (say 140 mg) should be given.

The maintenance dose of gentamicin must be adjusted in view of Mr R's marked renal impairment. Ideally, the maintenance dose should be calculated on the basis of Mr R's renal function and a knowledge of gentamicin pharmacokinetics; however, as long as Mr R's renal function can be estimated using the Cockroft and Gault equation (see answer 8), a maintenance regimen can be selected using one of several tables available. Mr R's serum creatinine is currently 170 micromol/L and his weight 67 kg. Therefore, his creatinine clearance can be estimated as 35 mL/min. The manufacturers of the gentamicin injection used recommend a dose of 80 mg 12-hourly for a patient with this degree of renal impairment. This would, therefore, be a reasonable regimen for Mr R to commence on.

13. Because at the start of treatment Mr R is febrile, dehydrated and neutropenic.

Febrile patients often have abnormally low serum gentamicin levels, possibly as the result of increased renal blood flow. Dehydration reduces the volume throughout which the drug can distribute, without affecting the ability of the kidneys to remove the drug, so that the drug's half-life will decrease. Neutropenic patients have been reported to have an increased volume of distribution of gentamicin, resulting in increased dilution of administered doses and prolonged half-life. The combination of these three factors will have an unpredictable, but possibly significant, effect on serum gentamicin levels.

14. Blood biochemistry should be scrutinised for signs of worsening renal function resulting from gentamicin toxicity and regular gentamicin assays should be insisted upon.

Gentamicin monitoring should start at the time of the third dose and be repeated every two to three days, with the aminoglycoside doses being adjusted, if necessary, to bring blood levels within the therapeutic range.

15. Yes.

It is too early to conclude that Mr R's febrile episode is not infective in nature. Negative blood cultures are of little significance in febrile neutropenics, where a causative organism is frequently never isolated during episodes of clinical sepsis. However, the fact that Mr R's fever is not settling suggests that the organism causing his condition may be resistant to the antibiotics in use. A frequent cause of infection in neutropenic patients with indwelling venous catheters is *Staphylococcus epidermidis*, a normal skin commensal. It is often resistant to first-line antibiotics and, unless especially asked for, is often not reported by hospital bacteriology laboratories (as it is considered to be a sampling contaminant, and only 6% of blood cultures containing this organism represent true staphylococcal bacteraemia). At this point it would thus be reasonable to carry out repeat blood cultures and commence empirical vancomycin treatment for *Staph. epidermidis*.

16. They are too high to be correct, and should be repeated.

The most likely explanation is that an inexperienced phlebotomist has withdrawn blood samples for assay through Mr R's Hickman line, which was still heavily contaminated from its use during drug administration. Repeat sampling is necessary using a peripheral vein.

17. No.

The fall in concentration of his blood electrolytes, urea, and creatinine probably represent increased dilution as dehydration is reversed.

18. No.

What Mr R is describing (a small group of tense vesicles, clustered around his waist *unilaterally*, whose appearance was preceded by a stabbing irritation) sounds more like the beginnings of a local herpes zoster infection (shingles), triggered by his immunosuppression, rather than prickly heat, which typically presents as a large area of *itchy* red papules distributed *bilaterally* and not associated with paraesthesias that precede the appearance of the rash. In an immunosuppressed patient, shingles may lead to a life-threatening generalised infection. Thus, the doctor looking after Mr R must be informed promptly of his symptoms so that anti-viral therapy can be started, if appropriate.

19. No. A dose of 300 mg twice daily is appropriate for Mr R.

Mr R's renal impairment requires that the dosage of this nephrotoxic and renally excreted drug be reduced from the normal adult dose of 2 g daily. Recalculating from the patient's current blood chemistry shows him to have a creatinine clearance of 39 mL/min. Using the dosage nomogram supplied by the drug's manufacturers it can be calculated that Mr R should be receiving a vancomycin dose of 630 mg/day. This could be administered as 150 mg four times daily; however, a dose of 300 mg twice daily reduces the risk of drug accumulation and is also more convenient, and should be recommended.

20. No. Vancomycin should never be given by rapid intravenous injection, as this can lead to the "red man syndrome" caused by widespread release of histamine within the body.

The syndrome is characterised by sudden and severe hypotension, flushing and/or rash on the face, neck, chest, and upper extremities, and, occasionally, by death from cardiac arrest or seizures. Administering vancomycin over at least one hour, as an infusion in saline or dextrose, usually prevents this problem. Restricting the infusion volume to 250 mL should avoid fluid-overloading Mr R, which is always a possibility in patients with impaired renal function.

21. Regular assays of Mr R's serum vancomycin levels should be performed.

Although the relationship between plasma concentration and toxicity is less clear for vancomycin than for the aminoglycosides, peak levels should be between 25 and 30 mg/L and trough levels in the range 5–10 mg/L.

22. Not initially.

At the time of starting acyclovir therapy Mr R's lesions were well localised. If oral treatment is successful in preventing the appearance of new lesions, then intravenous treatment is not indicated. However, if oral treatment does not halt the spread of Mr R's skin lesions, then intravenous treatment should be started without delay.

23. No.

There has been debate recently about the relative merits of cheap, but inconvenient, idoxuridine paints, and expensive, but convenient, acyclovir tablets for treating shingles in immunocompetent patients. The effect of either agent in such patients seems to be modest. However, Mr R is immuno-compromised, and so systemic treatment with acyclovir is mandatory to prevent dissemination of his infection. There is no evidence that adding topical idoxuridine to Mr R's treatment will confer any benefit.

24. No.

Mr R's vancomycin levels are in the therapeutic range and he is responding to treatment. However, there has been a modest elevation in his serum creatinine and urea levels since he commenced his vancomycin treatment. This may well be due to day-to-day variation in the patient, or in laboratory assay procedures. Alternatively, it may indicate that Mr R is suffering some renal toxicity from his vancomycin treatment. At present, this is not a cause for concern, when set against the risks of inadequate treatment. Treatment should be continued, and a close watch kept on vancomycin levels and renal function.

25. He should receive prophylactic antibiotic and antifungal therapy.

Mr R is no longer profoundly neutropenic; however, his neutrophil count is rising only very slowly. For this reason, a seven-day course of prophylactic antibiotics is indicated (e.g. ciprofloxacin 500 mg twice daily). Additionally, in view of his previous problems with candidal infections, suitable antifungal prophylaxis should be given, such as nystatin mouthwash 2 mL four times daily for seven days.

Mr R should be advised on when and how to take these medications (see answer 1); and told the importance of taking them even though he is no longer feeling ill. It should be impressed upon him that if he develops a temperature, sore throat, or skin rash, he should contact his general practitioner as a matter of urgency.

References and Further Reading

Anon., Aminoglycoside toxicity, *Lancet*, 1986, **1**, 670–671.

Benson J.M. and Nahata M.C., Clinical use of systemic antifungal agents, *Clin. Pharm.*, 1988, **7**, 424–438.

Blum R.A. and Rodvold K.A., Recognition and importance of *Staphylococcus epidermidis* infections, *ibid.*, 1987, **6**, 464–475.

Callender S.T. *et al.*, The lymphomas, in *Oxford Textbook of Medicine*, 2nd edn, Weatherall D.J., Ledingham J.G.G. and Warrell D.A. (eds), Oxford, Oxford University Press, 1987, 19.169–19.186.

Cockroft D.W. and Gault M.H., Prediction of creatinine clearance from serum creatinine, *Nephron*, 1976, **15**, 31–41.

Dekker A.W. *et al.*, Infection prophylaxis in acute leukaemia: a comparison of ciprofloxacin with trimethoprim-sulfamethoxazole and colistin, *Ann. intern. Med.*, 1987, **106**, 7–12.

Evans W.E., Schentag J.J. and Jusko W.J. (eds), *Applied Pharmacokinetics: Principles of Therapeutic Drug Monitoring*, 2nd edn, Spokane, Applied Therapeutics, 1986.

Guiot H.F.L. and van Furth R., Partial antibiotic decontamination, *Br. med. J.*, 1977, **1**, 800–802.

Hawthorn J.W. *et al*, Empirical antibiotic therapy in the febrile neutropenic cancer patient: clinical efficacy and impact of monotherapy, *Antimicrob. Agents Chemother.*, 1987, **31**, 971–977.

Jolleys J.A., Treatment of shingles and post-herpetic neuralgia, *Br. med. J.*, 1989, **298**, 1537–1538.

Marcus R.E. and Goldman J.M., Management of infection in the neutropenic patient, *ibid.*, 1986, **293**, 406–408.

McKendrick M.W. *et al.*, Oral acyclovir in acute herpes zoster, *ibid.*, 1529–1532.

Purvis J. and Reavley R., Oral candidiasis, *Pharm. J.*, 1989, **242**, 353–354.

Richards D.M. *et al.*, Acyclovir: a review of its pharmacodynamic properties and therapeutic efficacy, *Drugs*, 1983, **26**, 378–438.

Rozenberg-Arska M. *et al.*, Ciprofloxacin for selective decontamination of the alimentary tract in patients with acute leukaemia during remission induction treatment, *J. infect. Dis.*, 1985, **152**, 104–107.

Schimpff S.C., Overview of empiric antibiotic therapy for the febrile neutropenic patient, *Rev. infect. Dis.*, 1985, **7**, S734–S740.

Taylor W.J. *et al.* (eds), *Individualizing Drug Therapy*, 1st edn, New York, Gross, Townsend, Frank, 1981.

Tyler E.M. *et al.*, Management and prevention of amphotericin B-induced side effects, *Hosp. Pharm.*, 1988, **23**, 254–259.

MALIGNANCY-ASSOCIATED HYPERCALCAEMIA

Lindsay H. Smith

District Principal Pharmacist, Clinical Services Manager, Mount Vernon Hospital, Northwood, Middlesex

Day 1 Fifty-nine-year-old Mrs K was admitted following referral by her general practitioner. She had a two-week history of weakness, vomiting and general malaise. Her condition had deteriorated markedly over the last two days and she had become increasingly confused and drowsy.

Four years previously she had been diagnosed as having breast cancer, and had undergone a radical mastectomy and a course of radiotherapy. Following this she had remained well until six months ago, when bone metastases had been confirmed.

Her drug therapy on admission was:

Tamoxifen 20 mg orally twice daily (which she had been taking for the past six months to control disease progression)
Lactulose 15 mL orally daily
Bisacodyl 10 mg orally twice daily when needed for constipation
Metoclopramide 10 mg orally three times a day as required for sickness
Prochlorperazine 25 mg suppositories twice daily as required for sickness
Morphine sulphate slow-release tablets 120 mg twice daily

Mrs K's daughter had informed the general practitioner that Mrs K had required more than usual of her sickness and constipation medication over the last week.

On examination Mrs K looked pale, dazed, and thin. She was sweaty, physically very weak, and had pain in her left hip and groin.

Her serum biochemistry results were:

Sodium 139 mmol/L (reference range 135–143)
Potassium 3.7 mmol/L (3.6–5.2)
Urea 9.8 mmol/L (3.5–6.5)
Calcium 3.45 mmol/L (2.2–2.6)
Albumin 34 g/L (35–50)

Liver function tests were all within the normal range.

Intravenous fluid therapy was prescribed as follows:

Sodium chloride 0.9%, 1 L over eight hours, then
Glucose 4% with sodium chloride 0.18%, 1 L over eight hours, then
Sodium chloride 0.9%, 1 L over eight hours

1. What do Mrs K's laboratory results indicate? What are the most likely explanations for the abnormal results?

2. What should be taken into account when interpreting Mrs K's serum calcium level?

3. On the basis of her serum calcium level, should Mrs K's hypercalcaemia be classified as mild, moderate or severe?

4. What factors influence the choice of treatment for hypercalcaemia? What, if any, general guidelines may be applied to treatment?

5. Could Mrs K's other drug therapies be contributing to her hypercalcaemia and presenting symptoms?

6. Is her anti-emetic therapy appropriate? If not, what changes would you recommend?

Day 2 Mrs K was still drowsy and confused. Intravenous fluid therapy was continued as follows:

Glucose 4% with sodium chloride 0.18%, 1 L over eight hours, then
Sodium chloride 0·9%, 1 L over eight hours, then
Glucose 4% with sodium chloride 0.18%, 1 L over eight hours

Her anti-emetic regimen was changed to metoclopramide 10 mg, to be given by either the intramuscular or the intravenous route to control vomiting, followed by metoclopramide 10 mg orally three times a day.

7. Why was Mrs K commenced on intravenous fluid therapy?

8. Was the fluid therapy prescribed appropriate? If not, what changes would you recommend to the regimen? How should the fluid therapy be monitored?

9. What drug options are available for the acute treatment of hypercalcaemia? How is each thought to exert its hypocalcaemic effect, and when can this effect be expected to commence?

10. What side-effects are associated with each of these agents?

11. What monitoring would be required?

Day 3 No improvement was apparent in Mrs K's clinical condition, although her sickness and constipation were now controlled with regular medication.

Laboratory results showed that her serum calcium level had fallen to 3.31 mmol/L (2.2–2.6). Her serum albumin level was 32 g/L (35–50).

12. Which drug treatment would you recommend for Mrs K?

More intravenous hydration therapy was prescribed:

Sodium chloride 0.9%, 1 L over eight hours, then
Glucose 4% with sodium chloride 0.18% 1 L over eight hours

This was followed by an infusion of disodium pamidronate (APD).

13. How soon after administering disodium pamidronate therapy will its maximum effect be seen?

Day 6 Mrs K had become much brighter and less confused, and her appetite had improved. She no longer required regular anti-emetic therapy.

Serum biochemistry results were:

Sodium 138 mmol/L (135–143)
Potassium 3.9 mmol/L (3.6–5.2)
Urea 4.5 mmol/L (3.5–6.5)

Calcium 2.73 mmol/L (2.2–2.6)
Albumin 34 g/L (35–50)

Day 7 Mrs K was allowed home.

Day 21 Mrs K was readmitted via casualty. She had become increasingly weak and confused over the previous four days. Blood urea and electrolytes were requested.

Serum biochemistry results were:

Sodium 131 mmol/L (135–143)
Potassium 4.2 mmol/L (3.6–5.2)
Urea 6.4 mmol/L (3.5–6.5)
Calcium 3.28 mmol/L (2.2–2.6)
Albumin 36 g/L (35–50)

14. Is such a rapid relapse common?

15. What treatment would you recommend now?

Intravenous hydration therapy was started. In the first 24 hours Mrs K received 3 L of sodium chloride 0.9%. This was repeated in the following 24 hours. On the third day she was prescribed 2 L of sodium chloride 0.9% over 16 hours, followed by disodium pamidronate 30 mg in 250 mL of sodium chloride 0.9% over four hours.

In view of her quick relapse after her previous treatment with pamidronate, it was decided to commence Mrs K on oral maintenance hypocalcaemic therapy.

16. Is oral maintenance treatment likely to be effective in controlling her hypercalcaemia?

17. What drugs could be used? Which would you recommend for Mrs K?

Day 22 Mrs K was prescribed disodium etidronate 400 mg orally twice daily.

18. How should Mrs K's maintenance treatment be monitored?

19. How long should this therapy continue? What are the future therapeutic options for Mrs K?

Day 24 Mrs K's clinical condition had improved and it was decided to allow her home the next day.

20. What points would you cover when counselling Mrs K on her new medication?

Answers

1. Mrs K's laboratory results show that she has hypercalcaemia, an elevated serum urea level, and mild hypoalbuminaemia. The most likely explanation for these abnormal results is that she has malignancy-associated hypercalcaemia.

Malignancy-associated hypercalcaemia occurs in around one-third of patients with late-stage breast cancer. The underlying cause of hypercalcaemia associated with malignancy is unclear, although several possible explanations have been proposed including:

(a) the production of a parathyroid-hormone-type protein by the tumour, and

(b) the release of bone-resorbing cytokines from secondary bone tumours.

Mrs K's elevated serum urea level and mild hypoalbuminaemia are probably direct consequences of her hypercalcaemia. An increase in serum urea concentration can occur as a result of polyuria and vomiting induced by hypercalcaemia. Hypoalbuminaemia may also result from hypercalcaemia-induced vomiting.

2. Her serum albumin concentration.

The reason for this is that total (i.e. bound and unbound) serum calcium levels are measured in the laboratory, although only the unbound calcium is physiologically active. Changes in serum albumin concentration can alter the ratio of bound to unbound calcium within the total serum calcium level. This makes a true assessment of calcium status impossible unless the serum albumin concentration is also considered.

Some laboratories will report both the total serum calcium level and an albumin-adjusted value. Alternatively, adjustment of the serum calcium level can be made using the following formula:

$$Ca_{adj} = Ca_{obs} + 0.02(40 - alb)$$

Where Ca_{adj} is the adjusted calcium concentration (in mmol/L)

Ca_{obs} is the observed calcium concentration (in mmol/L)

alb is the serum albumin concentration (in g/L)

Mrs K's total serum calcium level was reported as 3.45 mmol/L, and her serum albumin concentration as 34 g/L. Using this formula her adjusted serum calcium can be calculated as 3.57 mmol/L.

3. Severe.

Serum calcium levels have been related to the degree of hypercalcaemia in the following manner:

(a) Mild hypercalcaemia – an adjusted serum calcium level above 2.6 mmol/L, but not greater than 3.0 mmol/L.

(b) Moderate hypercalcaemia – an adjusted serum calcium level of between 3.0 mmol/L and 3.5 mmol/L.

(c) Severe hypercalcaemia – an adjusted serum calcium level above 3.5 mmol/L.

4. (a) The degree of hypercalcaemia (as assessed from the adjusted serum calcium level),

(b) the severity of hypercalcaemic symptoms, and

(c) the ability to treat or control the underlying cause of hypercalcaemia.

The treatment needs of each patient should be individually assessed; however, some general guidelines may be applied. If the patient is asymptomatic and has mild hypercalcaemia, no immediate hypocalcaemic treatment is usually needed, but regular monitoring of the patient's serum calcium level and clinical condition are required, and adequate hydration must be maintained. If the hypercalcaemia is associated with malignancy, then non-urgent treatment may be advisable at this stage, if effective treatment of the underlying tumour is unlikely to be achieved.

For asymptomatic patients with moderate hypercalcaemia, non-urgent treatment is indicated, using rehydration alone or in combination with an agent such as an intravenous bisphosphonate. If hypercalcaemia is severe and/or the patient has marked hypercalcaemic symptoms, then acute hypocalcaemic treatment using rehydration and an appropriate hypocalcaemic agent is required.

5. Yes.

(a) Tamoxifen may produce hypercalcaemia during the initial stages of treatment of patients with bone metastases, and this could have contributed to Mrs K developing hypercalcaemia. The mechanism underlying this hypercalcaemic effect remains unclear. Mrs K's continued treatment with tamoxifen should be reviewed, since it also appears to be ineffective in controlling her disease progression.

(b) Prochlorperazine is a phenothiazine derivative which can produce sedation, and anticholinergic and extrapyramidal side-effects. Mrs K has recently increased her anti-emetic intake, and an increased use of prochlorperazine suppositories could be contributing to her symptoms of drowsiness and confusion.

(c) Metoclopramide has also been prescribed as

an anti-emetic for Mrs K. Drowsiness and confusion have occasionally been associated with its use at the doses prescribed; it could, therefore, have contributed to Mrs K's symptoms, although this is unlikely.

(d) Morphine sulphate may also have contributed to Mrs K's symptoms of drowsiness and confusion, if a recent dose increase had been made. In addition, a recent large dosage increase could have accounted for her increased need for anti-emetics and laxatives, although this is unlikely.

(e) Laxatives. The increased use of laxatives by Mrs K could have contributed to her dehydration and reduced her serum potassium level.

6. No. Mrs K requires parenteral metoclopramide therapy until her symptoms are controlled. Her prochlorperazine therapy should be discontinued.

The continued use of prochlorperazine suppositories by Mrs K to control her vomiting is inappropriate on two counts: firstly, they are probably contributing to her symptoms of drowsiness and confusion, making assessment of her clinical condition difficult; secondly, the effectiveness of treatment administered via the rectal route may be impaired by Mrs K's recently increased laxative use.

Mrs K therefore requires a parenterally administered anti-emetic to control her vomiting, the use of which is unlikely to contribute to her existing symptoms. Metoclopramide is available as a parenteral formulation for intramuscular or intravenous use, and this would be a suitable choice for her.

Once Mrs K's initial vomiting has been controlled, the metoclopramide tablets already prescribed should provide a suitable oral treatment.

7. To correct her presenting dehydration.

Dehydration commonly occurs in patients with hypercalcaemia as a result of polyuria and vomiting. Hypercalcaemia induces polyuria through the impaired action of antidiuretic hormone (ADH) on the renal collecting ducts. This is brought about by calcium-induced inhibition of the adenylcyclase-cyclic AMP mediating system. Inhibition of solute transport in the loop of Henle also occurs, and this contributes to the renal concentrating defect.

8. No. A regimen of sodium chloride 0.9% plus potassium chloride 20 mmol/L is more appropriate. Her serum electrolyte levels and fluid balance should be monitored closely during this therapy.

Mrs K's serum sodium and potassium levels on presentation were at the low end of their respective reference ranges, probably owing to losses incurred through vomiting. Her hydration regimen must thus ensure adequate replacement of these electrolytes to prevent deficiencies developing.

The regimen prescribed for Mrs K at present does not provide adequate replacement of these electrolytes. It contains no potassium, and includes glucose 4% with sodium chloride 0.18%, which provides a disproportionate replacement of fluid to sodium (each litre providing only 30 mmol of sodium) and so puts Mrs K at risk of developing hyponatraemia.

A more appropriate regimen for Mrs K would be 3 L of sodium chloride 0.9% (each litre providing 150 mmol of sodium) over 24 hours, with the addition of potassium chloride 20 mmol/L.

Regular measurements of serum electrolyte levels and fluid balance are required in patients receiving fluid and electrolyte replacement therapy. This enables adjustments to be made to the replacement regimen in order to prevent the development of electrolyte and hydration disturbances. In Mrs K's case, the risk of her developing a disturbance in her fluid and electrolyte balance has been increased, because electrolyte and fluid balance monitoring has not been undertaken during her rehydration therapy thus far.

9. A number of drug treatments are available for the acute treatment of hypercalcaemia. They vary in their ability to lower serum calcium levels, the methods by which they achieve this, and in their onset and duration of action.

(a) Frusemide given intravenously in large doses (80–120 mg every two to six hours), often combined with forced saline diuresis, can reduce serum calcium levels within four hours. This hypocalcaemic effect is thought to result from an enhanced renal excretion of calcium produced by the maintenance of high rates of sodium excretion. A direct action on the kidney, blocking renal calcium resorption, may also occur.

(b) Calcitonin is usually administered by subcutaneous or intramuscular injection in a dose of around 100 units every 12 hours for the treatment of malignancy-associated hypercalcaemia. However, doses of up to 8 units/kg every six hours have been employed. The intramuscular route is preferred when peripheral perfusion is inadequate.

Calcitonin seems to produce its hypocalcaemic effect in two ways: firstly, through the lowering of calcium resorption in the kidney; and secondly, through the inhibition of bone resorption. Calcitonin therapy produces a fall in serum calcium levels within two to four hours, but the effect is rarely sufficient to achieve normocalcaemia. After two to six days of treatment, resistance to the hypocalcae- mic effect has been observed, but this may be prevented in some cases by the co-administration of a corticosteroid.

(c) Plicamycin (mithramycin) may be given as a single infusion of 25 micrograms/kg in patients with normal hepatic and renal function. It substantially decreases serum calcium levels within 48 hours, producing normocalcaemia in 61–78% of patients. Where normocalcaemia is not achieved, additional infusions are usually successful. Patients with pre- existing hepatic or renal dysfunction require a reduction in dose to 12.5 micrograms/kg.

Plicamycin is an antitumour antibiotic which was found to lower serum calcium levels in patients treated with it for neoplastic disease. The most likely mechanism for its hypocalcaemic effect is inhibition of bone resorption.

(d) Bisphosphonates. The bisphosphonates are analogues of pyrophosphate which are thought to produce a lowering of serum calcium levels by inhibiting osteoclast-mediated bone resorption, in an action brought about by their adsorption onto hydroxyapatite crystals.

At present only two bisphosphonates are licensed for use: disodium etidronate and disodium pamid- ronate. The time to onset of their hypocalcaemic effect lies between 24 and 48 hours.

In uncontrolled studies intravenous disodium etidronate has produced normocalcaemia in over 75% of patients with malignancy-associated hyper- calcaemia. A dose of disodium etidronate of 7.5 mg/ kg in 250 mL of sodium chloride 0.9%, over two hours daily for three days, is currently recom- mended, although a dose reduction may be required in patients with renal impairment.

Intravenous disodium pamidronate has also pro- duced normocalcaemia in a high percentage of patients (over 90% in one recent study). Disodium pamidronate may be given as a single infusion of 15–90 mg (depending on the patient's serum cal- cium level), in sodium chloride 0·9% or glucose 5%. The infusion volume and the time required for its administration depend upon the dose given. Alternatively, the drug may be given as divided doses over two to four consecutive days.

In patients with severe hypercalcaemia, a combi- nation of disodium pamidronate and calcitonin (100 units every eight hours) has been used to provide a more rapid fall in serum calcium levels than is achieved with pamidronate therapy alone.

(e) Intravenous phosphates have been adminis- tered in widely varying doses (10 to 100 mmol daily) in the treatment of acute hypercalcaemia. The fall in serum calcium levels they produce is dose-depen-

dent and occurs within minutes of their administra- tion, reaching a minimum level after 12–24 hours, and lasting for one to two days.

Precipitation of calcium as calcium phosphate in bones and at other sites in the body is thought to account for the hypocalcaemic effect produced.

(f) Corticosteroids were widely used in the past but have little place in the treatment of acute hypercalcaemia today. Alone, they tend to be ineffective at reducing serum calcium levels except in some haematological malignancies. Where an hypocalcaemic effect does occur, it can take up to a week to be apparent.

Corticosteroids co-administered with calcitonin may be useful at preventing resistance developing to the hypocalcaemic effect produced by calcitonin.

10. As might be expected, different side-effects are associated with each treatment.

(a) Frusemide has been associated with severe electrolyte and fluid disturbances, and should only be used where facilities for intensive monitoring exist. It is unsuitable for patients with cardiac failure or renal insufficiency.

(b) Calcitonin causes transient nausea and vomiting in approximately 10% of patients. Ana- phylactic reactions can also occur, and skin testing is recommended in atopic individuals.

(c) Plicamycin is associated with a high incidence of side-effects. Most seriously, bleeding can occur, and treatment should be discontinued if epistaxis or other signs of haemorrhage are noted. Renal dys- function and hepatotoxicity have occasionally been reported at the doses employed for the treatment of hypercalcaemia, and transient elevations in liver enzyme levels occur in some 35% of patients at these lower doses. Other side-effects frequently encoun- tered include severe nausea and vomiting, anorexia, diarrhoea and stomatitis; less frequently, fever, weakness, depression, and dermatitis can occur.

(d) Bisphosphonates. Disodium etidronate can produce elevated serum creatinine levels and, occa- sionally, acute renal failure. During long-term use, inhibition of bone mineralisation may occur, which leads to an increased fracture rate. Other side- effects reported are diarrhoea, taste disturbance, and increased bone pain.

Disodium pamidronate can cause transient eleva- tions in body temperature, and also nausea. Unlike disodium etidronate it appears not to inhibit bone mineralisation, and renal dysfunction has not so far been reported.

(e) Intravenous phosphates have produced hypotension, a precipitous decrease in serum cal- cium, and acute renal failure, particularly where they have been administered too rapidly. Calcification of blood vessels, alveoli, myocardium, and kidneys have also occurred. A progressive deterioration in renal function can accompany the precipitation of calcium in the kidneys.

11. Before acute treatment of any sort is started, baseline measurements of serum calcium, albumin, urea and electrolyte levels are necessary, and these should be repeated regularly during the treatment period. For agents such as the bisphosphonates and plicamycin, where serum calcium levels continue to fall for several days or more after treatment, regular measurements need to be continued during this time. Specific monitoring is also required for specific therapies.

For frusemide, in addition to the above, fluid balance must be monitored, ideally via a central venous catheter, and serum magnesium levels should be included in the electrolyte determinations.

For frusemide, plicamycin, disodium etidronate, and intravenous phosphates, renal function monitoring is essential, so regular serum creatinine levels are also required. Regular monitoring of serum phosphate levels are also necessary when intravenous phosphates are used.

Finally, for patients treated with plicamycin, platelet count, prothrombin time, and bleeding time measurements are required before, during, and for several days after, treatment; regular liver function tests should also be performed.

12. Mrs K has an adjusted serum calcium level of 3.57 mmol/L and marked hypercalcaemic symptoms. She therefore requires acute treatment for her hypercalcaemia; of the agents previously considered, the bisphosphonate disodium pamidronate is the most suitable.

Both disodium etidronate and disodium pamidronate have been shown to reduce serum calcium levels effectively in malignancy-associated hypercalcaemia. They do not require repeated injections, nor are they subject to the limited hypocalcaemic effect and escape phenomenon seen with calcitonin. The bisphosphonates also cause fewer serious side-effects than plicamycin, frusemide, and the intravenous phosphates.

Of the two, disodium pamidronate is the bisphosphonate of choice for Mrs K, since it can be given as one single infusion, and, so far, has not been associated with the abnormalities in renal function seen with disodium etidronate.

On the basis of her serum calcium level and present experience with disodium pamidronate, a single infusion of 30 mg of pamidronate in 250 mL of sodium chloride 0.9% over four hours is appropriate for Mrs K.

13. Disodium pamidronate produces a maximum lowering of serum calcium levels four to five days after treatment is initiated.

14. Yes.

Recurrence of hypercalcaemia tends to occur 14 to 21 days after a single dose of disodium pamidronate, unless measures are taken to treat the underlying cause of the hypercalcaemia, or maintenance therapy is successfully introduced.

Unfortunately, treatment of the advanced malignancy suffered by Mrs K appears to be inadequate; nineteen days after receiving treatment with disodium pamidronate, Mrs K has had a relapse of her hypercalcaemia.

15. Intravenous hydration therapy and further treatment with disodium pamidronate.

Mrs K has marked hypercalcaemic symptoms and an adjusted serum calcium level of 3.36 mmol/L, which again warrants acute treatment. She previously responded well to pamidronate and treatment can be repeated.

It has been suggested that the effectiveness of disodium pamidronate may be decreased as the number of repeat treatments increases; however, the position is unclear at present, and awaits further study.

Following the acute treatment Mrs K should be considered for oral maintenance therapy, to help prevent a further recurrence of hypercalcaemia.

16. This is difficult to predict and depends largely on the patient's ability to tolerate oral treatment.

The drugs available at present tend to be low in efficacy or poorly tolerated. Several new oral bisphosphonates are under investigation and may improve the success of maintenance treatment in the future.

17. Three alternatives are currently available: oral phosphate therapy, corticosteroid therapy, and disodium etidronate therapy. The last is most appropriate for Mrs K.

(a) Oral phosphates have been used in doses of between 32 and 96 mmol daily to maintain acceptable serum calcium levels, but they are poorly tolerated, causing diarrhoea in many patients. Hyperphosphataemia may also be a problem.

(b) Corticosteroid therapy is better tolerated

than treatment with oral phosphates. Here again the doses used have varied widely (e.g. prednisolone 10–40 mg daily) but such therapy has only been found to be effective in a minority of patients. In most of these cases hypercalcaemia was due to granulomatous disease or a lymphoproliferative disorder.

(c) Disodium etidronate treatment is also often poorly tolerated, producing marked nausea. However, tolerance may be improved by giving the total daily dose (20 mg/kg/day orally) in several aliquots. Poor absorption can also limit the effectiveness of oral disodium etidronate, and it should be taken on an empty stomach.

Treatment with oral disodium etidronate is favoured for Mrs K, since corticosteroid therapy is unlikely to be effective and oral phosphates are unlikely to be tolerated. An additional factor in favour of disodium etidronate treatment is that Mrs K has already responded well to intravenous bisphosphonates.

A suitable oral regimen for Mrs K would be 400 mg of disodium etidronate twice daily. In addition to this, she must be advised to maintain a liberal fluid intake to prevent dehydration.

18. Mrs K's serum calcium, albumin, urea, and electrolyte levels should be monitored regularly.

Regular monitoring of these parameters should ensure that any elevation in her serum calcium level is detected before serious symptoms develop, and that dehydration and electrolyte disturbances are avoided.

It has also been suggested that serum alkaline phosphatase levels should be monitored in patients receiving oral maintenance treatment with disodium etidronate, as impairment of bone mineralisation produces elevated levels of serum alkaline phosphatase. However, secondary carcinoma of the bone can also produce raised levels of serum alkaline phosphatase, and this makes the value of measuring serum alkaline phosphatase levels questionable for monitoring disodium etidronate therapy in Mrs K.

19. Provided the oral disodium etidronate is effective and tolerated by Mrs K, then an initial treatment period of 30 days is recommended. Future therapeutic options depend on her response to this therapy.

If serum calcium levels remain clinically acceptable during these first 30 days of therapy, then treatment with disodium etidronate may be continued for up to 90 days. Treatment is not recommended beyond this time because of the increased risk of impaired bone mineralisation on the drug's long-term use, and because treatment for more than 90 days has been inadequately studied.

If Mrs K's maintenance treatment with oral disodium etidronate is ineffective, or has to be discontinued, then treatment with an oral phosphate could be tried. Beyond this the only option for Mrs K is for her to receive acute treatment intermittently when hypercalcaemia recurs.

20. The following should be covered when counselling Mrs K on her new medication:
(a) Disodium etidronate.

(i) It must be taken regularly, twice a day.

(ii) Eating should be avoided for two hours before and after a dose, since food in the stomach reduces the drug's effectiveness.

(iii) The tablets may be taken with water or fruit juice.

(b) General measures.

(i) Drink plenty of water.

(ii) Avoid mineral supplements and antacids high in calcium, and also vitamin D supplements. Ask the pharmacist for advice if buying over-the-counter products.

(iii) If previous symptoms return (i.e. weakness, fatigue, confusion, and nausea) contact your doctor immediately.

In most cases of malignancy-associated hypercalcaemia, intestinal absorption of calcium is suppressed. Dietary restriction of calcium (in the form of milk and milk products) is therefore likely to provide only minimal benefit, and is not necessary for Mrs K unless her intake is excessive.

References and Further Reading

Burns Schaiff R.A. *et al.*, Medical treatment of hypercalcaemia, *Clin. Pharm.*, 1989, **8**, 108–121.

Cuddy P.G., Fluid and electrolyte disorders – hypercalcaemia, in *Applied Therapeutics – the Clinical Use of Drugs*, Young L.Y. and Koda-Kimble M.A. (eds), Vancouver, WA, Applied Therapeutics, 1988, 603–608.

Heath D.A., Hypercalcaemia in malignancy, *Br. med. J.*, 1989, **298**, 1468–1469.

Prior F.G.R., How to design intravenous fluid therapy, *Pharm. J.*, 1989, **242 (Suppl.)**, HS36–HS38.

Ralston S.H. *et al.*, Treatment of cancer associated hypercalcaemia with combined aminohydroxypropylidene diphosphonate and calcitonin, *Br. med. J.*, 1986, **292**, 1549–1550.

Stevenson J.C., Current management of malignant hypercalcaemia, *Drugs*, 1988, **36**, 229–238.

SYMPTOM CONTROL IN TERMINAL CARE

Shelagh French

Staff Pharmacist, Drug Information, City Hospital, Nottingham

Day 1 Mr D, a 63-year-old engineer with a 20-year history of intermittent back pain, was admitted to the ward at the request of his general practitioner because of steadily increasing pain. He described it as a "terrible pain in the back", which was episodic, radiating down from both hips, through the buttocks, and down the backs of both thighs and calves to the soles of his feet. It was predominantly an ache but occasionally was worse, "like an electric shock". It was exacerbated by movement and certain body positions, and was preventing mobilisation.

Mr D had first presented two months earlier with constant severe pain which he described as "so bad that he could not bear to move". He was a long-standing pipe smoker and had a history of asbestos exposure at his place of work.

At that time he had undergone extensive investigations which are briefly summarised as follows. He had exhibited extreme tenderness over the T10 and L1 areas making all spinal movement impossible. A chest x-ray had revealed a 2–3 cm mass in the left main bronchus which was diagnosed on biopsy as a squamous cell carcinoma. A bone scan revealed evidence of metastatic deposits at T12, L4, and in the right femur and the second right rib. He had received a course of deep x-ray treatment (DXT), three to the chest and six to the back, with an excellent response and resumption of mobility.

On examination at the present admission Mr D appeared pale, with no obvious lymphadenopathy. Decreased expiration was noted on the right hand side of the chest and he had a dull right lung base. The main findings of significance were an abnormality of plantar reflexes, slight floppiness of the legs and wasting of the left quadriceps.

His medication had been changed two weeks previously, from morphine slow-release tablets to morphine mixture, and his drug regimen was now:

Morphine mixture 125 mg orally every four hours
Indomethacin 25 mg orally four times daily, after food
Senna tablets, two at night
Dextromoramide 5 mg orally when required for breakthrough pain

1. *What treatment options are available for squamous cell carcinoma of the bronchus?*

2. *Why did Mr D receive a course of DXT?*

3. *Why had indomethacin been prescribed for Mr D? Would you have recommended any other agent in preference?*

4. *Was it appropriate to change Mr D's morphine from slow-release tablets to morphine mixture?*

5. *Should morphine mixture ALWAYS be given every four hours?*

6. *Do you consider dextromoramide an appropriate choice for Mr D's breakthrough pain?*

7. *Should an anti-emetic always be prescribed with morphine therapy? Which anti-emetic would you recommend?*

8. *What problems might Mr D experience as a result of regular morphine therapy? What would you recommend to treat these side-effects?*

9. *What is the likely reason for the exacerbation in Mr D's pain that has caused this admission?*

The suggested diagnosis was that nerve root involvement was causing the increased pain and slight weakness. The plan was to treat the nerve root involvement, control the pain and maintain mobility.

The dose of morphine was increased, flurbiprofen substituted for indomethacin, and corticosteroid therapy initiated.

10. Why was steroid therapy considered appropriate?

11. Which steroid would you recommend for Mr D, and at what dose?

12. What side-effects may Mr D experience as a result of long-term corticosteroid therapy?

Mr D's drug therapy was now as follows:

Morphine mixture 150–200 mg orally every four hours
Flurbiprofen 100 mg orally twice daily after food
Lactulose 20 mL orally twice daily
Senna tablets, two to four at night
Dexamethasone 16 mg orally daily, reducing quickly

13. Would you recommend the use of an H_2-receptor blocker to protect Mr D against peptic ulcer?

Day 3 The pain was improved but Mr D was still suffering from occasional pain on movement. He was feeling much more cheerful. The plan was to continue the steroid therapy and monitor carefully for its effects.

Day 4 Mr D was comfortable and cheerful, although he still had some pain in the lumbar region. His dexamethasone dose was reduced to 12 mg orally daily.

Day 6 Mr D complained of a sore mouth, particularly on eating, and drinking hot liquids. On examination, the oral mucosa was noted to be red and sore with white adherent plaques. This was diagnosed as thrush.

14. Why was it likely that Mr D would develop a candidal infection of the mouth?

15. What would you recommend to treat the infection and why? What other suggestions would you make to improve mouth care, and Mr D's comfort?

Day 7 The dexamethasone dose was reduced to 8 mg orally daily.

Day 8 Mr D was stable but still complaining of a recurrent stabbing pain. Tumour infiltration of the nerve was suspected.

16. What is the cause of this opiate-unresponsive pain?

17. What types of drug treatment are effective for this sort of pain? What is the rationale for their use?

Day 9 Carbamazepine was introduced at a low dose of 100 mg orally twice daily, to be gradually increased according to response, up to a maximum of 400 mg orally three times daily.

18. What other treatment options are available for intractable pain?

Day 12 Mr D's pain stabilised on this regimen, although he was not completely pain-free. He was comfortable, cheerful, and mobile, and anxious to return home. He was discharged to the care of his general practitioner on the following medication:

Morphine mixture 200 mg orally every four hours
Flurbiprofen 100 mg orally twice daily after food
Lactulose 20 mL orally twice daily
Senna tablets, two to four at night
Dexamethasone 2 mg orally once daily
Carbamazepine 200 mg orally three times daily

The general practitioner was to review the medication, and Mr D was also going to be followed up by a Home Care Sister, in order to ensure that he would be kept under close surveillance, and his treatment modified in the light of changes to his condition.

It will be important to ensure that Mr D can cope with everyday tasks, and maintain his mobility. His prognosis is poor, and his condition is likely to deteriorate, so his medication may require frequent adjustments in order to provide adequate symptom control. It is also important that the needs of the family caring for Mr D are taken into account, so that they can cope with his deteriorating state. However, the main aim would be to provide a good quality of life through effective analgesia and appropriate symptom control, as required.

19. When is a syringe driver appropriate for pain control?

20. What contributions can a pharmacist make to improving medication acceptability and compliance in patients receiving terminal care?

Answers

1. Surgery and radiotherapy.

Squamous cell carcinoma is a non-small-cell lung cancer. Localised disease that is peripheral in the chest, less than 3 cm in diameter and without nodal involvement is curable by surgery or radiotherapy (90% disease-free at three years). However, most patients present with disseminated disease; at this stage radiotherapy is the mainstay of treatment for symptom control. Chemotherapy is experimental and controversial, and prolongation of survival is unlikely.

2. Mr D received DXT as a palliative therapy to shrink his bone metastases, and hence relieve his bone pain and reduce compression of the spinal cord and nerve roots.

At presentation Mr D had evidence of extensive metastatic disease, with deposits at T12, L4, the right femur, and the right second rib. Some tumours, particularly primary breast, kidney, lung, and prostate, are likely to metastasise to the bone, producing pain which is often severe, particularly on pressure or movement. This pain is difficult to relieve. As the metastases grow, they also cause extensive destruction of the bone, with fractures and compression of the spinal cord and nerve roots. The symptoms then vary from pain in the affected area to paraplegia.

Radiotherapy is the treatment of choice for bone metastases, but it may not always be practical, for example, in a patient suffering from multiple rib metastases.

3. Mr D was prescribed indomethacin to help control his severe bone pain caused by multiple metastases. Although a suitable choice when therapy was initiated, an alternative agent such as flurbiprofen should now be evaluated.

If radiation therapy is impractical, or not fully effective, or in the period during which the beneficial effects of DXT are awaited, treatment with non-steroidal anti-inflammatory drugs (NSAIDs) is appropriate.

It is thought that as metastases grow in skeletal deposits they produce both bone destruction (osteolysis) and bone formation (osteosclerosis). Most, but not all, bony metastases produce an osteolytic prostaglandin derivative, probably PGE_2. This causes resorption of the surrounding bone and sensitisation of nerve endings to painful stimuli; it is this that accounts for the severe pain associated with bony metastases. Inhibitors of prostaglandin synthesis are usually effective in relieving this pain, which is only partly opiate-responsive.

In theory any NSAID could be used, and the choice often depends on a compromise between efficacy and toxicity. Aspirin is cheap and effective but many patients cannot tolerate the full dose of 4 g per day which is often necessary (dyspepsia may occur in up to 25% of patients). An alternative is benorylate, which provides 2.3 g aspirin and 1.94 g paracetamol in each 4 g dose. The gastric tolerance of benorylate is certainly better than that of aspirin, but some patients may develop fullness in the ears, or tinnitus, which limits its usefulness. The NSAIDs can all cause gastro-intestinal upset and bleeding, skin rashes, reduced renal perfusion, increased water retention, and antagonism of antihypertensive therapy. Indomethacin is particularly associated with these side-effects, and, in addition, can produce bizarre central nervous system effects, especially in elderly women. Other alternatives to indomethacin include flurbiprofen, diflunisal, diclofenac, and naproxen. All are reasonably well tolerated. If a patient does not respond to, or cannot tolerate, one type of NSAID it may be worthwhile changing to another from a different class. For this reason it is worth changing Mr D from indomethacin to flurbiprofen therapy.

4. Yes, because Mr D's analgesic requirement was increasing.

Although MST® slow-release morphine tablets are useful for pain control in stable patients, they may not be ideal for restabilising patients whose analgesic requirements are changing. After a single dose of MST, plasma levels of morphine rise to a peak in three to four hours, whereas a peak plasma level is achieved one hour after a dose of morphine solution; hence it is easier to control pain quickly with four-hourly doses of morphine solution. The new dose required is usually found by increasing the previous dose by 25–50%, then reassessing. When the symptoms are fully controlled, slow-release morphine can be re-instituted by direct conversion (i.e. MST dose = total daily dose of morphine in solution divided by two). The contribution of dextromoramide, or other drugs being used for breakthrough pain, should also be taken into account when calculating the new morphine dosage requirement.

5. Morphine sulphate solution should usually be prescribed to be administered every four hours, but there are a few exceptions.

Four-hourly morphine solution is indicated for the relief of chronic pain. Occasionally, in the very elderly (over 80 years of age), it may be possible to give it less often. Very rarely, it may be given every three hours, but careful investigations of the pain to ensure that all other appropriate drug and non-drug measures have been considered should be carried out first.

The main reason why six doses per day may not be prescribed is to avoid the dose in the middle of the night. The four-hourly regimen may be modified by stopping the 2 a.m. dose, and increasing the 10 p.m. dose by 50–100%; however, this may not be possible in patients receiving doses of morphine above 100 mg every four hours.

6. Yes, although another approach could have been used.

Dextromoramide is a potent opiate agonist analgesic (orally, 10 mg morphine is approximately equivalent to 5 mg dextromoramide) but it has a short duration of action of only about three hours. It is therefore of no value for regular dosing, but it does have a place as "top-up" medication, for example at dressing changes or for breakthrough pain when analgesic requirements are not fully stabilised. In such situations it can be given sublingually. Some patients do describe a euphoric "lift" with dextromoramide.

An alternative strategem would have been to prescribe a single dose of morphine solution, equivalent to a normal four-hourly dose, to be taken when required.

7. No. However, when morphine therapy dose cause nausea and vomiting, haloperidol is usually an effective anti-emetic.

Vomiting with morphine is a side-effect that occurs mainly in the first few days of treatment, or when a dose is increased. In addition, only about two-thirds of patients taking morphine will experience this side-effect. If nausea and vomiting do occur, tolerance usually develops after five to seven days. If the dose is then increased, it may recur until tolerance again develops. It has been suggested that this side-effect could be associated with fluctuations in plasma levels of morphine, and that slow-release products may be associated with a lower incidence of nausea and vomiting, but this is still debatable.

The major, but not the only, mechanism of morphine-induced nausea and vomiting is stimulation of the chemoreceptor trigger zone in the brain stem, which involves dopamine D_2 receptors. If nausea and vomiting are not due to any other cause, then haloperidol is considered by many to be the anti-emetic of choice, given in a dose of 1.5 mg at bedtime.

Sometimes morphine can precipitate vomiting by other mechanisms (e.g. through vestibular disturbance, delayed gastric emptying, or as a consequence of constipation). Vestibular disturbance should respond to cyclizine or hyoscine therapy, and delayed gastric emptying to metoclopramide or domperidone. Very occasionally, nausea and vomiting are so severe that it is necessary to prescribe an alternative narcotic analgesic.

8. There are many myths surrounding the regular use of morphine. Drowsiness, tolerance, addiction, and respiratory depression are not inevitable consequences of regular morphine therapy.

(a) Tolerance to the analgesic effects of morphine is not a problem when the drug is used regularly as prophylactic therapy in individually titrated doses, and many patients remain on the same dose for weeks or months. In rare cases the dose may be reduced. Increases in dose should only be necessary as a result of changes in the patient's underlying condition.

Tolerance does however occur to some of the side-effects of morphine therapy, and this can be useful. Drowsiness, like nausea and vomiting, tends to be a problem in the first few days of treatment, or after a dose increase, but patients should be encouraged to persevere with their medication until tolerance does occur, usually in three to seven days. Occasionally, drowsiness indicates that the dose of morphine is too high and a dose reduction is necessary.

(b) Respiratory depression should not occur in patients if a dose has been carefully titrated against pain. However, great care is needed if a patient has undergone another pain-relieving procedure, such as DXT for bone metastases, as this may reduce the pain stimulus to respiration and necessitate a reduction in morphine dosage to avoid respiratory depression.

(c) Addiction is not a problem in terminal care patients. Psychological addiction does not occur in this context. Physical dependence can occur over a long period of time, and if the pain is removed by other means, morphine therapy should be gradually, not abruptly, withdrawn.

(d) Constipation always occurs with morphine therapy, and tolerance to this side-effect does not develop. Mr D must receive regular laxatives, which ideally should include a stool softener (such as lactulose or docusate sodium) plus a peristaltic stimulant (such as senna). Typical doses are lactulose 20–30 mL orally twice daily, plus senna tablets, one to four at night. Alternatively, co-danthrusate capsules (one to four at night, or even more) may be necessary. Co-danthramer suspension is again available, but many patients find the texture and taste unpleasant.

(e) Other side-effects associated with morphine therapy include confusion and postural hypotension, which are particularly noted in the elderly and can be managed as for drowsiness. Sweating may also occur. This is sometimes, but not always, helped by prednisolone or dexamethasone therapy.

9. It is likely that Mr D has increasing pain due to nerve root compression.

Secondary deposits in the spinal vertebrae are the most common cause of nerve root compression. The compression occurs because the tumour is surrounded by inflammation and oedema, which exerts pressure on veins and lymphatics causing localised swelling. The pain of nerve root compression is typically described as a constant ache in the initial stages, although later the patient may suffer intermittent shooting pains.

10. Because corticosteroids reduce perineural oedema.

By reducing the inflammatory swelling around the tumour, the effective tumour mass is reduced, the compression alleviated, and the pain relieved. There is also some experimental evidence that systemic steroids have an effect on both nerve membranes and synaptic transmission.

11. Dexamethasone, 16 mg daily in divided doses.

Dexamethasone or prednisolone are both useful for this indication, but dexamethasone is preferable because it causes less water retention than prednisolone and, milligram for milligram, it is more potent (0.75 mg dexamethasone is equivalent to 5 mg prednisolone).

Dexamethasone should be prescribed initially in a dose of 12–24 mg daily, in order to reduce perineural oedema quickly. Once a response has been noted, the dose should be reduced over several days to the lowest dose that will control the symptoms. If a definite improvement is not seen in 10–14 days, dexamethasone therapy should be tailed-off gradually and discontinued.

12. Mr D may experience a number of side-effects.

Dexamethasone in the dose prescribed will cause adrenal suppression if used for more than seven days, so the dose must not be discontinued abruptly. Corticosteroid therapy is weakly linked with peptic ulceration, with the risk depending on the dose and duration of therapy. Patients with advanced cancer are thus at risk of developing ulcers because of the large steroid doses used, but most authorities would consider that the benefits of such therapy outweigh the risks. Steroids should always be given with food, to try to minimise gastric upset, although this strategy may not be effective.

Steroids increase susceptibility to infection, produce hypokalaemia, and cause fluid retention and impaired glucose tolerance. On the positive side they can increase appetite and elevate mood, although in some patients the stimulant effect is exaggerated and a frank psychosis may occur. It has been reported that taking the last dose no later than 6 p.m. may avoid insomnia, but this is uncertain.

13. No.

There is conflicting information from various studies in animals and man concerning the effectiveness of H_2-receptor blockers in preventing the gastro-intestinal side-effects of corticosteroids. At present, there is no overwhelming evidence that they are useful, although they are often prescribed.

14. He is debilitated, and his immune system is depressed by corticosteroid therapy.

Patients like Mr D, with a terminal malignancy, are generally debilitated and have a reduced oral intake. Although *Candida* can be found in the mouth of many such patients, a definite candidiasis is usually the result of a reduction in immunity, most often caused by steroid therapy. It is unlikely to be the result of cross-infection. Other factors, such as reduced fluid intake, mouth-breathing, and anticholinergic side-effects associated with sedative or anti-emetic therapy can all contribute to poor oral hygiene.

Oral candidiasis not only makes eating and drinking difficult, but can also severely reduce the patient's quality of life. It usually presents as redness or soreness of the mouth, with white adherent patches, and/or inflammation at the corners of the mouth (angular cheilitis).

15. Nystatin liquid 200,000 units every four hours for seven days.

Nystatin liquid is an effective oral anticandidal agent, in a dose of 1–5 mL every four hours, although therapy may have to be continued for two weeks. It may, however, be unsuitable for patients who are weak, as they can find it difficult to hold the suspension against the lesions for long enough for it to be effective. Nystatin pastilles or amphotericin lozenges can be suitable alternatives, but some patients' mouths may be too dry to suck these products comfortably. Miconazole gel is a palatable alternative if the above situations apply. It can be smeared around the mouth and onto the lesions, and hence stays in contact with them for longer.

Oral ketoconazole, 200 mg daily for seven days, is an alternative systemic antifungal that is rapidly effective for oral candidiasis. Ketoconazole use is associated with serious hepatotoxicity, although the effect appears to be dose-related, in most cases occurring after 14 days' therapy with an approximate incidence of 1 in 10,000. However, the possibility of heptotoxicity should not preclude ketoconazole use in advanced cancer; this small but serious risk is usually outweighed by the benefits of treating a severe oral *Candida* infection which might otherwise significantly reduce a patient's quality of life.

Ketoconazole must be given with food for maximum absorption. It is an enzyme inhibitor and can interact with other drugs, including some used in terminal care. Antacids, anticholinergics and H_2-receptor blockers may reduce its absorption, and such agents should be taken not less than two hours after ketoconazole. The effects of phenytoin may be enhanced by ketoconazole use. Fluconazole is an alternative to ketoconazole, although considerably more expensive. Like ketoconazole, it may interact with phenytoin.

Mouth care in general may be helped by small modifications to therapy, for example, by changing drugs known to cause a dry mouth to ones less likely to do so (e.g. phenothiazines to butyrophenones, tricyclics to mianserin). A dry mouth may be helped by artificial saliva solutions, such as Glandosane®. A dirty, although not infected, mouth may be cleaned in a number of ways: for example, by physical debridement with a soft brush or swab and cleansing solution; with an effervescent mixture, such as a 1 g Vitamin C tablet held on the tongue; by hydrogen peroxide; or, if the patient can co-operate, by chewing unsweetened pineapple chunks. If the patient has dentures, they should be soaked in 1% sodium hypochlorite solution (for metallic dentures, use povidone-iodine solution). If the mouth is painful, benzydamine solution, undiluted or diluted 50%, either as a mouthwash or applied by a swab, may be useful. Alternatively, simple teething gels are effective.

16. The pain is probably due to tumour infiltration of the nerve. This pain is often resistant to high-dose opiates, and its underlying mechanism is still not fully understood.

One theory suggests that pain following nerve injury is not the result of simple transmission in the spinothalamic tract, and is therefore not necessarily susceptible to conventional analgesic drugs, or to the interruption of the nociceptive pathway. There may be changes at the dorsal horn level of the spinal cord. This type of pain is given the term neuropathic or deafferentation pain, and may have many causes. It may be that the metastatic lesion first produces nerve compression, resulting in a pain susceptible to analgesics, but further unrelieved compression leads to nerve damage, sensory loss, and, in some, development of deafferentation pain. However, the exact mechanism is not known and may not be the same in all cases.

17. Many different classes of drugs have been used to treat this type of pain, even though the aetiology of it is not fully understood. There are thought to be many neurotransmitters, neuromodulators, facilitators, and inhibitors at the first synapse in the dorsal horn, which could be involved in pain, and this probably explains the diversity of drugs used.

The anticonvulsants appear to be useful for severe stabbing or shooting pain. Carbamazepine 50 mg orally three times daily, increased slowly to 400 mg orally three times daily, phenytoin 100 mg orally three times daily, sodium valproate 200 mg orally twice daily, and clonazepam 500 micrograms orally twice daily, increasing to 1 mg orally three times daily, have all been used. The exact mode of action in pain is unclear, but may involve suppression of spontaneous activity in damaged nerve fibres.

Where nerve involvement is characterised by a burning sensation and local hypersensitivity, a tricylic antidepressant may be useful. This can produce an effect within days, rather than the two weeks required for an antidepressant effect. Amitriptyline, imipramine, clomipramine, dothiepin and mianserin have all been shown to be effective. They act on the monoamine pathways that descend from the brainstem, and have an inhibitory action at the dorsal horn level. Two of the main transmitters involved are serotonin and noradrenaline; inhibition of re-uptake at the synapses by antidepressants would potentiate the inhibitory effect of the descending pathways (i.e. the intrinsic pain-suppressing system). Cholinergic involvement may also be important.

More recently, the Class 1 oral anti-arrhythmic local anaesthetics, such as mexiletine, flecainide, and tocainide, have been used effectively. They enter the cerebrospinal fluid and may exert their effects on central synapses. Alternatively, through a sodium-channel blocking mechanism, they may block activity in hyperexcitable nerve membranes in pain-producing foci.

Finally, clonidine given epidurally (and often followed by oral therapy) may be effective by inhibiting adrenergic transmission in the spinal cord. Baclofen, L-tryptophan, and naloxone have also been used.

Unfortunately, not all the nerve pains will respond to the usually effective drugs, and it may be necessary to try several agents with different modes of action.

Carbamazepine would be a suitable drug to start with for Mr D, in a trial of about six weeks. It can cause considerable drowsiness and dizziness on initiation of therapy, but these side-effects can be minimised by starting the drug at a low dose, preferably with the first dose at night; for example, 100 mg orally twice daily, increasing gradually, according to the response, up to 400 mg orally three times daily.

18. If conventional analgesic therapy, including epidural and intrathecal therapy, does not control the pain, there are still many effective approaches that can be used. These include nerve blocks, cordotomy, and pituitary ablation.

Some authors would advocate the use of these techniques much earlier in therapy; however, such techniques are not universally available. They are all highly specialised, and are beyond the scope of this case study.

19. When oral therapy is no longer possible.

The continuous subcutaneous administration of drugs via a syringe driver is convenient and practical, but it should only be used when oral medication is no longer possible, (for example, because of severe nausea and vomiting, dysphagia, bowel obstruction, severe weakness, or coma) and regular injections become necessary. It may also be used in the last few days of life, although most patients can and should be maintained on oral medication during this time. When it must be used, it provides a useful way of combining analgesic, anti-emetic, and antispasmodic drugs in an infusion given over a 24-hour period.

20. A pharmacist can make many contributions to optimising the terminal care of patients, but to contribute fully, it is vital to be aware of that individual patient's problems.

Many patients are confined to bed, and may take all their medication in a semirecumbent position. Care must be taken when large tablets and capsules are prescribed for such patients, as these formulations are liable to stick in the oesophagus. This is particularly important if the drug is also irritant, as many patients may be unable to tolerate the large amount of fluid required to prevent prolonged oesophageal transit time, with resultant oesophageal irritation. If suspensions are used, a careful check on their formulation must be made, to ensure that the patient does not receive a large volume of sorbitol, which may cause diarrhoea. The same considerations should be applied to patients with a history of radiotherapy or surgery to the head, neck or chest, to those with strictures or compression of the oesophagus, and to patients with swallowing difficulties.

Sublingual medication may appear to be a useful alternative in some patients, but the problem of a dry mouth, often as a result of anticholinergic medication, can make this route uncomfortable or impossible. The bitter taste of opiates taken by this route can, however, be improved, for example; if a mint is sucked at the same time.

The rectal route is not ideal for many patients, especially these with gastro-intestinal or gynaecological malignancies, or where movement is difficult or causes pain.

Finally, pharmacists must be alert to the problems of compliance. Some patients may be on many different types of medication for various symptoms and, especially if medication has recently been changed, may be unsure of the reasons for each one. A medication card, giving the names of the medicines, their purpose, any special instructions, and the times each should be taken, can help to ensure the patient is fully informed. The card can also be shown to any doctor or nurse who visits, and changes to medication can be clearly highlighted. The pharmacist should also ensure that the patient, or their carer, can manipulate all the containers (often a mixture of boxes, bottles, droppers, oral syringes, etc.), and should rationalise them, via compliance aids, if necessary.

References and Further Reading

Dickson R.J., Pain unresponsive to high dose opiate drugs, *Palliative Med.*, 1989, **3**, 61–64.

Glynn C., An approach to the management of the patient in deafferentation pain, *ibid.*, 15–21.

McQuay H.J., Pharmacological treatment of neuralgic and neuropathic pain, *Cancer Surv.*, 1988, **7**, 141–159.

Oliver O.J., Syringe drivers in palliative care: a review, *Palliative Med.*, 1988, **2**, 21–26.

Page C.M., Terminal care at home, *Prescribers' J.*, 1988, **28**, 8–13.

Regnard C.F.B., *A Guide to Symptom Relief in Advanced Cancer*, 2nd edn, Manchester, Haigh and Hockland, 1986.

Saunders C. (ed.), *The Management of Terminal Malignant Disease*, 2nd edn, London, Edward Arnold, 1984.

Tempest S.M., The control of terminal pain in malignant disease, *Pharm. Update*, 1987, **3**, 302–306.

Twycross R.G. and Lack S.A., *Therapeutics in Terminal Care*, Beaconsfield, Beaconsfield Publications, 1984.

Twycross R.G. and Lack S.A., *Oral Morphine in Advanced Cancer*, Beaconsfield, Beaconsfield Publications, 1984.

HUMAN IMMUNODEFICIENCY VIRUS DISEASE AND THE ACQUIRED IMMUNODEFICIENCY SYNDROME

PART I—Herpes Simplex Infection, Oral and Oesophageal Candidiasis, and Cytomegalovirus Infection

Janet Clarbour

Staff Pharmacist (HIV Drug Co-ordinator), St Stephen's and Westminster Hospitals, London

Day 1 Thirty-three-year-old Mr I attended his local Sexually Transmitted Diseases (STD) clinic, with a six-day history of pain on defaecation. His past medical history included syphilis two years earlier, two episodes of gonorrhoea over the past five years, and anal herpes six months previously. Mr I stated that he was single, homosexual, and was not taking any regular drug therapy.

Examination revealed a red mucosa with several well-defined ulcers around the anal margin. Swabs for viral cultures were taken and a standard STD work-up was carried out, which included tests for chlamydia, gonorrhoea, and syphilis.

A diagnosis of anal herpes was made, and a five-day course of oral acyclovir, at a dose of 200 mg five times daily, was prescribed. Human immunodeficiency virus (HIV) testing was discussed, and pre- and post-test counselling by the health advisor was arranged.

HIV testing by enzyme-linked immunoabsorbent assay was subsequently positive, and Mr I was advised to attend the HIV clinic at three-monthly intervals, to monitor for HIV-associated problems.

1. Was the dose of acyclovir appropriate for Mr I's herpes simplex infection?

2. Should maintenance acyclovir therapy be prescribed?

Month 12 Mr I had been well over the previous year, but routine examination of his oral cavity revealed white plaques with surrounding areas of inflammation.

His drug therapy consisted of oral acyclovir 400 mg twice daily (which had been started following a seven-day course of 400 mg orally five times daily for a repeat attack of anal herpes he had suffered ten months previously).

On direct questioning, Mr I admitted to some soreness of his mouth, but was otherwise asymptomatic. Swabs were taken for fungal culture, in order to confirm the diagnosis of oral *Candida* infection. Amphotericin lozenges were prescribed to be sucked four times daily for two weeks.

3. Are there any factors that might have precipitated Mr I's candidal infection?

4. Is topical anti-candidal therapy appropriate for Mr I?

One week later Mr I returned, complaining of worsening mouth soreness, and a loss of taste which was affecting his appetite. Results of the previous week's swabs confirmed *Candida albicans* infection, and white candidal plaques were still evident in his oral cavity. Ketoconazole 200 mg orally twice daily for one month was prescribed.

5. What baseline tests should be carried out before prescribing ketoconazole?

6. Is ketoconazole the most appropriate systemic antifungal agent for this patient?

7. Would you recommend prophylactic antifungal therapy after treatment of the acute candidal infection?

Month 14 Mr I returned to clinic with a recurrence of oral *Candida* infection, and was prescribed continuous ketoconazole therapy (200 mg orally twice daily).

Month 18 Mr I attended the clinic complaining of dysphagia and heartburn. Examination of the oral cavity showed typical candidal plaques. Mr I said he had been fully compliant with his medication (acyclovir and ketoconazole) but admitted taking large amounts of antacids over the previous weeks, which had been prescribed by his general practitioner for heartburn.

A presumptive diagnosis of oesophageal and oral candidiasis was made. This also constituted a diagnosis of Acquired Immunodeficiency Syndrome (AIDS) for Mr I, as a presumptive diagnosis of oesophageal *Candida* infection, in the presence of positive laboratory evidence of HIV, constitutes one of the Communicable Diseases Centre definitions of AIDS. (Candidiasis of the oesophagus diagnosed definitively, even in the absence of a positive HIV test, also constitutes an AIDS diagnosis, provided other causes of immunodeficiency can be excluded.)

An endoscopy was arranged for Mr I. This showed ulcers in the oesophagus characteristic of *Candida* infection; the ulcers were biopsied. Antifungal therapy was changed to fluconazole, and Mr I's prescription on discharge after the endoscopy was as follows:

Fluconazole 50 mg orally once daily
Acyclovir 400 mg orally twice daily
Co-trimoxazole 960 mg orally twice daily
Zidovudine 100 mg orally four times daily, to be increased to 250 mg orally four times daily after two weeks

Mr I's T4 count at this time was 191 cells/mm^3 (reference range 700–1200, although HIV disease is usually indicated by a count of less than 500). This further indicated progression of his HIV disease.

8. What symptoms might distinguish oesophageal candidiasis from heartburn?

9. What factors may have contributed to the failure of ketoconazole therapy?

10. What drugs may affect the efficacy of ketoconazole therapy?

11. Was it appropriate to change Mr I's antifungal therapy?

12. Why have zidovudine and co-trimoxazole been prescribed? Is the zidovudine dosing regimen appropriate?

Month 25 Mr I had attended clinic at monthly intervals, in order to monitor his HIV disease and associated drug therapy. He had remained well until this visit, when he complained of painless blurred vision. Examination by a trained ophthalmologist revealed retinal haemorrhage, with exudate in the right eye characteristic of cytomegalovirus (CMV) retinitis. An urgent admission to hospital was arranged for treatment of the CMV infection.

13. What agents are available for the treatment of CMV infection? What are their advantages and disadvantages?

14. What information would you need in order to advise on choice of therapy for Mr I's CMV retinitis?

Mr I's serum biochemistry and haematology results on admission were:

Sodium 138 mmol/L (reference range 135–144)
Potassium 3.9 mmol/L (3.1–4.4)
Calcium 2.2 mmol/L (2.15–2.55)
Albumin 35 g/L (30–42)
Urea 4.9 mmol/L (2.2–7.4)
Creatinine 91 micromol/L (60–115)
White blood cells (WBC) 2.3×10^9/L (4–11×10^9)
Haemoglobin 11 g/dL (13–18)
Platelets 238×10^9/L (150–400×10^9)
Liver function tests within normal limits

Discussion with Mr I established that he wished to continue with zidovudine therapy if possible. Foscarnet therapy was commenced, and Mr I's other therapies (fluconazole, acyclovir, co-trimoxazole, and zidovudine) continued unchanged.

15. Would you have recommended foscarnet therapy for Mr I? How should it be administered?

16. What laboratory results should be monitored during foscarnet therapy, why, and how frequently?

Serum biochemistry results (where significantly different from those on admission) were:

Day 5 Creatinine 100 micromol/L (60–115)
Day 7 Creatinine 110 micromol/L
Day 9 Creatinine 135 micromol/L

Ophthalmic examination on day 7 of the admission showed that Mr I was responding to therapy. There was no further deterioration in his right eye lesions and slight improvement in his visual acuity. A follow-up examination for day 21 of therapy was arranged.

In view of Mr I's rising serum creatinine level, CMV treatment was changed to intravenous ganciclovir, at a dose of 5 mg/kg twice daily.

17. Would you have recommended this course of action? Is the dose of ganciclovir appropriate?

18. Can Mr I's other drug therapies continue as before?

19. What laboratory results should be monitored during ganciclovir therapy, why, and how frequently?

After discussion with medical staff, Mr I chose to continue with zidovudine therapy while receiving ganciclovir, despite the risk of haematological toxicity on combined treatment, as zidovudine was the only drug therapy that was effective against his underlying HIV disease.

Close monitoring of laboratory results was recommended; these (where significantly different from those on admission) were as follows:

Day 13 WBC 2.1×10^9/L $(4–11 \times 10^9)$
  Creatinine 130 micromol/L (60–115)
Day 15 WBC 2.0×10^9/L
  Creatinine 108 micromol/L
Day 17 WBC 1.7×10^9/L
  Creatinine 98 micromol/L
Day 19 WBC 1.5×10^9/L

20. What recommendations would you make regarding changes in therapy, and why?

Day 21 Mr I's therapy had been continued unchanged. His WBC count was now 1.3×10^9/L, and ophthalmic examination showed his retinitis to be in remission.

21. Is maintenance therapy for Mr I's CMV disease indicated?

22. What ganciclovir maintenance regimen would you recommend?

Day 23 Mr I was discharged. His discharge prescription and serum biochemistry and haematology results were as follows:

Zidovudine 250 mg orally four times daily
Co-trimoxazole 960 mg orally twice daily
Acyclovir 400 mg orally twice daily
Fluconazole 50 mg orally once daily
Ganciclovir 300 mg intravenously five times a week

WBC 1.1×10^9/L $(4–11 \times 10^9)$
Creatinine 100 micromol/L (60–115)

His body weight was 60 kg.

In view of his latest laboratory results, discontinuation, or at least dose reduction, of zidovudine therapy was recommended. This was discussed with the patient, and zidovudine was temporarily discontinued (and removed from Mr I's take-home drugs) to allow his WBC count to recover.

23. What points would you cover when counselling Mr I on his take-home drugs?

Month 30 Mr I had been seen weekly initially, and then monthly once his WBC count had stabilised at around 2×10^9/L. His CMV retinitis showed signs of reactivation after three months, so it was decided to increase the ganciclovir therapy to 300 mg daily. This had brought Mr I's retinitis into remission; however, his WBC count had again started to fall.

24. What options regarding drug therapy are now available, and what is Mr I's prognosis?

Answers

1. Yes.

Standard doses of acyclovir are usually adequate for the treatment of herpes simplex infections in the early stages of HIV disease, when patients are not severely immunocompromised (T4 counts usually greater than 300–400/mm^3). However, as HIV infection progresses, and immune function deteriorates, higher doses are usually required, such as 400 mg five times a day for seven to ten days. Higher doses are also recommended where malabsorption is present, i.e. in HIV-related gut disorders.

2. No. Maintenance acyclovir therapy is indicated for the prevention of herpes infections in immunocompromised hosts. In early HIV disease this is not always necessary, as the immune system is relatively intact.

Maintenance acyclovir therapy is not generally prescribed after the first herpes attack in early HIV disease. However, if repeated attacks occur at frequent intervals, as is often the case, then maintenance therapy is indicated. Doses of 200–400 mg orally twice daily are usually adequate, but if there are still recurrences, this dose may be increased to 200–400 mg three or four times daily, or to whatever is necessary to prevent recurrence.

3. No. There are not always precipitating factors for candidal infections in HIV disease.

A precipitating factor, such as recent broad-spectrum antibiotic or corticosteroid therapy, may be implicated, but in many cases oral candidiasis appears as immune function deteriorates as a result of progression of HIV infection. It is commonly seen in a previously well, HIV-infected patient presenting with their first opportunistic infection, or in a patient whose immune function is worsening, as evidenced by a fall in the T4 count to below 300/mm^3 without a concurrent opportunistic infection.

Oral candidiasis can be asymptomatic, although patients commonly complain of loss of taste and of a sore mouth, especially during or after eating acidic foods.

4. Yes.

Topical antifungal therapy is useful when candidiasis is confined to the oral cavity, there are no precipitating factors, and the patient is otherwise well. Mr I satisfies all these criteria, and a trial of oral amphotericin therapy is thus indicated. However, systemic antifungal therapy is often required in HIV disease, especially when patients have evidence of other HIV-associated problems. For example, oral *Candida* infection in a patient with *Pneumocystis carinii* pneumonia (PCP) treated with broad-spectrum co-trimoxazole therapy is very unlikely to respond to topical antifungal treatment.

5. Liver function tests.

Ketoconazole has been associated with hepatotoxicity, and it is thus important that baseline liver function tests are carried out, and that liver function is monitored regularly as long as therapy is continued. Mr I must also be questioned about past liver disease, as this may predispose him to hepatotoxicity. Any irregularity in Mr I's liver function must be investigated, as not only would it exclude treatment with ketoconazole, but it may represent an HIV-associated condition (such as atypical mycobacterial infection, or lymphoma).

6. Yes.

Three systemic antifungals are currently available: itraconazole, ketoconazole and fluconazole. Their pharmacokinetic and toxicity profiles differ, as does their cost. Ketoconazole is least expensive, but has the disadvantages of hepatotoxicity and twice-daily dosing. Itraconazole seems free from hepatotoxicity, and can be given once daily, but is much more expensive, and (at the time of writing) is not licensed for the treatment of oral candidiasis. Fluconazole is similar in cost to itraconazole, is also given once daily, and is predominantly renally cleared. It appears to be less hepatotoxic than ketoconazole, and to be more specific for fungal P450-type enzymes, and so it does not display many of the drug interactions shown by the former two agents, especially in the lower doses used for oral *Candida* infections; however, some interactions are now being reported as the usage of fluconazole increases.

Each hospital will formulate its own policy regarding the use of these agents, but, provided regular monitoring of liver function is carried out, and the patient is not receiving concurrent therapy with drugs known to interact with ketoconazole, this drug is often used as first-line systemic therapy, as there is more experience with this agent.

7. No. As with acyclovir, maintenance antifungal therapy is not always required.

If precipitating factors are present, or if the patient is more severely immunocompromised than Mr I is at present, then it can be indicated even after the first attack, as most patients with HIV-associated oral *Candida* infections will experience a relapse within three-months of a course of antifungal therapy. As the antifungal drugs are not without toxicity, it is usually down to the patient and his doctor to decide whether continuous therapy is prescribed (to prevent the recurrence of oral candidiasis), or whether the patient is supplied with a course of antifungal therapy to start when symptoms become apparent (i.e. to manage repeat attacks when they occur).

If, following discussion, Mr I is not keen to take continuous ketoconazole therapy as it is not strictly necessary, he should be reminded to attend the clinic if he experiences any symptoms that could indicate a repeat attack, and he should be reassured that such an attack could be treated promptly.

8. The timing of the pain in relation to eating.

Patients with oesophageal candidiasis often complain of dysphagia and pain that is worsened by eating. On further questioning, the pain can be linked not directly to ingestion of food, but to the action of swallowing. White candidal plaques are also usually present in the oral cavity.

In simple heartburn, pain is also associated with food intake, but it commonly occurs after meals, when pain is experienced because of reflux oesophagitis, or gastric irritation resulting from increased stomach acidity in the presence of food.

9. Mr I's high antacid consumption, or the fact that he may suffer from achlorhydria and/or malabsorption.

(a) Antacid consumption. Ketoconazole requires an acid environment for maximal absorption. Reduced drug absorption occurs during concomitant therapy with drugs that reduce gastric acidity, such as H_2-receptor blockers, antacids, and anticholinergic agents.

It is likely that Mr I's antacid therapy reduced his ketoconazole absorption, thus reducing its efficacy and allowing the candidal infection to break through. However, Mr I's presentation to his general practitioner with "heartburn" may actually have been symptoms of oesophageal *Candida* infection, and may thus have indicated ketoconazole failure even before the introduction of antacid therapy.

(b) Achlorhydria. HIV disease is associated with reduced gastric acidity, and this would also result in reduced absorption of ketoconazole.

(c) Malabsorption. HIV disease is associated with diarrhoeal manifestations, and malabsorption even in the absence of diarrhoea, and these factors may also have contributed to reduced absorption and failure of ketoconazole therapy.

10. Drugs that may interact with ketoconazole (other than those discussed in the previous answer) are: anticoagulants, rifampicin, phenytoin, and cyclosporin.

Both rifampicin and phenytoin may reduce the effectiveness of ketoconazole (and may themselves be affected) by altering hepatic metabolism. Both drugs are often used in HIV disease: rifampicin and rifampicin-like compounds for mycobacterial infection, and phenytoin as an anticonvulsant when fitting is a complication of central nervous system manifestations of the disease.

11. Yes.

If administration of antacids had been discontinued, it is possible that the ketoconazole may have cured the oesophageal *Candida* infection; however, it seems more likely that the symptoms of oesophageal candidiasis were present before the administration of antacids, and had led Mr I to consult his general practitioner with "heartburn". It can thus be assumed that other factors (such as achlorhydria) were responsible for the failure of ketoconazole therapy in Mr I, and a change to a drug that does not require an acid environment for absorption is therefore appropriate. Itraconazole also requires an acid environment for absorption, but fluconazole appears not to, and so is the alternative of choice.

12. (a) Zidovudine.

Zidovudine therapy has been prescribed in the hope that, by preventing further replication of HIV, further destruction of the immune system will be prevented or delayed. It is common practice in many hospitals specialising in HIV disease to introduce zidovudine therapy after an AIDS diagnosis, or in an HIV-infected individual at high risk of progressing to AIDS. Mr I now has an AIDS diagnosis; even in the absence of this, he would be at high risk of progressing to AIDS, because of a T4 count below 200/mm^3. It is therefore appropriate to offer him zidovudine therapy, provided there are no contra-indications, such as a low haemoglobin level or WBC count, as zidovudine is the only licensed anti-retroviral drug currently available.

Mr I must be told of the risks associated with zidovudine use (predominantly the haematological and long-term muscular side-effects).

The zidovudine dosage regimen prescribed for Mr I is appropriate. It is usual to introduce zidovudine at low doses (100 mg orally four times daily) in an attempt to minimise some of the subjective side-effects that are common on introduction of therapy (such as gastro-intestinal intolerance, and headache), and to increase this to standard doses after a few weeks. A dose of 250 mg orally four times daily is now the accepted standard used by most centres at the time of writing.

(b) Co-trimoxazole.

Co-trimoxazole therapy has been prescribed as prophylaxis against the opportunistic infection PCP. Even though Mr I is receiving zidovudine therapy, he is still highly susceptible to opportunistic infections. PCP is the commonest opportunistic infection in HIV disease, and is still associated with considerable morbidity and mortality, especially if not treated promptly. Since PCP prophylaxis is generally non-toxic, it makes sense to prevent the infection occurring in the first place by offering primary prophylaxis.

Anti-retroviral therapy and PCP prophylaxis, are discussed further in case study 22.

13. There are two drugs routinely used in the treatment of CMV disease: ganciclovir (previously known as DHPG) and foscarnet. CMV immunoglobulin (passive immunotherapy with CMV antibodies) has also been used in the treatment of CMV infections in bone marrow transplant patients.

Ganciclovir is a nucleoside analogue closely related in structure and mode of action to acyclovir, but with activity against additional members of the herpes group of viruses, including CMV. Its main drawback is dose-related bone marrow suppression, which is enhanced by concomitant use of bone marrow suppressive drugs such as zidovudine. Foscarnet is a pyrophosphate analogue which inhibits herpes viruses and some retroviruses, including HIV. Its main drawbacks are nephrotoxicity and altered serum calcium levels (hypo- and hypercalcaemia have been reported).

Both drugs have to be given intravenously. Good comparative trials have not been carried out, and data on their relative efficacies are not available. Different centres will express a strong prefence for a particular drug, often depending on the site of CMV infection (CMV disease occurs in many sites, commonly the eye, lung, or gut). We do not believe that there are significant differences in efficacy between the two drugs in the treatment of CMV retinitis, and the choice is thus usually dependent on patient factors.

14. (a) Concurrent and recent drug therapy,
     (b) full blood count,

   (c) serum calcium level (corrected for albumin), and
   (d) serum creatinine level.

A patient with an abnormal calcium level, preexisting nephrotoxicity, or concurrent or recent treatment with other nephrotoxic drugs (such as an aminoglycoside or pentamidine) should not be prescribed foscarnet, but should receive ganciclovir therapy. Concurrent or recent intravenous pentamidine therapy is also a contra-indication to foscarnet therapy, because the combination has resulted in life-threatening hypocalcaemia. Since both drugs have long half-lives it is possible that the same interaction could result if the therapies were given within a short time of each other.

Conversely, a patient with poor bone marrow reserve should not receive ganciclovir. It is advisable for patients receiving ganciclovir not to receive concomitant zidovudine therapy. Ideally, zidovudine therapy should be discontinued for the duration of the treatment with ganciclovir; however, many patients are reluctant to stop zidovudine therapy, and, with careful monitoring, it may be possible for a patient to receive both drugs on the understanding that if problems of bone marrow suppression occur, one or both drugs must be stopped. Generally, the patient will opt to stop zidovudine rather than ganciclovir therapy, as the latter is preventing further sight deterioration, which is important to the patient's quality of life.

15. Yes. It may be administered by intermittent or continuous intravenous infusion, preferably through a central line.

Mr I has no specific contra-indications to either ganciclovir or foscarnet therapy. Although his WBC count and haemoglobin levels seem low, these are relatively normal for someone with HIV disease, which can be associated with leucopenia and anaemia even in the absence of other causative factors, and such levels do not contra-indicate ganciclovir therapy. A low WBC count is well tolerated by patients with HIV disease. They appear not to become susceptible to infections commonly seen in other leucopenic patients, unless the WBC count drops considerably lower, i.e. below 1×10^9/L.

If Mr I wishes to continue zidovudine therapy, then foscarnet is probably the best choice for him, since it is unlikely to affect his haematopoietic system.

Foscarnet, supplied in 500 mL infusion bottles, can be administered by intermittent or continuous intravenous infusion. Continuous infusion, after a bolus loading dose, is the recommended method of administration, because of the drug's short serum half-life. However, the pharmacokinetics of foscarnet are extremely complicated: it is sequestered in bone, and has a long terminal half-life. Recent evidence from the USA suggests that three-times-daily intermittent dosing is as effective as continuous infusion; however, nursing staff may prefer a continuous infusion, which requires little intervention once set up.

Infusions of foscarnet can cause thrombophlebitis if administered peripherally. It should thus be recommended that administration is through a central line; where this is not possible, a 1 in 2 dilution of the infusion solution using an equal volume of 5% dextrose or dextrose-saline (via a piggy-back method) is recommended. Normal saline is also compatible with foscarnet, but since the foscarnet infusion is high in sodium, this could result in sodium overload; therefore, dextrose solutions are generally preferred.

16. Serum creatinine, calcium, and phosphate levels.

As previously discussed, nephrotoxicity is the main problem with foscarnet therapy. Serum creatinine levels should be monitored at least three times a week during an acute course of treatment, and more frequently if any increase is reported. It is important to look for a trend of rising creatinine, rather than a one-off result, which could be erroneous. The dose of foscarnet needs to be adjusted if there is a significant change in the serum creatinine level, since it is predominantly excreted unchanged by the kidneys (the data sheet contains a table of the recommended foscarnet dose according to renal function). Therapy should be stopped if a significantly rising serum creatinine level is seen.

Other laboratory results to monitor include serum phosphate and calcium levels. Hypocalcaemia, which can be life-threatening, is the other important adverse effect to recognise, and Mr I must be encouraged to report any tingling or loss of sensation in the extremities as these may indicate hypocalcaemia. Although it should be remembered that these symptoms may occur in the absence of hypocalcaemia, they nevertheless provide a useful warning to check the serum calcium level. It must always be remembered to correct the reported serum calcium level for any deficit in albumin, which is common in HIV disease.

If the serum calcium level drops but is still within the normal range, oral calcium supplements may enable foscarnet therapy to continue. If the calcium level drops more acutely, or is below the normal range, foscarnet therapy should be halted and the calcium level corrected using intravenous calcium treatment, before any decisions regarding further foscarnet therapy are taken. Each individual patient's circumstances must be discussed, and consideration given to whether to discontinue foscarnet therapy, by weighing up the risks and benefits of continued treatment.

17. Yes. Mr I's renal function is deteriorating, probably as a result of foscarnet-associated nephrotoxity.

Foscarnet therapy needs to be discontinued, since – if it is causing the deterioration in renal function – the situation is likely to get worse if therapy is continued.

The introduction of ganciclovir to replace foscarnet therapy is necessary for Mr I, in order that he completes the three weeks of treatment generally regarded as the optimum course required to bring about remission of CMV retinitis.

Ganciclovir is renally cleared, and requires dose adjustment when the patient's serum creatinine level exceeds 125 micromol/L. Mr I's serum creatinine level just exceeds this, but as his renal function is likely to return to normal quickly on discontinuation of foscarnet therapy, dosage adjustment is probably not necessary, and the usual ganciclovir dosing regimen of 5 mg/kg twice daily is appropriate. However, as it is possible that Mr I's renal function could deteriorate further even after foscarnet therapy is stopped (because of foscarnet's long half-life, and also because there may be other factors contributing to, or causing, his renal problems), continued monitoring of Mr I's renal function is indicated, with adjustment of his ganciclovir dose when appropriate.

18. As Mr I's renal function has deteriorated, the dosage regimen of any concurrent therapy that is renally excreted or has nephrotoxic potential must be re-evaluated. In addition, the question of whether zidovudine therapy should continue must be addressed.

Zidovudine is hepatically metabolised; acyclovir, whilst being renally cleared, is remarkably non-toxic. Both acyclovir and co-trimoxazole therapy would require much worse renal function before a dose reduction is necessary. Fluconazole is renally cleared, but dosage adjustment is only necessary if the creatinine clearance falls below 40 mL/min. (Mr I's creatinine clearance [male, age 35, weight 65 kg], calculated by the method of Cockcroft and Gault, is 57 mL/min.)

The only other alteration in drug therapy that should be considered, in view of the commencement of ganciclovir therapy, is the temporary cessation of zidovudine, as discussed in answer 13.

19. Full blood count monitoring is necessary during ganciclovir therapy. Renal function should also be monitored (see answers 14 and 17).

Monitoring should be carried out on alternate days, at least initially, especially if zidovudine therapy is continued, because it is very likely that Mr I's renal function and full blood counts may alter, given the circumstances discussed.

20. The need for concurrent ganciclovir and zidovudine therapy should be re-evaluated

Mr I's renal function is slowly improving, as shown by the reduction in his serum creatinine levels, and thus no dose adjustments for renal impairment (as discussed in answer 17) are necessary. However, as anticipated, Mr I's WBC count is falling during combined therapy with zidovudine and ganciclovir. If this were to fall much further, Mr I may become susceptible to infection. Consideration should thus be given to stopping ganciclovir therapy (as Mr I has now had 19 of 21 days of anti-CMV treatment), or to stopping zidovudine therapy. If the ophthalmic appointment can be brought forward, and the retinitis is not yet in remission, zidovudine discontinuation is recommended, since continued anti-CMV therapy would be indicated; however, the medical staff may decide to continue both therapies until the ophthalmic examination in two days time, as his WBC count is unlikely to fall below the critical level of 1×10^9/L in this time, and it may psychologically affect Mr I if his drug therapy is altered.

21. Yes. CMV retinitis commonly reactivates within weeks of discontinuing ganciclovir therapy (foscarnet therapy may be associated with longer remission periods), and maintenance treatment is usually offered to keep the retinitis in remission.

Maintenance therapy for CMV infections of other sites is not usually indicated, because of much longer remission periods. Maintenance therapy with ganciclovir is complicated, as it must be given intravenously.

22. Optimum maintenance regimens have not been worked out, but we find a single daily infusion of ganciclovir 5 mg/kg on five days a week to be suitable in most cases.

Regular monitoring of the patient's eye condition and relevant laboratory parameters, together with the juggling of therapy to obtain maximal efficacy and minimal toxicity for a given individual, are necessary. Sometimes an increase in dose to 5 mg/kg every day is necessary to maintain remission.

23. (a) General points.

Mr I's drug therapy is being given to prevent opportunistic infections occurring or recurring. Thus Mr I must be advised not to stop his therapy without consulting the doctor, and to take the medications at the prescribed times. Other general counselling points – such as what to do in the event of missed doses, side-effects to be aware of, action to take in the event of such side-effects occurring, and what to do if vomiting occurs soon after taking a dose – must also be covered. Patient information leaflets covering these points for each medicine are extremely useful for patients such as Mr I, for whom polypharmacy is common. Other than ganciclovir, Mr I's drug therapy is not unique to HIV disease, and thus specific details of these counselling points will not be discussed here.

(b) Ganciclovir maintenance therapy.

The main area of counselling for Mr I is with regard to his maintenance ganciclovir therapy, which must be administered intravenously, usually through a Hickman line. Many patients can be taught to self-administer ganciclovir doses; however, some will need support and help from a district nurse or general practitioner. If Mr I is willing and able to administer his drugs through his Hickman line, he must be instructed in the care of the line; such instruction includes recognition of potential infection, such as fever and/or reddening around the central line site both of which must be promptly investigated in someone like Mr I, who is receiving therapy that predisposes him to neutropenia.

Pharmaceutical aspects (such as the reconstitution and dilution of ganciclovir, the storage of reconstituted ganciclovir vials, heparinisation of the line, and compatibility of ganciclovir with the heparin solution) must all be covered. The techniques are usually taught by nursing staff on the ward before discharge. Reinforcement of this with written information on aspects of drug administration and care of the line are invaluable, and it is important that the pharmacist contributes to such documentation.

24. Zidovudine therapy should not be re-started, as Mr I's WBC count is falling on ganciclovir therapy alone. Somehow a balance must be achieved between controlling the retinitis and preventing drug toxicity.

The dose of ganciclovir could be reduced, but this is likely to cause the retinitis to become active again. Some centres have attempted intravitreal injections of ganciclovir, in an attempt to reduce systemic toxicity with the drug, but the technique is complicated and can cause retinal detachment. Alternatively, maintenance foscarnet therapy could be attempted, with careful monitoring of renal function. Foscarnet was previously associated with nephrotoxicity in Mr I, but this may not occur with the lower doses used for maintenance therapy.

The various options must be discussed with the patient, and a joint decision made regarding his future management.

The prognosis following a diagnosis of CMV retinitis is generally poor. CMV infection is a late complication of HIV disease and is associated with poor residual immune function. This makes other opportunistic infections likely. Although CMV is only manifesting as retinitis in Mr I, it is likely that it has disseminated to other sites.

Mr I may decide to opt for no further active management of his retinitis, and his quality of life may well be improved once he is freed from the responsibilities of daily intravenous drug administration.

Acknowledgement

With thanks to Dr Don Smith, AIDS Research Registrar, St Stephen's Clinic, for his helpful comments and for reviewing this case study.

References and Further Reading

Dismukes W.E., Azole antifungals: old and new, *Ann. intern. Med.*, 1988, **109**, 177–179.

Fletcher C.V. and Balfour H.H., Evaluation of ganciclovir for cytomegalovirus disease, *DICP Ann. Pharmacother.*, 1989, **23**, 5–11.

Glatt A.E. *et al.*, Treatment of infectious complications of human immunodeficiency virus, *New Engl. J. Med.*, 1988, **318**, 1439–1448.

Jacobson M.A. and Mill J., Serious cytomegalovirus disease in the acquired immunodeficiency syndrome (AIDS), *Ann. intern. Med.*, 1988, **108**, 585–594.

Merigan T.C. and Lane H.C. (eds), Cytomegalovirus infection and treatment with ganciclovir, *Rev. inf. Dis.*, 1988, **10 (Suppl.** 3).

Purdy B.D. and Plaisance K.I., Infection with the human immunodeficiency virus: epidemiology, pathogenesis, transmission, diagnosis and manifestations, *Am. J. Hosp. Pharm.*, 1989, **46**, 1185–1209.

Youle M. *et al.*, *AIDS – Therapeutics in HIV Disease*, Edinburgh, Churchill Livingstone, 1988.

CASE STUDY *22*

HUMAN IMMUNODEFICIENCY VIRUS DISEASE AND THE ACQUIRED IMMUNODEFICIENCY SYNDROME

PART II—Pneumocystis carinii *Pneumonia and Cerebral Toxoplasmosis*

Sarah Fitt

HIV Pharmacist, Dulwich Hospital, London

Day 1 Thirty-four-year-old Mr H, who was known to be antibody-positive for the human immunodeficiency virus (HIV), was admitted as an emergency. He presented with a seven-day history of increasing shortness of breath which was worse during the day. He had had a dry non-productive cough but no haemoptysis, and had suffered sweats over the last few nights. His appetite over the past few days had decreased, and his weight had dropped from approximately 65 kg to 56 kg over the past few weeks.

On examination he was noted to have a temperature of 39°C, a pulse of 125 beats per minute and a respiratory rate of 35 per minute. He was very short of breath, with poor lung expansion and shallow rapid breathing; however, his chest was clear and there was no bronchial breathing.

A chest x-ray was requested, which showed diffuse bilateral shadowing with no signs of consolidation.

His arterial blood gases on admission (on 40% oxygen) were:

PaO_2 7.2 kPa (reference range 11.9–13.2)
$PaCO_2$ 4.1 kPa (4.8–6.3)
HCO_3 21 mmol/L (22–30)
pH 7.42 (7.35–7.45)

His haematology results on admission were:

White blood cells (WBC) 2.4×10^9/L (4.5–10×10^9)
Haemoglobin 9.8 g/dL (13–18)
Platelets 297×10^9/L (150–600×10^9)

Because Mr H was known to be HIV-positive, a diagnosis of either *Pneumocystis carinii* pneumonia (PCP) or another atypical pneumonia was considered a strong possibility.

1. How should Mr H be treated to cover for PCP and atypical pneumonias?

2. Would you recommend the use of steroids to help manage Mr H's hypoxia?

3. What additional therapies would you recommend to prevent the side-effects and toxicity associated with high-dose co-trimoxazole therapy?

Day 2 A bronchoscopy and transbronchial biopsy were performed, and washings were sent for histology. Although some centres use the method of induced sputum as the first-line investigation of suspected PCP (a method that involves the patient nebulising 3% saline, and the resulting sputum being collected for examination), there are varying reports of this technique's success; patients who have a negative sample after an induced sputum test thus go on to have a bronchoscopy.

The chest x-ray was reviewed, and it was decided that PCP was the most likely diagnosis.

Arterial blood gases (on 60% oxygen) were:

PaO_2 11.6 kPa (11.9–13.2)
$PaCO_2$ 3.28 kPa (4.8–6.3)
HCO_3 30.3 mmol/L (22–30)
pH 7.46 (7.35–7.45)

Haematology results were:

WBC 3.0×10^9/L ($4.5–10 \times 10^9$)
Haemoglobin 10.5 g/dL (13–18)
Platelets 364×10^9/L ($150–600 \times 10^9$)

Day 3 Results of the transbronchial biopsy confirmed the diagnosis of PCP, and therefore acquired immunodeficiency syndrome (AIDS).

Mr H's temperature was now 37°C. He was feeling better, and eating, but he was still short of breath and tired.

His drug therapy was:

Co-trimoxazole 35 mL (3.6 g) intravenously twice daily
Hydrocortisone 100 mg intravenously four times daily
Folinic acid 15 mg orally once daily
Chlorpheniramine 4 mg orally three times daily if required
Metoclopramide 10 mg orally three times daily if required

Later that night the on-call houseman was asked to see Mr H, as his respiratory rate had increased to 50 per minute on 60% oxygen and he had a temperature of 38.5°C.

On examination Mr H was noted to have a regular pulse of 96 beats per minute, and his blood pressure was 160/80 mmHg.

His arterial blood gases (on 60% oxygen) were:

PaO_2 8.5 kPa (11.9–13.2)
$PaCO_2$ 3.57 kPa (4.8–6.3)
HCO_3 22.4 mmol/L (22–30)

4. Could Mr H's raised temperature and increased respiratory rate be drug-related? If so, what is most likely to be causing the problem?

5. Would you recommend any changes to Mr H's drug therapy?

Mr H's therapy was amended. When he was reviewed a few hours later it was noted that his temperature had dropped to 37.2°C, and his respiratory rate to 20 per minute.

Day 6 Mr H had improved both clinically and radiologically. On the ward round it was decided to decrease his dose of steroids, and to add dapsone 100 mg orally once daily to his regimen.

6. How should dapsone therapy be monitored?

Day 10 Mr H was apyrexial, eating, and ready to go home.

Day 14 Mr H was discharged on:

Dapsone 100 mg orally once daily
Trimethoprim 400 mg orally three times daily
Folinic acid 15 mg orally once daily

His steroid therapy had been discontinued. This

treatment was to be continued for seven more days, and he was then to be seen at the out-patient clinic with a view to starting zidovudine therapy and prophylaxis against PCP.

Discharge haematology results were:

WBC 2.1×10^9/L ($4.5–10 \times 10^9$)
Haemoglobin 10.2 g/dL (13–18)
Platelets 212×10^9/L ($150–600 \times 10^9$)

7. What general points would you cover when counselling Mr H on his discharge medication?

8. What type of PCP prophylaxis is most appropriate for Mr H?

9. Why is zidovudine therapy indicated for Mr H?

10. What are the side-effects associated with zidovudine therapy?

Day 100 Mr H had remained well for three months, but he now presented to out-patients complaining of double vision and difficulty in walking. He was referred to the in-patient unit for further assessment.

His drug therapy on admission was:

Zidovudine 250 mg orally four times daily
Pentamidine (nebulised), 300 mg once a fortnight

On examination Mr H was noted to be lethargic but apyrexial, and he had no photophobia or neck stiffness. A computer-assisted tomography (CT) scan showed multiple lesions in the left cerebellar hemisphere and right occipital lobe. A provisional diagnosis of toxoplasmosis was made.

11. What is the first-line treatment for cerebral toxoplasmosis in HIV disease?

12. What are the possible side-effects associated with this therapy?

Day 104 On examination Mr H now had hyperthermia, hypotension, bradycardia, and paraesthesia of both feet, all of which were indicative of his *Toxoplasma* infection.

Day 110 Mr H was feeling much better and was responding well to treatment, which comprised:

Sulphadiazine 2 g orally four times daily
Pyrimethamine 25 mg orally once daily
Folinic acid 15 mg orally once daily
Zidovudine 250 mg orally four times daily
Pentamidine (nebulised), 300 mg once a fortnight

However, his haematology results showed a WBC of 2.5×10^9/L ($4.5–10 \times 10^9$), containing 30% (40–70%) neutrophils and 50% (20–45%) lymphocytes.

13. What are the possible causes of Mr H's neutropenia?

14. What action would you recommend?

Day 111 Mr H was now pyrexial, and had a widespread maculopapular rash.

15. What is the most likely cause of his rash and pyrexia?

16. What action would you recommend?

As Mr H's haematology results had improved, zidovudine therapy was re-started, and he was discharged on:

Dapsone 100 mg orally once daily
Pyrimethamine 25 mg orally once daily
Folinic acid 15 mg orally once daily
Zidovudine 250 mg orally four times daily
Pentamidine (nebulised), 300 mg once a fortnight

His haematology results on discharge were:

WBC 3.8×10^9/L (4.5–10×10^9)
Haemoglobin 9.5 g/dL (13–18)
Platelets 185×10^9/L (150–600×10^9)

Day 118 Mr H was reviewed on the ward. His WBC was now 4.5×10^9/L (4.5–10×10^9) and his haemoglobin level was 7.9 g/dL (13–18).

17. What might be the cause of Mr H's anaemia?

18. Could you recommend any alternative therapies to treat Mr H's toxoplasmosis?

Day 128 Mr H's drug therapy was:

Spiramycin 1 g orally four times daily
Pyrimethamine 25 mg orally once daily
Folinic acid 15 mg orally once daily
Zidovudine 250 mg orally four times daily
Pentamidine (nebulised), 300 mg once a fortnight

A routine assessment of his liver function tests (LFTs) revealed:

Alkaline phosphatase 303 iu/L (30–110)
Aspartate transaminase 72 iu/L (5–40)
Gamma-glutamyl transferase 559 iu/L (0–65)

19. What is the most likely cause of this increase in Mr H's LFTs?

20. How should Mr H be managed now?

Mr H was discharged on:

Zidovudine 250 mg orally four times daily
Pentamidine (nebulised), 300 mg once a fortnight
Pyrimethamine 50 mg orally once daily
Folinic acid 15 mg orally once daily

Unfortunately, this maintenance therapy for toxoplasmosis proved ineffective, and Mr H relapsed after six weeks. However, he was treated successfully with full-dose sulphadiazine therapy, despite his previous problems, and has now been maintained on sulphadiazine 500 mg orally four times daily and pyrimethamine 25 mg orally once daily, together with folinic acid, zidovudine and inhaled pentamidine therapy as before, for the last nine months, and has remained well.

Answers

1. Co-trimoxazole, at a dose of 120 mg/kg/day intravenously, in two doses, plus erythromycin 1 g intravenously four times daily.

Co-trimoxazole is highly effective in the treatment of AIDS-related PCP, and a 21-day course of treatment is usually recommended. It is well absorbed from the gastro-intestinal tract, so it can be given orally in mild to moderate cases of PCP (at the same daily dose), but, because of the potential severity of PCP infection and the side-effect of gastro-intestinal intolerance, it is usually given intravenously.

Toxicity can be a problem with the high doses required to treat PCP, so while Mr H is receiving co-trimoxazole therapy it is important to monitor his haematological values, and liver and renal function. In addition, drug levels can be measured, if required.

Each dose of co-trimoxazole is usually administered in 1 L of dextrose 5% over one hour, but it can be given in other fluids (such as sodium chloride 0.9%), and over longer periods of time to prevent fluid overload. If fluid restriction is required, co-trimoxazole can be given in a dilution of 1 in 10, as opposed to the 1 in 25 dilution usually recommended.

In cases of severe hypoxia where PCP is suspected, it is important not to wait for a diagnosis before commencing treatment. Often early intervention increases the likelihood of a successful outcome.

HIV patients are also more susceptible to bacterial chest infections, so it is important when treating Mr H to consider other possible causes of chest infection (such as *Legionella* or *Mycoplasma*) until a definitive diagnosis is reached. Co-trimoxazole is a suitable antibiotic for most bacterial chest infections, but the addition of erythromycin therapy covers atypical pneumonias such as *Legionella*. Erythromycin is usually given intravenously in such circumstances, at a dose of 1 g four times daily in 250 mL of 5% dextrose over one hour. While Mr H is on erythromycin therapy, his liver function needs to be monitored regularly.

2. Mr H's severe hypoxia warrants the use of intravenous steroid therapy.

The use of steroids in immunocompromised patients has been the subject of considerable controversy in the last few years; however, in HIV patients with PCP and severe hypoxia, there is increasing evidence that, by reducing inflammation in the alveoli, gaseous exchange is improved, hypoxia is reduced, and the need for mechanical ventilation is prevented. However, the use of steroids in some centres has been associated with an increased incidence of viral and bacterial infections, such as cytomegalovirus and the unmasking of tuberculosis. Clearly a balance has to be achieved between reducing hypoxia and preventing further infection, by using short courses of high-dose corticosteroids.

As Mr H's hypoxia is life-threatening, it is appropriate to start him on intravenous hydrocortisone at a dose of 100 mg four times daily. However, this therapy should be reviewed regularly.

3. Anti-emetic and antihistamine therapy, plus folinic acid supplements, should be co-prescribed.

Mr H should be prescribed metoclopramide at a dose of 10 mg orally three times daily, and chlorpheniramine 4 mg orally three times daily. Initially both drugs can be given when required for nausea and rashes respectively, but they should be given regularly if the side-effects become more severe. If vomiting occurs the drugs should be given intravenously. Mr H should also be prescribed folinic acid 15 mg daily orally.

If extrapyramidal side-effects occur with metoclopramide therapy, then domperidone can be substituted, as it does not cross the blood–brain barrier. Domperidone can be given orally at a dose of 10–20 mg every six hours, or rectally at a dose of 60 mg every six hours, if vomiting is a problem. Terfenadine at a dose of 60 mg orally twice daily, can be given if chlorpheniramine therapy causes unacceptable drowsiness.

High-dose co-trimoxazole therapy is associated with an increased incidence of adverse reactions, such as nausea, vomiting, rash, fever, and bone marrow suppression. Trimethoprim is a dihydrofolate reductase inhibitor and causes neutropenia and thrombocytopenia, especially at high doses. As Mr H's WBC was low on admission he should be started on folinic acid therapy to prevent any further drop, which would increase the chance of him suffering a secondary bacterial infection. Concurrent folinic acid administration does not antagonise co-trimoxazole's antiprotozoal effect, as protozoan cells do not take up the folinic acid as well as mammalian cells, while mammalian cells are more sensitive then protozoan cells to folinic acid.

4. Yes. In our experience, the most likely cause of Mr H's problem is the high-dose co-trimoxazole therapy, in particular the sulphamethoxazole portion of the drug.

Sulphonamides are well known to cause this reaction, especially in HIV patients where immune response is altered. The sudden onset of Mr H's symptoms suggests a drug reaction, rather than another infection or non-response to present therapy; however, the only way of distinguishing the cause is to withdraw the agent thought to be responsible and observe Mr H for any sign of improvement.

5. Yes. Discontinue co-trimoxazole therapy and commence treatment with intravenous trimethoprim at a dose of 20 mg/kg/day; dapsone 100 mg orally once daily should be added once Mr H has recovered from his drug reaction. In addition, the dose of steroids could be increased if his symptoms become more serious.

Trimethoprim on its own has good activity against PCP, but it has been shown that the anti-PCP activity is increased when trimethoprim is given in conjunction with a sulphonamide (as in co-trimoxazole), or with dapsone.

Pentamidine is widely used for the treatment of PCP, at a dose of 4 mg/kg/day intravenously. However, there are a number of serious side-effects associated with intravenous pentamidine therapy, including severe hypotension, hypoglycaemia, renal failure, and hepatitis. For these reasons it is not the first choice of alternative therapy for Mr H.

A number of experimental therapies are available for patients who do not respond to, or cannot tolerate, the above drugs. These include trimetrexate, which is a derivative of methotrexate, and a very powerful dihydrofolate reductase inhibitor. Trimetrexate is given by intravenous bolus at a dose of 30 mg/m^2/day for 21 days, with intravenous folinic acid 20 mg/m^2 every six hours for 23 days.

Another alternative is eflornithine, which is an inhibitor of ornithine decarboxylase, an enzyme which is active against parasitic cells rather than human cells. It must be given by continuous intravenous infusion at a dose of 400 mg/kg/day for 14 days. There have been reports of the success of this regimen when other therapies have failed.

The combination of intravenous clindamycin 600 mg four times daily with oral primaquine 15 mg daily has also recently been reported to be useful in severe PCP cases that have not responded to other therapy.

Finally, inhaled pentamidine has been used in mild cases of PCP at a dose of 600 mg daily for 14 days, but there are varying degrees of success with this therapy.

6. A full blood count should be carried out regularly.

Dapsone therapy can induce a number of haema-tological toxicities so regular haematological monitoring is essential. Although the dose of 100 mg daily prescribed for Mr H is appropriate for this indication, it is fairly high; it would therefore be useful to check Mr H's glucose 6-phosphate dehydrogenase (G6PD) status before starting treatment, as dapsone is more likely to cause methaemaglobinaemia and haemolytic anaemias in G6PD-deficient patients. However, it could be argued that, as Mr H has already been on a high dose of sulphonamide, and as dapsone is chemically related to the sulphonamides, this is unlikely to be a problem. If Mr H is G6PD-deficient, then alternative therapy should be prescribed to treat his PCP (e.g. intravenous pentamidine).

7. A number of general points should be discussed.

(a) It is important to emphasise that the discharge therapy is a course of treatment that must be completed.

(b) Mr H should be told that any side-effects (such as rashes or nausea), or any change in health (such as breathlessness or cyanosis) must be reported.

(c) As Mr H has been successfully treated for PCP, it is important that a relapse does not occur; it should be explained that this is to be achieved by starting PCP prophylaxis at his next out-patient appointment.

8. There are a number of choices available to prevent recurrence of PCP. Inhaled pentamidine therapy is most appropriate for Mr H.

Co-trimoxazole in a dose of 480 mg orally twice daily has been used widely for PCP prevention in other groups of immunocompromised patients (e.g. after renal transplant); however, in HIV patients this regimen has been associated with a high incidence of adverse reactions, such as rashes, bone marrow suppression, and nausea. In addition, relapses have been reported at this dose, so doses of 960 mg twice daily, or 960 mg twice daily on three days a week, have been used. There is also concern that such therapy may sensitise the patient to the drug, with the result that if high-dose co-trimoxazole therapy is required at a later date, it will not be tolerated.

Another option is the use of Fansidar® (sulfadoxine 500 mg, pyrimethamine 25 mg) which, because of its long half-life, only has to be given twice weekly. Again there are the problems associated with using sulphonamides, plus the relatively high incidence of Stevens-Johnson syndrome seen in patient groups treated with this drug. There have also been reports of PCP relapse during Fansidar prophylaxis.

Dapsone 50 mg orally daily has been used for PCP prophylaxis, as it is relatively cheap compared with some of the other alternatives; however, there is an increased risk of the drug causing anaemia when it is given with zidovudine.

Inhaled pentamidine is now being used widely for PCP prophylaxis. This involves the patient nebulising 300 mg of pentamidine once every fortnight. Because this route of administration results in low pentamidine blood levels, a lower incidence of systemic side-effects is seen with inhaled therapy than with intravenous pentamidine administration. The main side-effects of inhaled pentamidine are cough, bronchospasm, and a metallic taste. This method of prophylaxis also has the advantage that it only needs to be administered once a fortnight.

Because of Mr H's reaction to high-dose co-trimoxazole therapy, inhaled pentamidine is probably the most appropriate method of prophylaxis for him. In this centre, patients are taught by the HIV pharmacist to self-administer nebulised pentamidine on the in-patient ward. All patients inhale 1 mL of nebulised salbutamol (1 mg) in 2 mL of normal saline, to prevent possible bronchospasm; ten minutes later they inhale 300 mg of nebulised pentamidine in 5 mL of water, using a Turret nebuliser driven by an 8 L/min air compressor. This normally takes about 20 minutes. If the patient is happy with the procedure, then all the equipment is provided for self-administration at home.

9. To slow the advance of HIV disease.

As Mr H is now obviously severely immunocompromised, and by a diagnosis of PCP has AIDS, he needs to start zidovudine therapy. At this centre, patients are offered zidovudine therapy at an earlier stage in their HIV disease, but Mr H had declined the drug in the past.

Zidovudine is the only anti-HIV agent available at the time of writing that is licensed for the treatment of AIDS and severely immunocompromised patients. It has been shown to increase patient survival times significantly, by preventing further destruction of the immune system, and thereby reducing the number and severity of opportunistic infections. Zidovudine's use in earlier HIV disease, to prevent disease progression, is also being investigated, as there is thought to be improved response to the drug when the immune system has relatively better function; however, there is then the possibility of drug resistance occurring.

Before zidovudine is prescribed a full blood count needs to be performed, as the drug is contra-indicated in patients with a very low neutrophil count or low haemoglobin level, because of its potential to cause haematological toxicities. Mr H's renal and hepatic function should also be checked.

The doses of zidovudine used vary from centre to centre. The data sheet recommends 200 mg every four hours, but a 250 mg capsule is available, so a regimen of 250 mg four times daily is used widely. To reduce the incidence of side-effects a low dose can be prescribed initially, for example, 100 mg orally four times daily, gradually increasing to a full dose of 250 mg orally four times daily over two to three weeks. If haematological problems occur during drug use, then a lower dose can be used. In the future, lower doses may be found to be just as effective as the initially recommended doses of up to 1200 mg daily.

10. There are a number of side-effects associated with zidovudine therapy.

Two to three weeks after starting therapy, the patient may complain of nausea, myalgia, and headaches. Four to eight weeks after starting the drug, haematological toxicity may occur (in the form of anaemia and/or neutropenia), so careful monitoring of the blood count is required over this period. During the first three months, a full blood count should be carried out once a fortnight, and thereafter monthly. Long-term side-effects of zidovudine therapy (such as myopathy, drug resistance, and rebound meningio-encephalitis on cessation of therapy) are still being evaluated. Many patients are anxious about starting zidovudine therapy because of these side-effects, and they often need to be given a lot of explanation and reassurance.

Chronic paracetamol administration has been associated with an increased incidence of neutropenia, so an alternative analgesic should be recommended if necessary for chronic use, although intermittent doses of paracetamol are not likely to cause neutropenia.

11. Sulphadiazine 2 g orally four times daily, pyrimethamine 25 mg orally once daily, and folinic acid 15 mg orally once daily. After six to eight weeks, the doses can be reduced, and the drugs continued as maintenance therapy.

The combination of a sulphonamide and a folate antagonist is the most effective regimen against toxoplasmosis, which is a protozoal infection like PCP. Thus, despite the fact that Mr H has a previous history of an adverse reaction to a sulphonamide, he should be started on this combination. While he is being treated with this regimen for toxoplasmosis it is probably not necessary to continue his inhaled pentamidine therapy (though patients are often quite keen to continue because so few problems occur during treatment).

12. Sulphadiazine is a first-generation sulphonamide which is not very soluble, so an adequate fluid intake is required during therapy to prevent crystalluria (and hence to maintain adequate renal function). Side-effects include nausea, rashes, and blood dyscrasias. Pyrimethamine can also cause skin rashes and depression of haemopoiesis when given long-term, as it is a potent folate antagonist.

13. In our experience, the most likely cause of neutropenia is the combination of zidovudine and sulphadiazine, as these agents have an additive toxicity on the bone marrow.

Other possible causes include HIV disease affecting the bone marrow, and zidovudine therapy alone. However, HIV-induced neutropenia tends to be a more chronic problem, and zidovudine-induced neutropenia usually occurs earlier in treatment. Pyrimethamine therapy can also cause neutropenia, although the co-administration of folinic acid should prevent this. However, the dose of folinic acid (15 mg) prescribed for this indication is fairly arbitrary.

14. As Mr H is suffering from a life-threatening cerebral infection, his need for sulphadiazine treatment is greater than for zidovudine therapy, so the zidovudine should be stopped until his neutrophil count has improved.

Although Mr H's neutrophil count is $1.0 \times 10^9/L$, which is still within normal limits for administering zidovudine therapy, it is likely that continued co-administration of the two drugs will lead to a severe neutropenia, and place Mr H at risk of opportunistic bacterial infections. Zidovudine therapy can be re-started when Mr H's dose of sulphadiazine is reduced to the maintenance level after his six-week course of therapy, by which time his neutrophil count should have risen.

15. Sulphadiazine therapy.

Sulphadiazine, like other sulphonamides, is well known to cause rashes, especially in HIV patients. Mr H has been on therapy for ten days, which is when drug-induced rashes tend to occur; the appearance of an erythematous maculopapular rash, similar to his previous drug rash with co-trimoxazole, suggests a drug-related problem.

16. Stop sulphadiazine treatment and start dapsone therapy at a dose of 100 mg daily.

As in PCP, dapsone therapy has been shown to be active against toxoplasmosis, although its efficacy is not as well proven for this indication.

17. The combination of zidovudine and dapsone therapy.

This combination is known to cause a greater incidence of anaemia than either zidovudine therapy alone, or zidovudine plus pyrimethamine or other myelosuppressive drugs.

18. Spiramycin or clindamycin.

Alternative treatments for *Toxoplasma* infection have been used with varying degrees of success. Spiramycin is a macrolide antibiotic used to treat congenital toxoplasmosis at a dose of 1 g orally four times daily during pregnancy. Its efficacy in HIV-related toxoplasmosis has not been well established, because of its low penetration of the cerebrospinal fluid. Another option is clindamycin, which can be given orally or intravenously at a dose of 300–600 mg four times daily. Like spiramycin, the efficacy of clindamycin in HIV-related toxoplasmosis is not well proven; there is also a risk of pseudomembranous colitis associated with its use.

19. Spiramycin is excreted in bile and is probably responsible for the rise in LFTs noted, although other drugs, obstruction, or HIV disease could also be responsible.

If an ultrasound of the liver shows no obstruction, then withdrawal of the suspected drug is the next step, in order to see if there is any improvement. If there is no subsequent drop in Mr H's LFTs, a liver biopsy will be needed to exclude infection or tumours.

20. If Mr H's liver function improves following spiramycin discontinuation, the drug should not be re-prescribed. Instead, maintenance therapy with pyrimethamine should be started.

There are now very few therapeutic options left. However, Mr H has had four weeks of therapy, and he is clinically significantly improved, so his dose of pyrimethamine could be increased to 50 mg daily in an attempt to provide maintenance treatment against further *Toxoplasma* infection. His folinic acid therapy should be continued at the same dose.

References and Further Reading

Corkery K.J. *et al.*, Aerosolised pentamidine for treatment and prophylaxis of *Pneumocystis carinii* pneumonia: an update, *Respir. Care*, 1988, **33**, 676–685.

Fischl M.A., Treatment and prophylaxis of *Pneumocystis carinii* pneumonia, *AIDS*, 1988, **2 (Suppl. 1)**, S143–S150.

Gilson R. Clinical aspects of AIDS, *Med. Int.*, 1988, **57**, 2344–2352.

Langtry H.D. and Campoli-Richards D.M., Zidovudine: a review, *Drugs*, 1989, **37**, 408–450.

MacFadden D.K. *et al.*, Corticosteroids as adjunctive therapy in treatment of *Pneumocystis carinii* pneumonia in patients with acquired immunodeficiency syndrome, *Lancet*, 1987, **1**, 1477–1479.

Mills J., *Pneumocystis carinii* and *Toxoplasma gondii* infections in patients with AIDS, *Rev. infect. Dis.*, 1986, **8**, 1001–1010.

Pinching A.J., Prophylactic and maintenance therapy for opportunist infections in AIDS, *AIDS*, 1988, **2**, 335–343.

Weller I.V.D., Treatment of infections and antiviral agents, in *ABC of AIDS*, 1st edn, Adler M.W. (ed.), London, BMJ Publications, 1987, 33–36.

Youle M. *et al.*, *AIDS — Therapeutics in HIV Disease*, Edinburgh, Churchill Livingstone, 1988.

RHEUMATOID ARTHRITIS

Elizabeth A. Kay

Director of Clinical Pharmacy, Leeds General Infirmary

Day 1 55-year-old Mrs S was admitted from clinic. She was complaining of increasing pain and stiffness in the joints of both hands, feet, wrists, shoulders, and knees. Rheumatoid arthritis (RA) had been diagnosed 18 months previously but recently her problems had increased, with severe early morning stiffness lasting four to five hours and occasionally all day. Her previous medical history was unremarkable, but RA had affected her maternal grandmother. Her medication included enteric-coated aspirin 3.6 g/day orally (in divided doses), and indomethacin suppository 100 mg at night; in addition, she had been taking 'white indigestion mixture' recently.

On examination Mrs S looked unwell and tired, and was found to have two spongy lumps below her left elbow. She had gross swelling of the metocarpophalangeal (MCP) and proximal interphalageal (PIP) joints in both hands, and these joints were hot and tender to touch, and felt 'boggy'. Her other affected joints showed a reduced range of movement, and she complained of difficulty in completing daily tasks such as brushing her hair. In addition she exhibited some guarding and tenderness in the abdomen, and complained of rectal soreness with some fresh blood loss on toilet tissue.

Her serum biochemistry and haematology results were:

Haemoglobin 10.1 g/dL (reference range 12–16)
Mean cell volume 75 fL (76–96)
Mean cell haemoglobin concentration 0.32 g/dL (0.32–0.36)
Haematocrit 0.32 (0.36–0.47)
Platelets 580×10^9/L ($150–450 \times 10^9$)
Erythrocyte sedimentation rate (ESR) 65 mm/hour (0–20)
Serum iron 8 micromol/L (11–29)
Total iron binding capacity 55 micromol/L (54–80)
Ferritin 19 microgram/L (12–220)
Albumin 30 g/L (35–55)
Aspartate transaminase 50 iu/L (11–35)
Alkaline phosphatase 15 KA (4–13)

Sero-positive rheumatoid factor (sheep cell agglutination test for IgM antibody): greater than 1/1049 (normal: less than 1/32)

X-rays showed erosions on the second and third MCPs and PIPs of both hands.

Mrs S was instructed to take complete bed rest, and resting splints were made for both hands. Both knees were injected using aseptic technique. The joints were first drained to remove effusion fluid; lignocaine 2% (1 mL) was then injected into each joint, followed by triamcinoline hexacetonide 40 mg. The acromoclavicular joints of both shoulders were also injected using the same procedure, but the dose of steroid was reduced to 20 mg. The pharmacist was asked to record Mrs S's drug history; and in the meantime her non-steroidal anti-inflammatory drugs (NSAIDs) were continued as before.

1. What are the aims of treatment for Mrs S?

2. What poor prognostic signs of RA does she exhibit?

3. Was the initial management appropriate?

4. What information would you be looking for from her drug history?

5. Would you recommend that her treatment with NSAIDs be modified?

Day 5 Mrs S was feeling a little better following the rest.

Endoscopy had demonstrated mild gastritis but no evidence of ulceration. The drug history revealed that Mrs S had tried a large number of prescribed NSAIDs over the previous 18 months, and had also taken Nurofen® (ibuprofen 200 mg) which she had purchased from her local pharmacy. Mrs S felt that naproxen had been better than most NSAIDs and this was therefore commenced in a dose of 500 mg orally twice a day. She was advised to avoid over-the-counter analgesics. The team considered that Mrs S required disease-modifying antirheumatic drugs (DMARDs) and commenced the base-line investigations.

6. Would you recommend that Mrs S be prescribed prophylaxis against peptic ulceration?

7. Which disease-modifying agent would you choose and why?

8. What base-line data should be collected before therapy commences?

Day 10 Mrs S was prescribed penicillamine 125 mg orally daily.

Her haematology and urinalysis results were:

Haemoglobin 10.4 g/dL (12–16)
ESR 55 mm/hour (0–20)
Urinary protein less than 0.1 g/24 hours (less than 0.1)

9. Should Mrs S receive corticosteroids at this stage?

10. When should her dose of penicillamine be increased?

11. When should she expect to respond to penicillamine?

12. How should Mrs S's clinical response be monitored?

Day 38 Mrs S had improved substantially. She was receiving regular physiotherapy to improve her muscle tone and increase her range of joint movement. She was taking penicillamine without adverse effects, and she said that the naproxen seemed to be helping. She had no further problems with indigestion. She was considered fit for discharge and was to return to an out-patient appointment in three months. Her general practitioner agreed to carry out the necessary monitoring tests.

13. How should penicillamine therapy be monitored biochemically?

14. What points would you cover when counselling Mrs S on her therapy?

Month 4 Mrs S was seen in the out-patient department. She felt that she had deteriorated since discharge and once again was having significant problems with morning stiffness and pain. She was unwilling to be readmitted, and so it was decided to leave the naproxen unchanged, but to increase further her dose of penicillamine from 500 to 625 mg orally daily. Her knees were injected with triamcinolone hexacetonide as before, and she was ordered to take more rest. The monitoring of her blood and urine had shown no evidence of adverse effects, although her disease was noted to be active.

Haematology results were:

Haemoglobin 9.4 g/dL (12–16)
ESR 79 mm/hour (0–20)
White cell count 6.5×10^9/L (4–10×10^9)
Platelets 590×10^9/L (150–450×10^9)

Urinalysis revealed nothing abnormal.

Month 7 Mrs S was reviewed. Her RA continued to cause significant problems. She complained of mouth ulcers which she had had for several weeks. They were not relieved by Bonjela® and were now making her depressed.

15. Why might Mrs S have mouth ulcers?

16. What therapy changes would you recommend?

17. How should gold therapy be instituted?

18. How should gold therapy be monitored?

19. Would cytotoxic agents be appropriate for Mrs S?

20. Would combination therapy with DMARDS be more effective?

Answers

1. To reduce pain and stiffness, to improve functional ability, and to prevent deformity.

2. Mrs S has many features that indicate a poor prognosis for the disease. It is important to recognise these, since their presence should result in early intervention with disease-modifying therapy.

(a) Insidious onset of disease which has not really settled since first presentation;
(b) early involvement of large joints;
(c) active disease persisting beyond one year;
(d) early radiographic appearance of erosions;
(e) early appearance of nodules (the fibrous lumps noted below her elbow);
(f) positive rheumatoid factor in the first year;
(g) the following haematological abnormalities:

(i) Severe anaemia of chronic disease. This anaemia is characterised by a low haemoglobin with normocytic, normochromic red cells. The serum ferritin is normal, and serum iron is low with a low or normal iron binding capacity (transferrin). This is unlike iron-deficiency anaemia, which is characterised by hypochromic red cells, low ferritin, low serum iron and raised iron binding capacity. Anaemia of chronic disease occurs in inflammatory conditions, and, although there are normal iron stores in the bone marrow, these cannot be utilised. The only way to treat it is with disease-modifying therapy.
(ii) Raised ESR.
(iii) Raised platelet count (due to inflammatory disease).
(iv) Slight abnormalities in liver enzymes (these could, however, be due to treatment with indomethacin).

3. Yes.

Rest is a key but controversial component in settling inflamed joints, and those in favour of it will continue bed rest until inflammation subsides (two to three weeks). Intra-articular injections of corticosteroids can be very effective at relieving pain and swelling in inflamed joints. They do not help all patients, and the duration of effect can vary from a few days to several months; the reasons for this are unknown. Methylprednisolone acetate or triamcinolone hexacetonide are of roughly equal efficacy. The dose used should increase with the joint size. Knees are larger joints than shoulders, and the injection volume is usually 2 mL. Potential complications include introduction of infection, crystal synovitis (an inflammatory response to the presence of crystals in the joint space, which subsides after 24 hours), and tendon rupture.

4. (a) The names, doses, efficacy and side-effects of all previous NSAIDs;
(b) any other therapy prescribed for Mrs S's RA or other medical conditions;
(c) any other medication obtained over the counter, or from other sources; and
(d) how and when Mrs S takes her prescribed medication.

5. Yes. Naproxen 500 mg orally twice daily after food should be prescribed in lieu of her present NSAID therapy.

Changes in Mrs S's NSAID therapy are required for several reasons. Firstly, co-administration of aspirin with indomethacin reduces serum levels of the latter. This and other combinations of NSAIDs should be avoided. Combination therapy is no more effective than a single agent at optimal dose and it increases the incidence of adverse effects. Secondly, Mrs S's present medication includes both antacids and enteric-coated aspirin. Antacids increase urinary pH and thus increase renal clearance of salicylates; however, the administration of small oral doses of antacid is unlikely to affect the enteric coating of the aspirin. Thirdly, Mrs S has experienced local side-effects to rectally administered indomethacin and she should thus not be prescribed suppositories in future. Finally, she exhibits some signs of gastro-intestinal side-effects, which require further investigation, probably by endoscopy.

Mrs S's drug history should be used to help select more appropriate NSAID therapy. Factors to take into consideration include drug efficacy, side-effects, dosage regimen, drug interactions, and cost.

(a) Efficacy. All NSAIDs are more effective than placebo and at least as effective as aspirin. Studies comparing different agents are frequently poorly designed, and therefore difficult to interpret. The variation in response to NSAIDs between patients is greater than that between drugs, and therefore patient preference is important. Approximately ten per cent of RA patients will not respond to any NSAID.

(b) Side-effects. All NSAIDs cause side-effects, which are mostly related to the inhibition of prostaglandin synthesis. The dose and duration of NSAID therapy are important determinants of the side-effects experienced. NSAIDs with longer serum half-lives may be more toxic. Ibuprofen seems to be the least toxic. Pro-drugs such as fenbufen are metabolised to an active component after absorption. These agents produce fewer local adverse effects, but their systemic effects are no different to other NSAIDs. Adverse effects include gastro-intestinal bleeding and perforation (which especially affect elderly females), decreased renal function presenting as fluid retention which may progress to acute renal failure (which especially affects those with pre-existing renal impairment), and bronchospasm (affecting five per cent of asthmatics). Other side-effects less clearly related to prostaglandin inhibition affect the skin, liver and bone marrow. NSAIDs can also cause idiosyncratic effects, such as headaches and dizziness with indomethacin, and diarrhoea with mefenamic acid.

Animal studies have shown that, with one or two exceptions, most NSAIDs accelerate experimental osteoarthritic changes in the joints. How this occurs remains uncertain, but it is probably due to inhibition of proteoglycan synthesis. It is therefore possible that NSAIDs may actually cause joint damage in some patients.

(c) Dosage regimen. Once-daily dosage enhances compliance, although RA sufferers are usually highly compliant patients. The recommended frequency of dosing is based on NSAID plasma levels; however, less frequent dosing schedules are often effective, probably because the clearance of NSAIDs from synovial fluid is slower than that from plasma. When an NSAID with a long half-life, such as piroxicam, is prescribed in a single daily dose, it is important to ensure that the peak levels of the drug in synovial fluid coincide with the time of maximum patient discomfort. When early morning stiffness is the greatest problem, the long half-life NSAIDs are often more effective if taken at bedtime.

(d) Drug interactions. All NSAIDs increase the risk of bleeding from the gastro-intestinal tract in patients taking oral anticoagulants. Some NSAIDs, such as aspirin and azapropazone, interact with anticoagulants, and all NSAIDs interact with diuretics, antihypertensives, lithium and methotrexate. None of these will be relevant to Mrs S.

(e) The newer NSAIDs tend to be the more expensive.

Overall, the best choice of NSAID is generally an established agent, such as ibuprofen, ketoprofen, or diclofenac, which has a known adverse reaction profile. The NSAID selected should be tried for two weeks at the maximum recommended dose before it is dismissed as ineffective. In a hospitalised patient, response can be particularly difficult to assess because of other therapeutic interventions such as joint injections.

In Mrs S's case, naproxen therapy was felt to be appropriate on the basis of her drug history. A number of NSAIDs had already been tried, and most had been ineffective, even at maximum dose. Side-effects had not been a major problem in the past. Naproxen was felt by Mrs S to be the most effective drug she had tried to date and therefore it was re-prescribed. The experience of the author suggests that naproxen is often the NSAID of choice, because many patients find it has the best balance of efficacy to toxicity.

6. No. Mrs S should be advised to take her naproxen after food, and to stop taking ibuprofen purchased over the counter.

The mechanism of gastric damage from NSAIDs remains uncertain, but direct mucosal irritation as well as a systemic effect through inhibition of the enzyme cyclo-oxygenase is involved. The site of peptic ulceration is also unclear, with some studies reporting a prevalence of NSAID-induced gastric ulcers, and others an equal incidence of gastric and duodenal ulceration.

Cytoprotection of the gastric mucosa is maintained by prostaglandin E_2, through the production of mucus and the release of bicarbonate. Histamine H_2-receptor blockers and cytoprotective agents such as misoprostol and enprostil have been advocated for prophylaxis against ulceration.

A double-blind placebo-controlled study of 297 RA patients, which evaluated the prophylactic effect of ranitidine 150 mg twice a day against endoscopically proven gastric and duodenal ulceration from a variety of NSAIDs, showed a significant reduction in the incidence of duodenal ulceration but not gastric ulceration. The protective effects of misoprostol were studied in a double-blind, placebo-controlled study of 420 patients with osteoarthritis. Gastric ulcers occurred less frequently in the misoprostol group than the placebo group (p less than 0.001), but duodenal ulcers were rare and there was no difference in incidence between the misoprostol and placebo groups (2.5% versus 3.6%).

The results of these studies have lead to a recommendation that patients taking NSAIDs should receive both misoprostol and histamine H_2-receptor blockers, so that protection against both gastric and duodenal ulcers is provided. This approach is difficult to justify on the grounds of drug costs, and it remains unclear whether life-threatening complications can be successfully avoided using this approach. Furthermore, the use of misoprostol is associated with diarrhoea which can affect up to 80% of treated patients, and the agent is an abortifacient. Misoprostol therapy is also expensive. Since elderly patients (females particularly) are most at risk from NSAID-induced ulceration, it has been recommended that the combination of misoprostol plus a histamine H_2-receptor blocker be reserved for this group of patients.

7. Penicillamine 125 mg orally daily.

Disease-modifying (or 'second-line') therapy should commence without delay in a patient like Mrs S, who has poor prognostic signs. These drugs rarely induce remission but they slow the rate of disease progression. They have minimal anti-inflammatory activity and are therefore used in addition to NSAIDs. The available agents include penicillamine, gold salts (injection and oral), chloroquine and hydroxychloroquine, and sulphasalazine. Cytotoxic agents also have a disease-modifying effect.

Penicillamine and sodium aurothiomalate seem to be slightly more effective, but more toxic, than the antimalarials, sulphasalazine, and auranofin. Since Mrs S has active disease with poor signs, either sodium aurothiomalate or penicillamine would be appropriate. As penicillamine is an oral preparation, this is the agent of choice for Mrs S.

8. White blood cell count, platelet count, and 24-hour urinary protein measurement.

9. No.

Because of the side-effects associated with their long-term use, and because of disease rebound on withdrawal, oral corticosteroids should be reserved for:
(a) patients unresponsive to other treatments,
(b) the elderly with very active disease, and
(c) the house-bound breadwinner of a family.

Corticosteroids may also be given intravenously in large bolus doses (e.g. methylprednisolone 500 mg–1 g, three doses on alternate days). This form of therapy should only be given to patients commencing DMARDs; it has no place in the routine management of the disease. There is some evidence that bolus therapy speeds the response to DMARDs by approximately four to six weeks; however, it is associated with serious toxicity. Cases of myocardial infarction following corticosteroid bolus therapy have been reported, and the bolus dose should always be administered over at least 45 minutes to reduce the risks of myocardial ischaemia. Although Mrs S would be suitable for this therapy, it seems preferable to avoid it.

10. Every four to 12 weeks, the dose should be increased by 125 mg per day.

The usual maintenance dose of penicillamine is 500–750 mg per day, in a single early-morning dose. The disease does not respond more quickly if rapid dose increases are instituted.

11. After four to six months of therapy.

Response to all DMARDs is delayed, usually for up to four to six months. There is some evidence of a more rapid response to methotrexate therapy.

12. Mrs S's response to her DMARD therapy can be monitored by laboratory tests, her subjective opinion of the therapy, and by objective measurements.

Effective treatment will be shown by the following:
(a) a decrease in ESR, increase in haemoglobin, and a very slow decrease in rheumatoid factor titre;
(b) decreased early morning stiffness, decreased pain, increased mobility, an improved feeling of well-being; and
(c) decreased time to walk 50 yards, increased grip strength, decreased swelling of finger joints (measured using jewellers' rings), and decreased Ritchie index.

13. By full blood counts and proteinuria estimations every one to two weeks for eight weeks, then monthly, and also in the week following a dosage increase.

Withdrawal of treatment should occur if:
(a) Mrs S's platelet count falls below $120 \times 10^9/L$,
(b) her white blood cell count falls below $2.5 \times 10^9/L$, or
(c) three successive falls are noted within the normal range for these parameters.

Treatment may be re-started when counts return to normal, but should be stopped permanently if cell count falls recur. Thrombocytopenia affects approximately ten per cent of patients and usually occurs during the first six months of treatment. Agranulocytosis is much less common, and most cases occur during the first month of treatment.

If a proteinuria of greater than 1 g/24 hours is recorded, Mrs S should be monitored carefully, and treatment stopped if increasing amounts are noted. Proteinuria affects 5–26% of patients and primarily occurs in the first six to 12 months of treatment. The effect is usually reversible. If haematuria is noted, without a known cause, treatment should stop. Other measures of renal function are not required routinely.

Finally, it is useful to record Mrs S's haemoglobin

and ESR as measures of response to therapy. Also, Mrs S should be questioned about skin rashes or pruritis.

14. A number of points should be covered.

(a) The purpose of treatment and how it differs from NSAID therapy.

(b) The dose to take, and its timing (penicillamine should be taken on an empty stomach with water only; no food should be taken for at least one hour).

(c) The duration of time before a response can be expected.

(d) Potential side-effects and what to do should these occur.

(e) The monitoring requirements.

(f) The administration of other medicines. Mrs S should be advised not to take additional NSAIDs such as over-the-counter ibuprofen. She also should not self-administer iron tablets, and should avoid taking antacid mixtures within two hours of a dose of penicillamine.

(g) Sources of further information.

15. Mouth ulcers are a side-effect of penicillamine therapy which resolve upon discontinuation of treatment.

Reversible loss of taste is also a feature of penicillamine treatment. Other rare immunological or auto-immune disorders have been reported during long term therapy: these include myasthenia gravis, lupus erythematosus, Goodpasture's syndrome, and dermatomyositis. All necessitate treatment discontinuation.

16. Mrs S's disease-modifying therapy should be changed to sodium aurothiomalate.

Failure to respond to penicillamine does not lessen the likelihood of response to gold. Some believe that side-effects seen with penicillamine therapy predispose the patient to the same toxicity with gold therapy, but this is disputed. An advantage of the injectable preparation, sodium aurothiomalate, is that compliance is assured.

Oral gold, auranofin, is a completely different drug to sodium aurothiomalate. Studies suggest that auranofin is less effective than sodium aurothiomalate, although it is still associated with serious toxicity and therefore has rigorous monitoring requirements. Auranofin is not recommended for Mrs S.

Mrs S's NSAID therapy should remain unchanged.

17. An initial test dose of sodium aurothiomalate, 10 mg intramuscularly, should be administered; if there are no adverse effects, 50 mg should be given weekly for approximately 20 weeks, or until Mrs S 'responds'. At that time the injection frequency should be reduced to fortnightly or monthly.

Sodium aurothiomalate should be continued indefinitely in 'responders', unless toxicity occurs. The minimum effective dose is unknown, and neither response nor toxicity are related to serum gold concentrations.

18. A baseline full blood count and urinalysis should be performed as for penicillamine. Thereafter, monitoring of white blood cells, platelets, and urinary protein should occur at the same frequency as the injections. Mrs S should also be asked about skin rashes, pruritis and mouth ulcers.

19. Not at this stage in her disease.

Cytotoxic agents should be reserved for non-responders to other DMARDs because of their toxicity. Furthermore, there is mounting evidence that the incidence of neoplasia is increased in RA patients receiving cytotoxic therapy. For this reason these agents should, where possible, be reserved for older patients. Agents used include azathioprine, methotrexate, and cyclophosphamide. Should Mrs S not respond to gold therapy, she would require cytotoxic therapy, as it is unlikely that her disease could be controlled with either antimalarials or sulphasalazine.

20. Not on present evidence.

Studies investigating combination therapy with DMARDs have generally shown no greater response than to single drug therapy. Monitoring combination therapy is also difficult. Thus, until more information is available, single drug treatment should be used.

References and Further Reading

Anon., Which NSAID?, *Drug Ther. Bull.*, 1987, **25**, 81–84.

Anon., Misoprostol: ulcer prophylaxis at what cost?, *Lancet*, 1988, **2**, 1293–1294.

Dahl S.L., Rheumatic disorders, in *Applied Therapeutics – the Clinical Use of Drugs*, 4th edn, Young L.Y. and Koda-Kimble M.A. (eds), Vancouver, WA, Applied Therapeutics, 1988, 1775–1802.

Ehsanullah R.S.B. *et al.*, Prevention of gastroduodenal damage induced by non-steroidal anti-inflammatory drugs: controlled trial of ranitidine, *Br. med. J.*, 1988, **297**, 1017–1021.

Graham D.Y. *et al.*, Prevention of NSAID-induced gastric ulcer with misoprostol: multicentre, double-blind, placebo-controlled trial, *Lancet*, 1988, **2**, 1277–1280.

Kay E.A., Rheumatoid arthritis and osteoarthritis, *Pharm. J.*, 1988, **241**, 296–299.

TYPE II DIABETES

Judith Cantrill

Deputy Director of Pharmacy, Hope Hospital, Salford

Day 1 Mrs P, a 68-year-old housewife, was seen in the chiropody department. She had had a poorly healing ulcer on the plantar aspect of her left foot for three weeks. This had been cleaned and dressed daily by the district nurse. On examination, the area around the ulcer was found to be red, inflamed, and tender. The foot was swollen. She had been feeling generally unwell and lethargic for several months, but worse in the last week. The lesion on her left foot had been completely painless until one week ago.

Mrs P had been diagnosed as having Type II (non-insulin-dependent) diabetes three years earlier. The diagnosis had been made when she had presented with a gangrenous third toe on her right foot, which had been subsequently removed. At the same time she was also found to be hypertensive. Her only other complaints were of occasional ankle swelling and shortness of breath on exertion.

Her current drug therapy was:

Glibenclamide 15 mg orally in the morning
Co-amilozide 5/50 (amiloride hydrochloride 5 mg, hydrochlorothiazide 50 mg), two orally in the morning
Propranolol slow-release, 80 mg orally in the morning.

She lived with her husband, smoked 20 cigarettes a day and drank approximately 15 units of alcohol a week.

The chiropodist asked for the opinion of the diabetologist, who arranged for her admission the following day.

Day 2 Mrs P was admitted to hospital. On examination she was found to be pyrexial (temperature 38°C) and unwell. Her blood pressure was elevated (180/100 mmHg) and she was obese (weight 92 kg).

Her left foot was extremely swollen and very tender. The ulcer was approximately 3 cm wide and 1.5 cm deep and filled with pus. She had no pin-prick sensation over either foot, and absent reflexes at both knees and ankles. Her right foot felt colder

than the left, and the posterior tibial and dorsalis pulses were absent on the right. She had background retinopathy with microaneurysms in her right eye. She was also noted to have mild ankle oedema and some basal crepitations in both lungs.

Blood cultures and swabs of the ulcer site were sent to the microbiology department for culture and sensitivity, and an x-ray of her left foot was requested.

Her serum biochemistry and haematology results were:

Sodium 135 mmol/L (reference range 135–145)
Potassium 6.2 mmol/L (3.5–5.0)
Urea 22.7 mmol/L (2.5–7.5)
Creatinine 290 micromol/L (60–120)
Random blood glucose 22 mmol/L (3.5–10.0)
White cell count 15.6×10^9/L ($4.0–11.0 \times 10^9$)

Urine testing on the ward showed moderate amounts of protein and glucose, but no ketones.

1. What would be an appropriate choice of antibiotic(s) for Mrs P, and how should it be administered?

2. What factors might have contributed to the development of Mrs P's ulcer?

3. How should the ulcer be cleansed and dressed?

4. What other therapy may aid wound healing?

5. Why is insulin therapy indicated?

6. How should the insulin be administered and monitored?

7. Does Mrs P's hyperkalaemia require any treatment?

Day 5 Mrs P was apyrexial, and her foot was much less swollen and inflamed. Her blood glucose was well controlled on insulin, and ketones were absent from her urine. The x-ray of her foot showed no evidence of osteomyelitis.

On the ward round she was asked how she monitored her diabetes prior to coming into hospital. She replied that she used to test her urine with Clinitest® occasionally, but did not record her results. On questioning about dietary habits she admitted to eating biscuits and sweets. A request was made for the dietitian to see her.

Mrs P was prescribed oral antibiotics.

Serum biochemistry results were:

Sodium 137 mmol/L (135–145)
Potassium 4.5 mmol/L (3.5–5.0)
Urea 24.0 mmol/L (2.5–7.5)
Creatinine 285 micromol/L (60–120)
Glycosylated haemoglobin 11.4% (5.5–8.5)

Her urinary protein excretion was found to be 2.3 g/24 hours (less than 0.1) and her blood pressure was 175/105 mmHg.

8. What is the meaning of Mrs P's elevated glycosylated haemoglobin (HbA$_{1c}$)?

9. Why is Mrs P's urinary protein excretion elevated?

10. Was the combination of propranolol and co-amilozide appropriate antihypertensive therapy for Mrs P?

11. How should her hypertension be managed in the future?

12. How should her diabetes be managed at this stage of her hospital admission?

Day 14 Mrs P had remained apyrexial and her left foot now appeared normal in size and was not tender. The ulcer, although clean, was approximately the same size as on admission. It was decided to stop the antibiotics, mobilise the patient slowly, and observe the wound closely.

Her blood sugar was well controlled on her current insulin regimen. She had been seen by the dietitian, who reported that Mrs P had previously received very little dietary advice. The dietitian had also recommended a weight-reducing diet.

It was decided to plan for discharge the following week, and to change Mrs P back onto oral antidiabetic therapy.

13. What are the aims of treatment of diabetes in Mrs P?

14. What oral antidiabetic regimen would you recommend, and why?

15. How should Mrs P monitor her diabetes after discharge?

16. How should her ulcer be managed?

Day 20 Mrs P was discharged with an appointment for the diabetic clinic in six weeks' time.

Her discharge medication was:

Glibenclamide 20 mg orally in the morning
Captopril 12.5 mg orally three times daily
Frusemide 40 mg orally in the morning

She was also given a box of BM-Test 1–44®.

It was arranged for Doppler studies of Mrs P's legs to be carried out at an out-patient appointment.

17. What points would you cover when counselling Mrs P on her discharge medication?

18. What foot-care advice would be appropriate for this patient?

Week 9 The ulcer was now fairly clean but there was a small amount of pus at the base. Mrs P felt generally a little unwell and lethargic.

A random blood glucose estimation was found to be 15.3 mmol/L (3.5–10.0), and her glycosylated haemoglobin level was 11.3% (5.5–8.5). Her blood pressure was well controlled (160/85 mmHg) and her weight was 91 kg. The Doppler studies had demonstrated significant arterial occlusive disease in the right leg.

19. How should Mrs P's diabetes be managed now?

20. Would peripheral vasodilator therapy be of any value?

Week 13 Mrs P felt well and had noticed that she had much more energy. She was visiting the chiropodist regularly and the ulcer was almost healed. Her glycosylated haemoglobin level was now 8.9% (5.5–8.5).

Answers

1. Appropriate antibiotic therapy would be: ampicillin 500 mg intravenously every six hours, flucloxacillin 500 mg intravenously every six hours, and metronidazole 1 g rectally every eight hours.

Seemingly benign, superficial ulcers can progress to extensive cellulitis, osteomyelitis, and systemic toxicity. It is therefore imperative that infection is treated aggressively in the management of the diabetic foot. Even in moderately infected ulcers, therapy with a single antibiotic seldom provides adequate cover. Bacteriological cultures usually reveal two or three isolates from a single site. Aerobic Gram-positive organisms are the most prevalant, being present in 85% of cultures. These organisms are most commonly *Staphylococcus aureus*, *Staph. epidermidis* and *Streptococcus* spp. Gram-negative aerobes are present in about half the cases, most commonly *Proteus* spp. Anaerobic cultures are positive in about one-third of patients. A fetid odour emanating from the ulcer is particularly characteristic of the presence of anaerobic organisms.

Initially, broad-spectrum intravenous antibiotic therapy should be commenced, but not before appropriate swabs have been sent for culture and sensitivity. A combination of ampicillin, flucloxacillin and metronidazole usually provides appropriate initial therapy, and in a patient such as Mrs P, who is pyrexial and in whom bacteraemia is suspected, the parenteral route should be used initially. Therapy can be changed to the oral route once there is an adequate clinical response. Metronidazole can be administered rectally rather than parenterally, as there is near-complete absorption by this route, thus ensuring adequate blood levels.

2. Ischaemia, neuropathy, and lack of education.

Limb ischaemia is caused by a progressive decrease in the blood flow to the lower extremities. This predisposes to blistering and a tendency to infection. Ingrowing toenails, ill-fitting shoes, or even wrinkled socks are all common causes of foot injury to vulnerable skin. If the problem goes unrecognised, gangrene can quickly develop.

Absence of sensation may cause the patient with neuropathy to ignore the development of calluses (a sign of excessive pressure), or to be unaware of injury to the foot.

Mrs P has signs of both ischaemia (absent pulses) and neuropathy (absent pin-prick sensation). She will require advice about the prevention of future foot problems.

3. Sugar paste dressings are recommended. The wound should be cleansed with sterile, isotonic saline between dressings.

Sugar paste dressings exert an antimicrobial effect, principally through an osmotic action. Controlled trials of ulcer dressings are very difficult to perform, but there are several reports of success with these preparations. Following application, the paste is held in place with an absorbent pad. With all formulations, twice-daily application is desirable. The pastes rapidly absorb wound exudate, liquefy, and flow away from the ulcer, which acts to clean the wound. The use of sugar paste has not been shown to have a detrimental effect on diabetic control. There are a number of different formulations of sugar paste: one commonly used is in polyethylene glycol. Alternatively, preservative-free sugar can be applied directly to the wound. Dextranomer beads (Debrisan®) are also useful in the management of infected ulcers.

Alternatively, organic acid preparations can be used (e.g. Aserbine®). Skin tissues will absorb water and swell in an acid medium. Dead tissue, being less highly structured than living tissue, will swell to a greater extent. When an organic acid cream is applied to the ulcer surface, differential swelling occurs, which leads to separation of dead and healthy tissues. For best results the wound should be dressed twice daily. An organic acid solution should be used to remove slough and any remaining cream before the next dressing is applied.

In many situations, the most appropriate method of gentle cleansing at dressing changes is the use of a sterile solution of isotonic saline.

Eusol (calcium hypochlorite solution) has been used for many years in the management of infected wounds. However, when used in the packing or dressing of a wound, eusol has not been shown to be of any value as a desloughing agent. In addition, a number of studies have shown that hypochlorites can impair collagen synthesis, cause irreversible damage to the microcirculation, and increase the inflammatory response.

Hydrogen peroxide solutions may be of some value in dislodging small particles of debris from the depths of the wound; however, these solutions should not be used to irrigate closed cavities, as there is a danger that oxygen will pass into the blood stream and cause a life-threatening embolus.

Cetrimide and chlorhexidine are both active against Gram-positive, and (to a lesser extent) Gram-negative organisms. However, there are few clinical data to confirm their benefit in either preventing or treating infection. Cetrimide also has potentially useful surfactant properties, but it has been shown to have a markedly toxic effect upon fibroblasts.

4. Bed rest, and optimal control of blood glucose concentrations.

Complete bed rest is essential in the management of an infected foot ulcer. This alleviates the swelling and removes pressure from the foot. The heels should be protected, for example with a sheepskin dressing.

5. Because Mrs P is hyperglycaemic and has a febrile illness.

Insulin therapy is indicated for all diabetic patients with hyperglycaemia and a febrile illness. In this situation, insulin is the only means by which optimum blood glucose control can be obtained. If the blood glucose level remains even mildly elevated, infection is more likely to persist as a result of impaired leucocyte function.

6. The preferred method of administration is a continuous intravenous infusion of neutral insulin.

The infusion rate can be accurately controlled by means of a syringe pump. When this method is used, insulin is administered in a high concentration (e.g. 60 units in 60 mL 0.9% saline) and adsorption of insulin to plastic is not a significant problem. Insulin therapy should be initiated with an intravenous bolus of 10 units; this should be followed by an infusion of 0.1 units/kg/hour. Initially, blood glucose concentrations should be measured every two hours and the insulin dose adjusted accordingly. The aim should be to maintain Mrs P's blood glucose level between 4.5 and 11 mmol/L.

7. Yes. The co-amilozide therapy should be discontinued.

Mrs P's hyperkalaemia is associated with other signs of renal impairment (i.e. raised serum urea and creatinine levels). Co-amilozide contains a potassium-sparing diuretic and should not be administered to patients with renal impairment. Following co-amilozide discontinuation, Mrs P's serum potassium concentration should be monitored to ensure it returns to within the normal range. Specific therapy is only indicated if she exhibits signs or symptoms of hyperkalaemia: weakness, confusion, muscular paralysis, or electrocardiogram (ECG) changes. ECG changes are uncommon at potassium concentrations of less than 7 mmol/L.

8. Glycosylated haemoglobin (HbA$_{1c}$) provides objective evidence that Mrs P has had poor

glycaemic control over the previous six to eight weeks.

HbA$_{1c}$ is the name given to a sub-fraction of haemoglobin to which glucose binds. If the blood glucose is persistently high, the percentage that binds to haemoglobin is increased. This is an irreversible process and persists throughout the lifespan of the red blood cell. The measurement of HbA$_{1c}$ thus provides a means of assessment of overall blood glucose control over the preceding six to eight weeks. High levels are indicative of poor diabetic control, but HbA$_{1c}$ measurement provides no evidence of the fluctuations between high and low levels of blood glucose, and cannot be used for making day-to-day adjustments in treatment. In the out-patient and general practitioner settings, it has largely replaced the measurement of random blood glucose concentrations.

Mrs P had an elevated blood glucose level on admission to hospital, but this could have been explained by the presence of infection. However, the subsequent finding of an HbA$_{1c}$ of 11.4% is indicative of chronic, poor diabetic control.

9. Because of her underlying renal disease.

Normal subjects excrete up to 0.08 g of protein a day in the urine, amounts undetectable by usual screening tests. Proteinuria of more than 0.15 g a day is usually indicative of underlying disease, most commonly renal disease. After 15 years' duration of diabetes, up to 33% of patients have persistent proteinuria. Many patients with proteinuria also develop renal insufficiency, as judged by raised serum urea and creatinine concentrations. Hypertension and retinopathy also co-exist in the majority of diabetics with renal insufficiency. Mrs P has significant proteinuria at this time, but the test should be repeated to see if this is a persistent finding. She is also hypertensive and has a calculated creatinine clearance of approximately 25 mL/min.

10. No. Neither the propranolol nor the co-amilozide prescribed for Mrs P was appropriate.

The interaction between beta-blockers and diabetes is complex. The use of these agents is not absolutely contra-indicated, and each patient should be assessed individually, considering the following points.

(a) Beta-blockade inhibits beta-adrenergic-mediated insulin secretion; in Type II diabetes beta-blockers can impair insulin release and worsen glucose tolerance.

(b) Beta-blockers mask some of the symptoms of

hypoglycaemia (e.g. anxiety, tachycardia, tremor), but not all of them (e.g. sweating).

(c) Beta-blockers can elevate total peripheral resistance, causing vasoconstriction and reduced blood flow to most peripheral vascular beds. This may severely impair exercise tolerance and intensify intermittent claudication. Cardioselective agents are less likely than non-selective agents to exacerbate peripheral vascular disease.

(d) Both cardioselective and non-selective beta-blockers have been shown to elevate very low density lipoprotein (VLDL)-triglycerides and reduce high density lipoprotein (HDL) cholesterol levels, so should be used cautiously in diabetics with hyperlipidaemia.

(e) Cardiac failure due to coronary heart disease, hypertensive heart disease, and cardiomyopathy is frequent in the diabetic population. Beta-blockade can precipitate or exacerbate heart failure.

A beta-blocker was therefore not the optimum choice of antihypertensive therapy for Mrs P, who has chronic hyperglycaemia, peripheral vascular disease, and evidence of heart failure.

Diuretic therapy would appear to be a reasonable choice in a patient who has both hypertension and cardiac failure. However, the following points should be considered.

(a) In Type II patients who still depend on some endogenous insulin secretion, diuretic-induced hypokalaemia can impair insulin release and worsen glucose tolerance. Thiazide diuretics may also interfere with insulin action at a cellular level. Loop diuretics are less likely than thiazide diuretics to cause hyperglycaemia.

(b) Thiazide diuretics are effective when renal function is normal; however, when the serum creatinine level is significantly elevated, loop diuretics should be used.

(c) A potassium-sparing diuretic can be used to prevent diuretic-induced hypokalaemia in diabetics with normal renal function, but not in patients with renal failure who may have hypoaldosteronism and a tendency to potassium retention.

(d) Diuretics can also produce a reduction in HDL cholesterol, an increase in low density lipoprotein (LDL) cholesterol, and elevation of triglycerides. These lipid abnormalities may be transient and their long-term significance has yet to be established.

For Mrs P, the combination of a thiazide and a potassium-sparing diuretic is inappropriate. She has poorly controlled diabetes and renal insufficiency.

11. With an angiotensin-converting enzyme (ACE) inhibitor plus a loop diuretic, together with a weight-reducing diet and advice to stop smoking.

Co-existing hypertension and diabetes act as additive risk factors in the acceleration of vascular complications, which include cardiovascular disease, nephropathy, retinopathy, and peripheral vascular disease. It is therefore essential that Mrs P's hypertension is adequately treated by both pharmacological and non-pharmacological means. She should be strongly advised to lose weight and to stop smoking.

There are several pharmacological agents that can be considered.

(a) Alpha-adrenoceptor blockers. These agents can effectively reduce blood pressure in the diabetic patient without altering metabolic control. However, the side-effect of orthostatic hypotension may be a problem in the diabetic with clinical or subclinical autonomic neuropathy. Alpha-adrenoceptor blockers appear to have a beneficial effect on lipid profiles (an increase in HDL cholesterol and a decrease in triglycerides).

(b) Calcium-channel blockers. Because the process of insulin secretion from the pancreas is dependent on calcium entry into the beta cell, these agents may theoretically inhibit insulin release. However, there are only a few isolated case reports describing reversible deterioration in blood glucose control following the use of these agents.

(c) ACE inhibitors. There is now increasing evidence that ACE inhibitors may confer unique benefits in the management of diabetic nephropathy by reducing both systemic and intraglomerular arterial pressure. These agents can control hypertension and may slow the progression of renal disease, as assessed by a decline in urinary albumin excretion rate and improvement in glomerular filtration rate. They should, however, be used with caution in renal insufficiency as they can cause an acute deterioration in renal function, notably in patients with renal artery stenosis.

All three classes of drug are suitable for use in diabetic hypertension. However, Mrs P also has mild congestive cardiac failure and diabetic nephropathy. It is therefore appropriate to start her on captopril, with an initial test dose of 6.25 mg. In order to enhance the effect of captopril and minimise the dose required, frusemide 40 mg in the morning should be added to the regimen. The dose of captopril should be titrated until the desired hypotensive effect is achieved. A blood pressure of less than 160/90 mmHg would be desirable in Mrs P. Renal function and serum urea and electrolyte levels should be closely monitored following initiation of therapy.

12. By regular subcutaneous injections of insulin.

The infection is resolving and Mrs P has improved clinically. However, there is still infection present, and insulin therapy should be continued. The use of a continuous intravenous infusion is inconvenient for both the patient and the nursing staff. At this stage, insulin can be administered by *regular* subcutaneous injections. Good metabolic control is rarely achieved by the use of 'when required' subcutaneous injections.

The number of injections required varies from two to four daily, but at this stage it is probably most appropriate to use a four-times-daily regimen. One such regimen is: an injection of intermediate-acting insulin (e.g. isophane insulin) at bedtime, and injections of neutral insulin half-an-hour before each meal (i.e. three times daily). The daily dose of intravenous insulin that Mrs P has been requiring for the past few days should now be divided into four equal doses. The regimen should subsequently be adjusted according to response.

13. The aims of treatment for Mrs P are to:
    (a) keep her symptom-free,
    (b) improve and maintain her well-being,
    (c) prevent serious hypoglycaemia,
    (d) heal her foot ulcer, and
    (e) prevent the progression of complications.

Traditionally, Type II diabetes has been termed 'mild diabetes', and little thought has been given to the aims of treatment in these patients. However, the age- and sex-related mortality rates for these patients are twice those of their non-diabetic counterparts. Thus, more attention is now being focused on this group, who represent approximately 80% of the diabetic population.

14. Commence glibenclamide, but at an increased dose of 20 mg daily.

The treatment options are as follows:
(a) Continue with glibenclamide therapy. Mrs P had been treated with glibenclamide 15 mg in the morning prior to admission to hospital. This is the usual maximum recommended dose, but many patients are prescribed 20 mg in an attempt to improve control. Dividing the dose rarely improves control. Occasionally, higher doses have been reported to achieve improved control but this is usually short-lived.
(b) Change to another sulphonylurea. Glibenclamide is a potent sulphonylurea, and it is unlikely that there would be any benefit in changing to another agent.

(c) Add metformin to her drug regimen. In over 50% of patients, the addition of metformin to maximum doses of sulphonylureas achieves good metabolic control. However, metformin should be used with caution in patients with any disease that allows accumulation of the drug, or any disease that predisposes to the accumulation of lactate. Lactic acidosis is a very rare but potentially life-threatening complication of metformin therapy. Metformin is contra-indicated in Mrs P because she is suffering from impairment of renal function. Metformin is eliminated totally by the kidney, and will accumulate in a patient with renal insufficiency.
(d) Add guar gum to her drug regimen. Guar gum is an unabsorbable long-chain polysaccharide which delays absorption of carbohydrate from the intestine. Unfortunately it does not appear to achieve significant improvement in blood glucose profiles in many diabetic patients. This probably relates to unpalatability and poor compliance. The only way this product can achieve any significant benefit is if it is mixed in with the meal, but many patients find this unacceptable. If it is used, it should be initiated in small doses, which should be built up gradually in order to avoid gastro-intestinal disturbances.
(e) Change to insulin therapy. The incidence of secondary failure to oral hypoglycaemic agents is 5–6% per year. This is defined as a good initial response to oral agents, followed by a gradual decrease in effectiveness and eventual failure. These patients subsequently require treatment with insulin. There is often a great reluctance amongst both doctors and patients to initiate insulin therapy. As a result many patients continue on oral hypoglycaemic agents when the aims of treatment may be better achieved by the use of insulin therapy.

Finally, in addition to pharmacological therapy, it is essential that Mrs P be given dietary advice and encouraged to lose weight.

15. By home blood glucose monitoring.

Although urine glucose monitoring is adequate for most patients treated with oral hypoglycaemic agents, those who are heading for secondary failure should be encouraged to perform home blood glucose monitoring. Mrs P should be taught how to use the test strips, and when to do the tests, and should be provided with a booklet in which to record results.

16. With alginate dressings.

Mrs P requires a dressing that she or the district nurse can easily manage at home. Alginate dressings are haemostatic, highly absorbent, and biodegradable. The frequency of dressing changes will depend upon the condition of the wound. A clean, granulating ulcer will only require dressing twice weekly. The dressing is easily removed by irrigation with normal saline, which dissolves it.

There is also a wide range of foam, gel, and hydrogel dressings which may be equally effective. Consideration should be given to their cost, and availability on general practitioner's prescription.

17. (a) Glibenclamide.

(i) Can be taken as a single daily dose.
(ii) Take half-an-hour before breakfast.
(iii) Must be used in conjunction with dietary advice.

(b) Captopril.

(i) Take instead of propranolol.
(ii) It is being used to control high blood pressure and heart failure (ankle swelling and shortness of breath).

(c) Frusemide.

(i) May induce a diuresis (discuss appropriate timing).
(ii) Take instead of co-amilozide.
(iii) Helps captopril to work. Must take both.

(d) BM-Test 1–44®.

(i) Check technique has been taught.
(ii) Check that Mrs P has a monitoring book.

(e) General.

(i) Try to stop smoking.
(ii) When buying over-the-counter medication, inform the pharmacist about both hypertension and diabetes.

18. Detailed foot care advice is essential.

(a) Avoid extremes of heat;
(b) avoid walking barefoot;
(c) examine feet regularly;
(d) wear well-fitting footwear;
(e) report problems immediately;
(f) keep feet dry between the toes (use unscented talcum powder);
(g) don't let feet get dry and cracked (use moisturising lotion, but not between the toes);
(h) do not use iodine, epsom salts or corn remedies; and
(i) see a chiropodist regularly.

19. With insulin therapy.

Mrs P's diabetes is poorly controlled: she has a high random blood glucose level, and, more importantly, a persistently elevated glycosylated haemoglobin. In addition, she has not achieved any significant weight reduction, the ulcer has failed to heal, and she feels generally unwell. All of this is clear evidence that insulin therapy is now required. She should be commenced on twice-daily subcutaneous injections of insulin. This may be an intermediate-acting insulin (e.g. isophane insulin) alone, or a combination of intermediate and neutral insulins. If Mrs P requires combination therapy but has difficulty mixing the insulins, a fixed mixture preparation could be used. Although there is no proven clinical benefit, it is now standard practice to commence patients on human insulins. The dose should be calculated from her previous insulin requirements and then decreased a little to compensate for her extra mobility at home.

20. No.

The Doppler studies have demonstrated that Mrs P has significant arterial occlusive disease; however, vasodilators have not been proven to have any significant effect in arterial occlusive disease. This is particularly true in diabetic patients, in whom vasomotor activity is commonly absent.

Drugs such as calcium-channel blocking agents, prostaglandins, and oxpentifylline are not currently recommended for routine use in patients like Mrs P, but may hold promise for the future. Further deterioration of her peripheral circulation may be prevented by good control of her blood glucose level and hypertension, by weight reduction, and, most importantly, by her stopping smoking.

References and Further Reading

Anon., Looking after the elderly diabetic, *Drug Ther. Bull.*, 1987, **25**, 13–16.

Doran T. (ed.), *Diabetes Care – a Problem Solving Approach*, London, Heinemann, 1988.

Drury M.I., *Diabetes Mellitus*, 2nd edn, Oxford, Blackwell Scientific, 1986.

Hommel E. *et al.*, Effect of captopril on kidney function in insulin-dependent diabetic patients with nephropathy, *Br. med. J.*, 1986, **293**, 467–470.

Koda-Kimble M.A. and Rotblatt M.D., Diabetes mellitus, in *Applied Therapeutics – the Clinical Use of Drugs*, 4th edn, Young L.Y. and Koda-Kimble M.A. (eds), Vancouver, WA, Applied Therapeutics, 1988, 1663–1742.

Watkins P.J. *et al.*, Diabetic complications of non-insulin dependent diabetes, *Diabet. Med.* 1987, **4**, 293–296.

ANTICOAGULANT THERAPY

* Christopher Acomb and † Peter A. Taylor

* Director of Clinical Pharmacy, Bradford Health Authority, and † District Pharmaceutical Officer, Airedale Health Authority

Day 1 Mr W, a 52-year-old overlooker in the local wool mill, was admitted through his general practitioner with a red, swollen, left leg. He said that he had not knocked his leg but that 'it had just come up during the night'. He had taken some painkillers before going to his doctor.

His past medical history revealed that he had been started on co-amilozide 5/50 tablets (amiloride hydrochloride 5 mg, hydrochlorothiazide 50 mg) six months earlier for mild breathlessness on exertion. He had been treated for epilepsy in the past, but had not had any fits for over five years and was not currently taking any medication for this. He had been thinking of going back to his doctor because he had recently become more breathless, particularly at night.

On examination, Mr W was found to be short of breath with a regular pulse, and a raised jugular venous pressure. His left calf was inflamed and painful to the touch. When measured, his calf circumferences were: left leg 39.5 cm, right leg 38 cm. He was diagnosed as having a left deep-vein thrombosis (DVT) and mild left ventricular failure.

Mr W was prescribed:

Frusemide 40 mg orally each morning
Amiloride 5 mg orally each morning
Warfarin, loading dose to be given over three days
Heparin 40,000 units intravenously over 24 hours

1. Why does Mr W need both heparin and warfarin therapy?

2. What laboratory indexes would you check before starting oral anticoagulant therapy?

3. Was the dose and route of heparin prescribed for Mr W appropriate?

4. How is heparin treatment monitored in the laboratory?

5. What loading dose of warfarin would you recommend for Mr W? What factors did you take into account when making this recommendation?

6. How is warfarin treatment monitored in the laboratory?

7. Why is it important that a complete drug history is taken from Mr W?

Day 2 Mr W was slightly less breathless, although his leg was still swollen and painful. He was prescribed co-dydramol for the pain. His kaolin cephalin clotting time (KCCT) was reported as 120 s (reference range 30–40).

8. What changes in drug therapy would you recommend?

Day 4 Mr W was still a little breathless, and had now developed a cough with green sputum. He was diagnosed as having a chest infection and prescribed erythromycin 500 mg orally three times a day.

His KCCT was 85 s (30–40), and his prothrombin time (reported as INR) was 3.5 (2–4).

Heparin was continued at a dose of 30,000 units over 24 hours, and a maintenance dose of warfarin was prescribed.

9. How long should Mr W's heparin therapy be continued?

10. What maintenance dose of warfarin would you recommend? (Mr W's loading dose had been 7 mg daily for three days.) How should his therapy be monitored after the maintenance dose is initiated?

11. How long should Mr W's warfarin therapy be continued?

Day 5 Mr W's chest infection appeared to be improving and his leg was much better. His heparin therapy was discontinued.

Day 6 Mr W continued to do well; however, his INR was reported as 5.4 (2–4).

12. What are the possible causes of this high INR?

13. How should his high INR be managed?

Day 8 Mr W was doing very well, with both his chest and leg much improved. His INR was 2.9 (2–4), and it was decided to discharge him.

His discharge medication comprised:

Erythromycin 500 mg orally three times a day for one day, then stop
Frusemide 40 mg orally daily
Amiloride 5 mg orally daily
Warfarin 1.5 mg orally daily

14. What points would you cover when counselling Mr W about his warfarin therapy?

Day 12 On his visit to the out-patient clinic, Mr W's INR was found to be 2.6 (2–4), and his warfarin dose was continued at 1.5 mg orally daily for a further week.

Day 19 At Mr W's out-patient attendance the INR was found to have fallen to 1.8 (2–4).

15. What are the possible causes of Mr W's low INR?

Mr W was prescribed warfarin 2.5 mg daily.

Day 33 Mr W was admitted with epistaxis and haematuria. The only change in treatment was a prescription for azapropazone from his general practitioner two days before admission. The azapropazone had been prescribed for gout.

16. What are the probable causes of Mr W's problems? What action would you recommend?

17. What other drugs should be avoided or prescribed with caution and careful monitoring while Mr W continues to take warfarin?

Answers

1. Mr W requires anticoagulant therapy to prevent the extension of the clot that has formed in his leg. Intravenous heparin therapy provides an immediate anticoagulant effect until the slower-acting oral warfarin therapy exerts its full anticoagulant activity.

Heparin forms a complex with antithrombin III, which, in therapeutic doses, inhibits the action of thrombin and activated factor X. Warfarin is a vitamin K analogue and prevents the formation of vitamin K-dependent clotting factors II, VII, IX, and X.

Heparin acts rapidly and has a short half-life, so its action can be controlled quickly, but it must be given parenterally, which poses problems for treatment periods longer than a few days. However, Mr W will be at risk of further thrombosis for a number of weeks after this first incident.

In contrast, warfarin takes three to four days to exert its full anticoagulant effect, and is, therefore, not effective in limiting the extension of the thrombosis in the early phase. However, being orally active, it is very useful for long-term anticoagulant treatment.

2. A pre-treatment clotting screen should be carried out. Although other indexes (such as haemoglobin level, platelet adhesiveness, and liver function tests) are indicated in some patients, Mr W's history does not suggest that these tests are warranted in his case.

A pre-treatment clotting screen is essential to ensure that a patient has not already been anticoagulated, and that organic changes, such as liver disease, have not disrupted his clotting mechanism. Either of these conditions would mean an excessive response to the initial warfarin dose, but not necessarily the heparin dose.

There are other laboratory indexes that will help make anticoagulation safer, but they are not necessary for every patient, and they should only be carried out if there is evidence, either from a previous or a current medical history, that they may be abnormal. They include the following.

(a) A haemoglobin level. A patient with anaemia may have occult bleeding which would be exacerbated by anticoagulation. A baseline haemoglobin level would also be useful to detect bleeding in the future.

(b) A platelet level. Platelets are involved in the clotting process, and a thrombocytopenia would make the patient very prone to bleeding. However,

platelet counts can be deceptive, as it is the ability of platelets to adhere to one another, and not just the number of platelets, that determines their activity. This adhesiveness is seldom checked routinely, but such a measurement would detect the anti-platelet activity of non-steroidal anti-inflammatory drugs (NSAIDs).

(c) Liver function tests. The liver is involved in both the production of clotting factors and the metabolism of warfarin. Its normal function is therefore essential for safe anticoagulation.

Mr W only requires his INR to be measured. Although he may have a history of taking NSAIDs ('painkillers'), and there is thus a slight chance he may have had a gastro-intestinal bleed, he has given no history of dyspepsia and has no obvious signs of anaemia.

3. The route was appropriate but the dose was rather large.

The intravenous route for heparin is preferable to the administration of subcutaneous injections during the active treatment phase when effective anticoagulation is essential, as it gives much more rapid and controllable results. The subcutaneous route is useful for prophylactic therapy (e.g. during post-operative immobility).

Although, as the British National Formulary suggests, a dose between 20,000 and 40,000 units is commonly required, Mr W (who is aged 52, and not excessively large) probably requires only a middle-of-the-range starting dose, which should be adjusted appropriately once the effect has been measured. A starting dose of 30,000 units per day may have been more appropriate in this case.

Although bolus doses of heparin are recommended at the start of treatment, they are usually unnecessary. An infusion will result in steady-state levels within three to four hours, as heparin has a half-life of only one to two hours.

4. Heparin activity is estimated by a number of similar methods based on the thrombin time.

We use the KCCT, which has a normal value of 40 s, and which for effective anticoagulation should be elevated to 80–100 s. It should be noted that, at this level of activity, there may be interference of the thrombin time on the prothrombin time tests, and so tests measuring prothrombin time should be adjusted for heparin activity by the addition of protamine in the laboratory.

Heparin acts quickly and, having a short half-life, its activity can be assessed about four hours after an infusion has started, although in practice it is usually checked after about twelve hours. A similar time scale will apply after dose changes. Once-daily monitoring is necessary for patients on heparin therapy, although with some unstable patients monitoring may be increased to twice a day.

Treatment of excessive heparin activity is usually effected by stopping the infusion and ensuring, by repeating the KCCT, that the drug's activity is reducing. Protamine is only used for the treatment of haemorrhage following severe heparin overdose. The protamine dose is calculated by assuming that 1 mg of protamine will inactivate 80–100 units of heparin. Protamine itself has some anticoagulant activity and this, in addition to its potential for causing anaphylactoid reactions, means care must be taken if it is used.

5. Warfarin 7 mg daily for three days. This loading dose takes into account the fact that Mr W has left ventricular failure.

Warfarin is highly protein-bound, and has a long half-life. The administration of a loading dose thus reduces the time taken for the drug to achieve steady state.

The standard warfarin loading dose is 10 mg daily for three days. This should be reduced in certain conditions that may potentiate the action of warfarin. The following factors should be considered.

(a) Age. In general, the elderly are more sensitive to warfarin; it is recommended that a reduced loading dose is given to patients over 60 years of age.

(b) Body weight. Given that the volume of distribution is at least partially linked to body weight, a reduced loading dose should be given to patients weighing less than 60 kg.

(c) Plasma protein-binding capacity. This will be reduced in patients with low plasma protein levels, or in those already taking drugs that are highly protein-bound. Albumin is the principal plasma protein fraction that binds warfarin.

(d) Concurrent pathology. Some diseases, such as congestive cardiac failure, reduce the liver's ability to produce clotting factors and to metabolise warfarin effectively.

(e) Other drugs. Although already mentioned under plasma protein-binding, concurrent drug therapy can also interfere with warfarin activity at many other sites, and nearly all types of drug interaction have been reported.

In Mr W's case his loading dose should be reduced to 7 mg daily for three days, on the basis that his left ventricular failure may enhance the activity of warfarin. If he had had two or more of the above factors, then his loading dose should have been reduced to 5 mg daily for three days.

It should be noted that prescribers sometimes reduce the loading dose by giving 10 mg, 5 mg, and 5 mg over the three days. The first dose (10 mg) will often produce an exaggerated response on day 4, which makes calculation of the maintenance dose difficult and can lead to doses being missed because of the seemingly high INR.

6. Warfarin activity is monitored in the laboratory by measuring the prothrombin time.

The citrate in the blood sample is neutralised with excess calcium ions, and thromboplastin is added. The time taken for the sample to clot is then known as the prothrombin time. Comparing this with a sample containing no anticoagulant will give a prothrombin time ratio. Recently, the thromboplastin used in this test has been standardised so as to allow a patient to be controlled by any laboratory. This standardisation has resulted in the test being renamed the International Normalised Ratio (INR).

INR values in the range of 2.0 to 4.0 are accepted as being therapeutic, although subgroups within this range are used to cover the various indications for warfarin anticoagulation. In Mr W's case, a range of 2.0 to 3.0 would be appropriate to prevent an extension of his DVT.

7. A drug history is essential prior to starting oral anticoagulation therapy with warfarin or other coumarin derivatives because many drugs can interact with warfarin to a clinically significant extent.

Two important facts were elicited from Mr W's medication history. First, it was noted that Mr W has a history of epilepsy. On questioning, he indicated that he had been taking phenytoin some three months earlier. Phenytoin and other drugs that induce warfarin metabolism may exert their effect for up to six weeks after stopping therapy. This demonstrates that not only current medication, but also any other medication taken over the previous six weeks, should be considered in an effort to reduce potential complications of warfarin treatment.

Secondly, Mr W had referred to 'painkillers' he had taken at home. When questioned further, he said that he normally took Hypon® tablets, but as he had run out he had taken some of his wife's Veganin®. Both of these over-the-counter products contain aspirin. This means:

(a) that he should be counselled regarding their future use, as he will need to avoid aspirin and aspirin-containing products while he is taking warfarin; and

(b) attention should be given to the possibility that aspirin-induced low platelet activity might cause bruising or other minor bleeding, despite normal INRs, or that drug-induced gastro-intestinal erosions may cause more major bleeding complications.

8. Reduce his heparin dose to 30,000 units intravenously per day.

Mr W's KCCT is too high, and so a reduction in heparin dose is needed. This is an empirical dosage reduction, but experience suggests that it would be expected to give a KCCT of around 80 s.

It is not necessary to alter Mr W's analgesic therapy. Co-dydramol should not affect his warfarin activity, unlike co-proxamol (which can enhance warfarin activity).

9. Heparin therapy should continue until the desired effect of warfarin has been achieved.

The INR value on day 4 is the first indication of warfarin activity and is the level from which the maintenance dose of warfarin can be calculated. As Mr W's INR is already in the therapeutic range, his heparin therapy can be stopped in 24 hours, provided his leg is improving. However, some patients can have high INRs but still have coagulation problems because an imbalance in the clotting process has occurred. This may be seen as a worsening of the DVT. In such cases, heparin should be continued until it is certain that warfarin activity is fully established, which may mean a further two or three days of heparin therapy.

10. Warfarin 2.5 mg daily.

This dose is calculated using the method of Dobrzanski, which relates the maintenance dose to the cumulative loading dose over three days (in this case 21 mg, rounded down to 20 mg) and the INR achieved on the fourth day. This relationship can be seen on the following chart. Although many factors can affect this relationship, in general it does give a very good conservative estimate of the maintenance dose required.

To use the chart, the cumulative loading dose given prior to the time of INR measurement should be calculated. The horizontal line corresponding to the measured INR should then be followed to the point where it intersects with the vertical line headed by the cumulative loading dose. The value at the point of intersection represents the recommended maintenance dose.

INR	Cumulative warfarin dose (mg)						
	15	20	25	30	35*	40*	45*
2.0	3.5	4	5	5.5	6	7	7.5
2.2	3.5	4	4.5	5	5.5	6	6.5
2.5	3	3.5	4	4	4.5	5	5.5
3.0	2.5	3	3.5	3.5	4	4	4
3.5	—	2.5	3	3	3.5	—	—
4.0	—	—	3	3	3	—	—
4.5	—	—	2.5	3	3	—	—
5.0	—	—	2.5	2.5	3	—	—

* Values of cumulative dose exceeding 30 mg may be found when the INR has not been measured at the correct time. Such values should not normally be used.

Further monitoring should be carried out after two to three days, and then, depending on the results obtained, the interval can be increased – initially to weekly, and then to two-, four-, and even six-weekly. If a graph of INR against time is drawn, the slope will indicate the need for monitoring; for example, a sharp change in the slope of the graph would indicate the need for more frequent monitoring or intervention to prevent values going outside the agreed limits.

Changes in treatment, or in the patient's pathology, also necessitate more frequent monitoring. The overall aim must always be to ensure that sufficient monitoring is undertaken to enable adverse changes to be detected without inconveniencing the patient excessively.

11. Provided there is no recurrence of his DVT, for six months.

A first DVT with no complications is normally treated with warfarin for a period of three months, although some authorities feel that patients who have a thrombotic episode may well be predisposed to this condition for much longer. In the case of Mr W, his mild heart failure could have been a contributing factor; until this is controlled he will continue to be at risk (it was a spontaneous DVT). We would recommend at least six months' anticoagulant therapy and, if the DVT should recur, then continuous treatment.

12. There are a number of possible causes of the high INR, including changes in Mr W's fluid balance (as a result of frusemide therapy), worsening of his heart failure (no clinical signs), drug interactions, and failure to take the correct dose. However, the most likely explanation is an interaction between erythromycin and warfarin.

Erythromycin is known to inhibit the enzyme systems involved in warfarin metabolism (as do trimethoprim and ciprofloxacin), and is best avoided in patients anticoagulated with warfarin. If erythromycin therapy is necessary, a reduction of 50% in the dose of warfarin is required before the antibiotic is started. Weekly monitoring should also be recommended until the effect of the erythromycin is no longer seen, which may be two or three weeks after antibiotic therapy is stopped.

13. Omit one dose then recommence treatment with 1.5 mg warfarin orally daily.

The British National Formulary gives good guidance on the management of over-anticoagulation. Mr W has a high INR but no apparent bleeding, and the probable cause of the increase in INR is known. He should therefore have one dose of warfarin withheld to reduce quickly the risk of a bleed, and he should then continue treatment with a lower dose. Reducing the dose to approximately 50% of that previously suggested would be appropriate. His INR should be monitored after a further two days, and the dose re-adjusted if necessary.

When the erythromycin therapy is stopped, Mr W's hepatic enzyme systems will return to normal. However, this return will not be as sudden as the inhibition; monitoring should therefore continue at least weekly, and his dose of warfarin should be adjusted until he returns to his pre-erythromycin dose.

14. It is essential to counsel patients who have been prescribed warfarin for the first time. There is a large amount of information to be conveyed to such patients, and counselling requires a high level of skill and a substantial amount of time. We take the view that it is unethical for a patient on warfarin to be discharged from hospital without being counselled.

The major points to be covered include the following.

(a) What warfarin is, and what it does.

(b) Why the patient is taking warfarin, and how its action can help.

(c) How much to take, and how the dose can be described (i.e. the colour or strength of the tablet, and how dose changes may involve different combinations of the three strengths of tablet available).

(d) When to take the dose, what happens if a dose is missed, and the importance of regular dosing.

(e) What affects the action of warfarin: food (diets high in vitamin K in particular); social activities (smoking, drinking, travel, exercise); and other medicines, including over-the-counter products, and alternative medicines.

(f) Who to tell that you are on anticoagulant therapy (doctor, dentist, pharmacist).

(g) What symptoms to look for which may indicate too much anticoagulant activity (e.g. gum bleeding, bruising, blood in urine), what the significance of each might be, and what to do about it.

(h) Who to contact if there are problems or doubts about treatment.

(i) What to do about diseases that might occur during treatment (for instance, influenza).

(j) When to come to clinic, and why monitoring is important.

(k) What the treatment goals are (to help the patient visualise their therapy and therefore help in terms of compliance and co-operation).

15. His warfarin dose was not increased when his erythromycin therapy was stopped.

This is the most likely cause of Mr W's low INR. Assuming non-compliance at this stage would be inappropriate. The effect of hepatic enzyme inhibition may take a week or two to be fully reversed, so monitoring and small dose increases (in this case 0.5 mg aliquots) will be required during this time until the original activity is resumed.

16. Azapropazone therapy is the most likely cause of his problems; it should be withdrawn and replaced by alternative therapy if needed.

On admission Mr W was found to have a very high INR (greater than 7.0), which was most probably caused by the addition of azapropazone to his warfarin therapy.

Most NSAIDs have some anti-platelet activity and, as such, can enhance bleeding, although this does not affect the INR. Similarly, although many NSAIDs are protein-bound, the warfarin that is displaced by their concurrent binding is rapidly eliminated by the liver; at most, a small transient rise in INR (usually for no longer than a day or two) may be seen. However, like the classical reaction between phenylbutazone and warfarin (which is now fortunately rarely seen), azapropazone is not only capable of displacing a significant amount of warfarin from its protein-binding sites, but it can also inhibit hepatic enzyme activity very rapidly. This produces a very profound increase in free warfarin levels and, therefore, in anticoagulant activity. The use of azapropazone (or phenylbutazone) must thus be avoided wherever possible in patients already taking warfarin; however, the data sheet for azapropazone gives good guidance on its use if it is deemed necessary.

NSAIDs also affect the gastro-intestinal mucosa,

causing damage and some blood loss, and this will be enhanced in the presence of warfarin.

Mr W's acute symptoms of gout may indeed require an NSAID, but diclofenac would be a more appropriate choice, being potent enough to treat the pain, while having no effect on warfarin metabolism and only a small effect on the protein-binding of warfarin.

Colchicine, which is also used in the acute treatment of gout, is not a safe alternative for Mr W, as it too is likely to cause changes in response to his anticoagulant therapy.

The use of allopurinol for long-term prophylaxis of gout may also be considered, provided that increased monitoring of Mr W's warfarin therapy is undertaken while allopurinol therapy is being introduced, as this drug is also reported to have an effect on anticoagulant therapy. An increase in warfarin activity is likely, although the size of the response varies from patient to patient.

Finally, the diuretics taken by Mr W should be reviewed to see if improvements in control or choice could be made, as they are the likely cause of his acute episode of gout.

Whichever method is used to control Mr W's gout, more frequent monitoring of his anticoagulant treatment must be initiated.

17. Warfarin and related compounds interact with many different drugs. A comprehensive, but not exhaustive, list of compounds involved can be found in the British National Formulary.

Patients can vary quite markedly in their response to interactions, making it sometimes difficult to predict the outcome. For this reason it is important to:

(a) recognise known drug interactions before the interacting medicine is given, and initiate treatment changes that will avoid marked disruption of anticoagulant control;

(b) ensure that the patient (and their general practitioner) is aware of the problem of drug interactions, and that the clinic is informed before any new medication (including alternative and over-the-counter medicines) is started;

(c) remember that changes in the dose of concurrent medication may influence the anticoagulant effect;

(d) use the smaller range of medicines known to be safe in the presence of anticoagulants, rather than the much wider armamentarium usually available; and

(e) monitor patients carefully when medication is being changed.

It is very easy to recognise a drug interaction after a marked change in anticoagulant control has occurred. It is more beneficial to the patient if that change is anticipated and prevented.

References and Further Reading

Bourne J.G. and Pegg M., Pharmacy contribution to outpatient management of oral anticoagulation, *Pharm. J.*, 1987, **238**, 733–755.

Dobrzanski S., Predicting warfarin dosage, *J. clin. Hosp. Pharm.*, 1983, **8**, 247–250.

Frech A. *et al.*, Individualisation of oral anticoagulant therapy, *Drugs*, 1979, **18**, 48–57.

Hirsh J. *et al.*, Optimal therapeutic range for oral anticoagulants, *Chest*, 1989, **95 (suppl.)**, 55–115.

Reinders T.P. and Steinke W.K., Pharmacists' management of anticoagulant therapy in ambulant patients, *Am. J. Hosp. Pharm.*, 1979, **36**, 645–648.

Stockley I., *Drug Interactions: their Clinical Importance, Mechanisms and Management*, 1st edn, Oxford, Blackwell Scientific, 1981.

Taylor P. and Acomb C., *Oral Anticoagulants – Patient Care and Control*, Leeds University Press, UK Clinical Pharmacy Association, 1987.

INDEX